THIRD EDITION

Conditions in Occupational Therapy

Effect on Occupational Performance

Editors

Ben J. Atchison, PhD, OTR, FAOTA
Professor and Graduate Program Coordinator
Department of Occupational Therapy
Western Michigan University
Kalamazoo, Michigan

Diane K. Dirette, PhD, OT
Associate Professor
Department of Occupational Therapy
Western Michigan University
Kalamazoo, Michigan

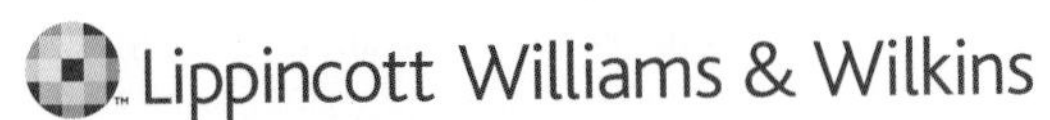
Lippincott Williams & Wilkins
a Wolters Kluwer business
Philadelphia • Baltimore • New York • London
Buenos Aires • Hong Kong • Sydney • Tokyo

Acquisitions Editor: Emily J. Lupash
Managing Editor: Andrea M. Klingler
Marketing Manager: Christen D. Murphy
Production Editor: Jennifer W. Glazer
Designer: Risa J. Clow
Compositor: International Typesetting and Composition
Printer: Data Reproductions Corporation

351 West Camden Street
Baltimore, MD 21201

530 Walnut Street
Philadelphia, PA 19106

Printed in the United States of America

First Edition, 1989
Second Edition, 2000

Library of Congress Cataloging-in-Publication Data

Conditions in occupational therapy:effect on occupational performance/editors, Ben J. Atchison, Diane K. Dirette.—3rd ed.
p. ; cm.
Includes bibliographical references and index.
ISBN-13: 978-0-7817-5487-3 (alk. paper)
ISBN-10: 0-7817-5487-9 (alk. paper)
1. Occupational therapy. 2. Occupational therapy—Case studies. I. Atchison, Ben. II. Dirette, Diane K.
[DNLM: 1. Occupational Therapy. 2. Mental Disorders. 3. Nervous System Diseases. WB 555 C745 2007]
RM735.C66 2007
615.8'515—dc22

2006014892

07 08 09 10
3 4 5 6 7 8 9 10

To my wife, Marcia, my best friend and life coach.

Ben Atchison

To my sister, Kathy, whose love and support always encouraged me to do better. I will miss you forever.

Diane Dirette

Preface

The goals of this textbook were the same in both the first and second editions: to provide a framework for students to learn about common conditions seen by occupational therapists and to facilitate the teaching and learning of conditions from an occupational therapy perspective. We thank Dr. Ruth Hansen for her significant contributions to the development of this framework and her significant contributions as first editor in the previous editions of this textbook.

The original goals of this book have not changed in this third revised edition of *Conditions in Occupational Therapy: Effect on Occupational Performance*. Although not all conditions that an occupational therapist will encounter are included, we discuss those most common to our practice.

All chapters have the same basic structure, including sections on etiology, incidence and prevalence, signs and symptoms, course and prognosis, and medical/surgical management. The information is synthesized from an occupational performance perspective, using language included in the Occupational Therapy Practice Framework. It is important to begin the occupational therapy process with an understanding of client factors, including body structures and functions associated with a given condition, and to examine the potential effect on the occupational performance areas.

In this edition, the Occupational Therapy Practice Framework language, which is the most current "language of the profession," is inserted. We are pleased to announce the addition of a chapter on anxiety disorders and major revisions across all chapters to ensure current information on all aspects of these selected conditions. Case studies have been updated and are included for each chapter.

There is a continuing discussion in our profession about whether occupational therapists "treat diagnoses." We do not propose that there be an emphasis on the treatment of a diagnosis. We understand and support a patient-first philosophy. We do, however, argue that there are specific factors that impact on the ability to perform occupational roles and functions that are unique to a given condition. These factors must be understood and analyzed regarding their relative impact on the patient's ability to participate and engage in daily activity.

Each chapter in this third edition provides the authors' interpretations of the effects of the condition on occupational performance. This analysis is not absolute. Those who use this book may disagree about the importance of various disabilities and the secondary changes that might occur. That process, however, is the key to our goal for publishing this book. We expect it to be a starting point for discussion and analysis of the condition and its impact on occupational performance.

Ben Atchison
Diane Dirette

Contributors

Ben J. Atchison, PhD, OTR, FAOTA
Professor and Graduate Program Coordinator
Department of Occupational Therapy
Western Michigan University
Kalamazoo, Michigan

Christine K. Urish, PhD, OTR/L, BCMH
Associate Professor
Department of Occupational Therapy
St. Ambrose University
Davenport, Iowa

David P. Orchanian, MPH, OTR
Clinical Faculty Specialist
Department of Occupational Therapy
Western Michigan University
Kalamazoo, Michigan

Diane K. Dirette, PhD, OT
Associate Professor
Department of Occupational Therapy
Western Michigan University
Kalamazoo, Michigan

Elizabeth L. Phillips, MSN
Doctoral Candidate
University of Michigan School of Nursing
Ann Arbor, Michigan

Gerry E. Conti, PhD, OTR
Department of Occupational Therapy
Wayne State University
Detroit, Michigan

Heather (Gallew) Javaherian, OTD, OTR/L
Assistant Professor
Department of Occupational Therapy
School of Allied Health Professions
Loma Linda University
Loma Linda, California

Jacqueline Eckert, MS, OTR
University of Michigan Medical Center
Ann Arbor, Michigan

Joanne Phillips Estes, MS, OTR/L
Assistant Professor
Department of Occupational Therapy
Xavier University
Cincinnati, Ohio

Joyce Fraker, MS, OTR
Department of Psychiatry
Ann Arbor VA Medical Center
Ann Arbor, Michigan

Kathryn Shangraw, MA, CCC-SLP
Kindering Center
Bellevue, Washington

Laura V. Miller, MS, OTR, CDI, CDRS
Drivers Rehabilitation Center of Michigan
Livonia, Michigan

Mary Steichen Yamamoto, MS, OT
Private Practice
Ann Arbor, Michigan

Paula W. Jamison, PhD, OTR
Assistant Professor
Department of Occupational Therapy
Western Michigan University
Kalamazoo, Michigan

Ruth Hansen, PhD, OTR, FAOTA
Professor Emeritus
Department of Occupational Therapy
Eastern Michigan University
Ypsilanti, Michigan

Thomas Zelnik, MD
Chair, Department of Psychiatry
St. Joseph Mercy Hospital
Clinical Assistant Professor
Department of Psychiatry
University of Michigan Medical Center
Ann Arbor, Michigan

Valerie Howells, PhD, OTR
Associate Professor
School of Health Sciences
Occupational Therapy Program
Eastern Michigan University
Ypsilanti, Michigan

Yvonne Russell Teske, PhD, OTR, FAOTA
Associate Professor
Department of Occupational Therapy
Shenandoah University
Winchester, Virginia

Contents

It is more important to know what kind of person has the disease than what kind of disease the person has.
—Sir William Osler (Address at Johns Hopkins University, February 1905)

1 Thinking Like An OT

Ruth Hansen, Diane K. Dirette, and Ben J. Atchison

Key Terms

Activity demands
Altruism
Client factors
Context
Dignity
Equality
Freedom
Justice
Truth
Prudence
Performance in areas of occupation
Performance skills
Performance patterns
Person-first language

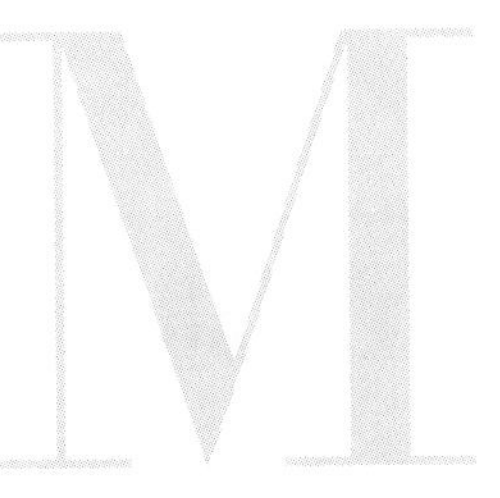

Melissa is an occupational therapy student beginning her first level II fieldwork experience. During the first week, she spent most of her time attending orientation sessions and observing as her supervising therapist treated patients. Now the time has come for patients to be assigned to her and for her to take responsibility for initiating treatment. When she receives her first referral, she reads the diagnosis and begins to decide what to do next.

How does a student learn to correlate general information about a diagnosis with the needs of a particular person and identify the problems that require occupational therapy intervention? How does a staff therapist set priorities for problems and decide which require immediate attention? How much problem identification can be done before the therapist actually sees the patient? How does a supervisor know when a student or therapist is doing a "good job" of screening referrals and anticipating the dysfunction that the patient might be experiencing? These are precursors to the actual intervention process and are essential to effective and efficient clinical reasoning, as described by Benamy (1).

The clinical reasoning procedure used by each health care professional is somewhat different. The information that is the main focus of intervention for a speech therapist will differ from that of a psychologist or a nurse. What makes occupational therapy unique among health care professions is that practitioners gather and use information to help people be self-sufficient in their daily activities. Such data gathering and analysis provide the therapist with the foundation for a treatment plan through a prioritized list of anticipated problems or dysfunctions for an individual.

To comprehend the unique aspects of occupational therapy requires an understanding of the core values, philosophical assumptions and domain of concern of the profession, and the language that is used to communicate information clearly and precisely.

Core Values of Occupational Therapy

The core values of occupational therapy are set forth in the document "Core Values and Attitudes of Occupational Therapy Practice" (2). Seven have been identified: **altruism, dignity, equality, freedom, justice, truth, and prudence**.

1. *Altruism* is the unselfish concern for the welfare of others. This concept is reflected in actions and attitudes of commitment, caring, dedication, responsiveness, and understanding.
2. *Dignity* emphasizes the importance of valuing the inherent worth and uniqueness of each person. This value is demonstrated by an attitude of empathy and respect for self and others.
3. *Equality* requires that all individuals be perceived as having the same fundamental human rights and opportunities. This value is demonstrated by an attitude of fairness and impartiality.
4. *Freedom* allows the individual to exercise choice and to demonstrate independence, initiative, and self-direction.
5. *Justice* places value on the upholding of such moral and legal principles as fairness, equity, truthfulness, and objectivity.
6. *Truth* requires that we be faithful to facts and reality. Truthfulness or veracity is demonstrated by being accountable, honest, forthright, accurate, and authentic in our attitudes and actions.
7. *Prudence* is the ability to govern and discipline oneself through the use of reason. To be prudent is to value judiciousness, discretion, vigilance, moderation, care, and circumspection in the management of one's affairs, to temper extremes, make judgments, and respond on the basis of intelligent reflection and rational thought (2).

These values are the foundation of the belief system that occupational therapists use as a moral guide when making clinical decisions.

Philosophical Assumptions

The philosophical assumptions of the profession guide occupational therapists in providing client-centered therapy that meets the needs of the client and society. These assumptions express our basic beliefs about the client and the context in which the client functions (3). These assumptions are:

- Each individual has a right to a meaningful existence: the right to live in surroundings that are safe, supportive, comfortable, and over which he or she has some control; to make decisions for himself or herself; to be productive; to experience pleasure and joy; to love and be loved.
- Each individual is influenced by the biological and social nature of the species.
- Each individual can only be understood within the context of his or her family, friends, community, and membership in various cultural groups.
- Each individual has the need to participate in a variety of social roles and to have periodic relief from participation.
- Each individual has the right to seek his or her potential through personal choice, within the context of accepted social constraints.
- Each individual is able to reach his or her potential through purposeful interaction with the human and nonhuman environment.
- Occupational therapy is concerned with promoting functional interdependence through interactions directed toward facilitating participation in major social roles (areas of occupational performance); and development of biological, cognitive, psychological, and social components **(client factors)** fundamental to such roles.
- The extent to which intervention is focused on the context, the areas of occupational performance or on the **client factors** depends on the needs of the particular individual at any given time.

Language

Although many language systems and mechanisms are available, we will discuss language from two perspectives. First, is a philosophical discussion of using person-first language. Second is the use of the *Occupational Therapy Practice Framework: Domain and Process* (4) that presents the professional language.

Person-First Language

In many cases, the literature and the media, both popular and professional, describe a person with a given condition as the condition—the arthritic, the C.P. kid, the schizophrenic, the alcoholic, the burn victim or the mentally retarded. All of these terms label people as members of a large group rather than as a unique individual. The use of person-first language requires that the person be identified first and the disease used as a secondary descriptor. For example, a woman, who is a physicist, is active in her church, and has arthritis; the fourth-grade boy, who is a good speller, loves baseball, and has cerebral palsy. The condition does not and should not be the primary identity of any person.

Consider the following: a father is introducing his son to his coworkers. Which of the following is the best introduction:

- "Hey, everyone, this is my retarded son, John."
- "Hey, everyone, this is my son, John, who is retarded and loves soccer and video games."
- "Hey, everyone, this is my son, John. He loves soccer and video games."

Of course, the third is the best choice. Yet it is common when describing a person who has a disability to emphasize the disability first. The consequence is a labeling process. "Although such shorthand language is commonplace in clinics and medical records, it negates the individuality of the person. Each of us is a person, with a variety of traits that can be used to describe aspects of our personality, behavior, and function. To use a disease or condition as the adjective preceding the identifying noun negates the multiple dimensions that make the person a unique individual" (5).

The Occupational Therapy Practice Framework

The professional language for the profession of occupational therapy was revised in 2002 and presented in a document entitled *Occupational Therapy Practice Framework: Domain and Process* (4). The Occupational Therapy Practice Framework (also referred to as the Practice Framework) replaced the *American Occupational Therapy Association's Uniform Terminology*, third edition (6). The Practice Framework outlines the language and constructs that describe the occupational therapy profession's domain of concern. The domain defines the area of human activity to which the occupational therapy process is applied. The process facilitates engagement in occupation to support participation in life. The focus of the process is on the use of and the enhancement of engagement in occupation. The specific aspects of the domain are outlined in the language of the Practice Framework.

The Framework is organized into six aspects—**performance in areas of occupation, performance skills, performance patterns, context, activity demands**, and client factors. Areas of occupation are broad categories of human activity that are typically part of daily life. The areas include activities of daily living, instrumental activities of daily living, education, work, play, leisure, and social participation. Performance skills are features of what a person does during an activity. These skills are separated into the categories of motor skills, process skills, and communication/interaction skills. Performance patterns are the habits, routines, and roles that a person adopts. Context refers to the conditions that surround the person. Those conditions include cultural, physical, social, personal, spiritual, temporal, and virtual contexts. Activity demands are the aspects of the task that influence the performance by the person. These demands include the objects used and their properties, space demands, social demands, sequencing and timing, required actions, required body functions, and required body structures. Client factors are the body functions and the body structures that reside within the person. See Figure 1.1 for an overview of the Practice Framework.

DOMAIN OF OCCUPATIONAL THERAPY

ENGAGEMENT IN OCCUPATION TO SUPPORT PARTICIPATION IN CONTEXT OR CONTEXTS

PERFORMANCE IN AREAS OF OCCUPATION
- ACTIVITIES OF DAILY LIVING (ADL)
- INSTRUMENTAL ACTIVITIES OF DAILY LIVING (IADL)
- EDUCATION
- WORK
- PLAY
- LEISURE
- SOCIAL PARTICIPATION

PERFORMANCE SKILLS
- MOTOR SKILLS
- PROCESS SKILLS
- COMMUNICATION/INTERACTION SKILLS

PERFORMANCE PATTERNS
- HABITS
- ROUTINES
- ROLES

CONTEXT
- CULTURAL
- PHYSICAL
- SOCIAL
- PERSONAL
- SPIRITUAL
- TEMPORAL
- VIRTUAL

ACTIVITY DEMANDS
- OBJECTS USED AND THEIR PROPERTIES
- SPACE DEMANDS
- SOCIAL DEMANDS
- SEQUENCING AND TIMING
- REQUIRED ACTIONS
- REQUIRED BODY FUNCTIONS
- REQUIRED BODY STRUCTURES

CLIENT FACTORS
- BODY FUNCTIONS
- BODY STRUCTURES

Figure 1.1 The domain of occupational therapy.

Each of these aspects has a relationship and influence on the others. The outcome is, of course, the ability to function and engage in occupations. Although at a given time you may focus on areas of occupation or client factors, the ultimate concern is whether the individual is able to perform necessary and desired tasks in daily life. For example, a therapist may evaluate a person's attention span, but not in isolation. Attention span is evaluated within the realm of the performance patterns and context of the person—the attention span required to work on an assembly line, to drive a car, to learn a card game, or to conduct a business meeting.

Once you know the diagnosis and age of the person, you can use this Practice Framework to examine systematically the deficits that occur in the client factors, as well as how these particular deficits can and do alter the person's ability to complete tasks in relevant areas of occupational performance. In other instances, you may focus primarily on the area of occupational performance or the contextual factors for the individual, without paying much attention to the underlying client factors that influence the performance areas. Definitions of all terms are provided in the glossary at the back of the book.

Organization and Framework of this Text

Whereas the primary purpose of this book is to describe the potential impact of a condition on occupational performance, the descriptions should not be considered prescriptive or exhaustive. It is necessary to understand common facts of these conditions, including etiology, basic pathogenesis, commonly observed signs and symptoms, and precautions. However, it is equally important to recognize that the effects of a condition on occupational well-being will also be dependent on contextual factors such as age, developmental stage, health status, and the physical, social, and cultural environment (7). Rather than viewing an individual as a diagnostic entity or as the sum of biological cells, the condition must be personalized.

The general organization of each chapter is the same. First, there is a detailed description of the etiology, information about incidence and prevalence, signs and symptoms, course and prognosis, and other information that is usually found in a medical or pathophysiology text. This book is unique because the authors have used these details to generate a description of the various aspects of occupational performance that might be affected. At the end of each chapter is a discussion of at least one case study. Cases provide a beginning point to discuss specific details about how the condition might impinge on the daily functioning of a person.

Occupational therapists have a unique and valuable view of an individual as an occupational being. All of us attach meaning to our lives and the lives of others through the activities and occupations that are part of our daily existence. Occupation, then, means more than just work. It is a much broader concept that refers to human involvement in activities that will result in productive and purposeful outcomes. It also includes participation in leisure, rest, and self-care activities that some may not consider productive and purposeful. For example, the occupations of a 3-month-old infant include those that could be categorized under the general headings of play or activities of daily living. Activities such as play exploration, socialization, and functional communication are critical at this age.

The complexity of occupation changes dramatically as the infant progresses toward preschool and school age. It is interesting to observe the rapid addition of new occupational roles and expectations as the child enters school. Many aspects of occupational development are emerging. For example, a 7-year-old child participating in classroom activities is involved in a type of work. Being on time, turning in assignments that are completed properly, good grooming, and getting along with others are all behaviors that will be important as the child approaches adulthood.

Adults are expected to assume, independently pursue, and maintain relevant occupations. Generally, adults spend the greater portion of their waking hours engaged in some type of work or instrumental activities of daily living. These occupations may be a job or vocation that is done for pay, organized volunteer activities, or home management. The percentage of time spent in each area is largely determined by the role the individual assumes. Additionally, adults spend a portion of their time exploring and performing leisure and social activities. Activities of daily living, sexual expression, grooming, and eating are also important for adults.

The basic tenets regarding occupational performance are that these tasks are critical and must be performed by the person or by others to survive. By engaging in various occupations the person develops, learns adaptive mechanisms, and meets individual needs. It is important to understand the influence of culture on adaptation. Cultural influences, such as institutions, rules, values, architectural design, art, history, and language, affect the ways and the extent to which a person uses adaptive mechanisms.

Conversely, illness, trauma, or injury can cause varying degrees of occupational dysfunction. The individual receiving occupational therapy is most often experiencing permanent, long-term changes in the ability to engage in everyday activities. The continuum between health and illness is dynamic. The individual's state of health or illness can be judged by the ability to engage in activities that meet both immediate and long-range needs, and to assume desired roles. Illness or disability is considered in relation to its effects on occupational performance and, therefore, the degree of occupational dysfunction that is experienced. These precepts are the foundation for the reasoning process described in this book. The combination of these assumptions or beliefs and the occupational performance structure is the frame that provides a unique occupational therapy perspective. Of course, this book cannot cover every condition that an occupational therapist will encounter in practice. We selected the conditions based on American Occupational Therapy Association (AOTA) survey data gathered in the late 1980s and the most recent data available from the 1990 AOTA Member Data Survey, Final Report, as well as feedback we received from individuals who read and used the first two editions of this textbook. We selected conditions representing the broad range of occupational therapy practice—mental health, physical rehabilitation, geriatrics, and pediatrics.

As an instructional tool, this book provides an opportunity to examine each condition closely. The reader is urged to use the information as a springboard for further study of the conditions included here and the many other conditions that occupational therapists encounter in practice. The analysis of the impact on occupational performance for a particular condition is dynamic, and the identification of the most important areas of dysfunction and, therefore, treatment will vary from practitioner to practitioner. Additionally, factors such as secondary health problems, age, gender, family background, and culture contribute greatly to the development of a unique occupational performance profile for each individual served.

The occupational performance approach to the identification of dysfunction described in this book can be used to examine the effects of any condition on a person's daily life. This process will enable the therapist to identify and set a priority for problems in occupational performance, which, in turn, will serve as the foundation for creating an effective intervention plan.

References

1. Benamy BC. Developing clinical reasoning skills. San Antonio, TX: Therapy Skill Builders, 1996.
2. Kanny E. Core values and attitudes of occupational therapy practice. Am J Occup Ther 1993;47: 1085–1086.
3. Mosey AC. Applied Scientific Inquiry in the Health Professions: An Epistemological Orientation. 2nd ed. Bethesda, MD: American Occupational Therapy Association, 1996.
4. American Occupational Therapy Association. Occupational therapy practice framework: Domain and process. Am J Occup Ther 2002;56: 609–639.
5. Hansen RA. Ethical implications. In: Hinojosa J, Kramer P, eds. Evaluation: Obtaining and interpreting data. Bethesda, MD: American Occupational Therapy Association, 2003.
6. American Occupational Therapy Association. Uniform Terminology for Occupational Therapy. 3rd ed. Am J Occup Ther 1994;48:1047–1054.

Recommended Learning Resources

American Occupational Therapy Association. Occupational therapy practice framework: Domain and process. Am J Occup Ther 2002;56:609–639.

Cerebral Palsy

Mary Steichen Yamamoto

Key Terms

Astereognosis
Ataxia
Athetoid (dyskinetic)
Clonus
Contracture
Deformity
Diplegia
Dysarthria
Graphesthesia
Hemiplegia
Homonymous hemianopsia
Hypertonicity (spasticity)
Hyperreflexia
Hypoxemia
Kernicterus
Kinesthesia
Kyphosis
Lordosis
Nystagmus
Primitive reflexes
Quadriplegia
Scoliosis
Strabismus
Topagnosia
Stretch reflex

Sigmund Freud, in his monograph entitled "Infantile Cerebral Paralysis," points out that a well-known painting entitled "The Lame" by Spanish painter Jusepe Ribera (1588–1656), which depicts a child with infantile **hemiplegia**, proves that cerebral paralysis existed long before medical investigators began paying attention to it in the mid-1800s (1). Freud's work as a neurologist is not generally well known and at the time that his monograph was published in Vienna in 1897, he was already deep into his work in the area of psychotherapy. However, he was recognized at the time as the prominent authority on the paralyses of children. Today, cerebral paralysis is known as cerebral palsy.

Cerebral palsy is not one specific condition but rather a grouping of clinical syndromes that affect movement, muscle tone, and coordination as a result of an injury or lesion of the immature brain. It is not considered a disease. Cerebral palsy is classified as and sometimes diagnostically referred to as a static encephalopathy. Static encephalopathy is permanent and unchanging damage to the brain. The developmental effects depend upon which part of the brain is involved and the severity of the damage. Static encephalopathies include other developmental problems that are not cerebral palsy, such as fetal alcohol syndrome, autism, mental retardation, and learning disabilities (2).

A child is considered to have cerebral palsy if all of the following characteristics apply:

1. The injury or insult occurs when the brain is still developing. It can occur anytime during the prenatal, perinatal, or postnatal periods. There is some disagreement about the upper age limit for a diagnosis of cerebral palsy during the postnatal period, but it generally ranges from 2 to 5 years of age (3,4).
2. It is nonprogressive. Once the damage has occurred, there is no further worsening of the child's condition or further damage to the central nervous system. However, the characteristics of the disabilities affecting an individual often change over time.
3. It always involves a disorder in sensorimotor development that is manifested by abnormal postural tone and characteristic patterns of movement. The severity of the impairment ranges from mild to severe.
4. The sensorimotor disorder originates specifically in the brain. The muscles themselves and the nerves connecting them with the spinal cord are normal. Although some cardiac or orthopaedic problems can result in similar postural and movement abnormalities, they are not classified as cerebral palsy.
5. It is a lifelong disability. Unlike some premature babies who demonstrate temporary posture and movement abnormalities during the first year of life, for children with cerebral palsy, these difficulties persist (5).

Etiology

Historically, birth asphyxia was considered the major cause of cerebral palsy. When British surgeon William Little first identified cerebral palsy in 1860, he suggested that a major cause was a lack of oxygen during the birth process. In 1897, Sigmund Freud disagreed, suggesting that the disorder might sometimes have roots earlier in life. Freud wrote, "Difficult birth, in certain cases is merely a symptom of deeper effects that influence the development of the fetus" (1). Although Freud made these observations in the late 1800s, it was not until the 1980s that research supported his views (6,7). In analyzing extensive data from a government study of more than 35,000 births, scientists discovered that less than 10% of the cases of cerebral palsy were a result of birth complications (8). The birth complications resulting in cerebral palsy are related to **hypoxemia** because of a reduction of umbilical or uterine blood flow (9). Table 2.1 lists specific risk factors related to intrapartum hypoxemia.

It is now known that in the majority of cases, the damage that results in cerebral palsy occurs prenatally. Congenital cerebral palsy that results from brain injury during intrauterine life is responsible for approximately 70% of children who have cerebral palsy (10). In most cases, however the specific cause is not known (10). There are a large number of risk factors that can result in cerebral palsy and the interplay between these factors is often complex, making it difficult to identify the specific cause. The presence of risk factors does not always result in a subsequent diagnosis of cerebral palsy. The presence of one risk factor may not result in cerebral palsy unless it is present to an overwhelming degree. Current thought is that often two or more risk factors may interact in such a way as to overwhelm natural defenses, resulting in damage to the developing brain. The strongest risk factors include prematurity

Table 2.1 CEREBRAL PALSY: CONTRIBUTING RISK FACTORS AND CAUSES

Preconception (parental background)
Biological aging (parent or parents older than 35)
Biological immaturity (very young parent or parents)
Environmental toxins
Genetic background and genetic disorders
Malnutrition
Metabolic disorders
Radiation damage

First Trimester of Pregnancy
Endocrine: thyroid function, progesterone insufficiency
Nutrition: malnutrition, vitamin deficiencies, amino acid intolerance
Toxins: alcohol, drugs, poisons, smoking
Maternal disease: thyrotoxicosis, genetic disorders

Second Trimester of Pregnancy
Infection: cytomegalovirus, rubella, toxoplasma, HIV, syphilis, chicken pox, subclinical uterine infections
Placental pathology: vascular occlusion, fetal malnutrition, chronic hypoxia, growth factor deficiencies

Third Trimester of Pregnancy
Prematurity and low birth weight
Blood factors: Rh incompatibility, jaundice
Cytokines: neurological tissue destruction
Inflammation
Hypoxia: placental insufficiency, perinatal hypoxia
Infection: listeria, meningitis, streptococcus group B, septicemia, chorioamnionitis

Intrapartum Events
Premature placental separation
Uterine rupture
Acute maternal hypotension
Prolapsed umbilical cord
Ruptured vasa previa
Tightened true knot of the umbilical cord

Perinatal Period and Infancy
Endocrine: hypoglycemia, hypothyroidism
Hypoxia: perinatal hypoxia, respiratory distress syndrome
Infection: meningitis, encephalitis
Multiple births: death of a twin or triplet
Stroke: hemorrhagic or embolic stroke
Trauma: abuse, accidents

Adapted from UCP Research and Educational Foundation. Factsheet: Cerebral Palsy: Contributing Factors and Causes. September, 1995.

and low birth weight (11). During the postpartum period, premature and low birth weight infants are at greater risk for developing complications, especially in the circulatory and pulmonary systems. These complications can lead to brain hypoxia and result in cerebral palsy. Intraventricular–periventricular bleeding and hypoxic infarcts that occur during this period also place the premature infant at increased risk (4). Additional risk factors that have more recently been identified include intrauterine exposure to infection and disorders of coagulation (8). Maternal infection is a critical risk factor for cerebral palsy, both during prenatal development and at the time of delivery. The infection does not necessarily produce signs of illness in the mother, which can make it difficult to detect. In a study conducted in the mid-1990s, it was determined that mothers with infections at the time of birth had a higher risk of having a child with cerebral palsy (12). Table 2.1 shows a more thorough list of risk factors.

In approximately 10% of children with cerebral palsy in the United States, the condition was acquired postbirth (10). The most common causes in the perinatal and early childhood periods include cerebrovascular accidents (CVAs), infections such as meningitis or encephalitis, poisoning, trauma such as near-drowning and strangulation, and illnesses such as endocrine disorders (4,10,13,14). Closed-head injury that occurs during this period is now classified as traumatic brain injury, even though the resulting impairments are very similar to cerebral palsy (4). The cause remains unknown in 20% to 30% of cases with an early onset of symptoms (4).

Incidence and Prevalence

Estimates of the incidence of cerebral palsy in the United States range from 1.5 to 4 per 1,000 live births (4,15). From 1991 to 1994, the Centers for Disease Control and Prevention (CDC) conducted a study that monitored children aged 3 to 10 years in Atlanta, Georgia. The overall rate of cerebral palsy was 2.8 per 1,000 children in metropolitan Atlanta (15). The United Cerebral Palsy Association estimated in 2001 that 764,000 children and adults in the United States show one or more symptoms of cerebral palsy. It is estimated that each year, 8,000 infants are diagnosed with cerebral palsy. Additionally, each year 1,200 to 1,500 preschool-age children are diagnosed with cerebral palsy (16).

There has been considerable advancement in obstetric and neonatal care during the past two to three decades. Many hoped these advancements would reduce the incidence of cerebral palsy. Unfortunately, the rate has increased slightly. This is probably a result of increased survival rates of very low birth weight and premature infants. Another factor may be the use of fertility treatments by older women that have resulted in an increase in the number of multiple births. Multiple births tend to result in infants who are smaller and premature and are at greater risk for health problems. On the average, they are half the weight of other babies at birth and arrive 7 weeks earlier (17). There is a 400% increase in the probability of cerebral palsy in twin births than in a single birth (17).

Signs and Symptoms

The early signs and symptoms common to all types of cerebral palsy are muscle tone, reflex and postural abnormalities, delayed motor development, and atypical motor performance (4).

Tone Abnormalities

Tone abnormalities include **hypertonicity** or spasticity, hypotonicity, and fluctuating tone. Fluctuating tone shifts in varying degrees from hypotonic to hypertonic. Muscle tone can be characterized as the degree of resistance when a muscle is stretched. For instance, when there is hypotonicity and the elbow is passively extended, there will be little to no resistance to the movement. With hypertonicity there will be increased resistance and it may be difficult to pull the elbow into full extension if there is a lot of hypertonicity. Most infants with cerebral palsy initially demonstrate hypotonia. Later the infant may develop hypertonicity, fluctuating tone, or continue to demonstrate hypotonia, depending on the type of cerebral palsy.

Reflex Abnormalities

With hypertonicity, reflex abnormalities such as **hyperreflexia**, **clonus**, overflow, enhanced **stretch reflex**, and other signs of upper motor neuron lesions are present (4). Retained primitive infantile reflexes and a delay in the acquisition of righting and equilibrium reactions occur in conjunction with all types of abnormal tone. When hypotonia is present, there may be areflexia, or an absence of **primitive reflexes**. These reflexes should be present during the first several months of life.

Postural Abnormalities

The presence of primitive reflexes and tone abnormalities causes the child to have abnormal positions at rest and to demonstrate stereotypical and uncontrollable postural changes during movement. For instance, a child with hypertonicity in the lower extremities often lies supine with the hips internally rotated and adducted and the ankles plantar flexed. This posture is caused by a combination of hypertonicity in the affected muscles and the presence of the crossed extension reflex. A child with hypotonicity typically lies with the hips abducted, flexed, and externally rotated because of low muscle tone, weakness in the affected muscles, and the influence of gravity.

Delayed Motor Development

Cerebral palsy is always accompanied by a delay in the attainment of motor milestones. One of the signs that often alerts the pediatrician to the problem is a delay in the child's ability to sit independently. While cerebral palsy is present at birth in all but the approximately 10% of cases, it is often not recognized until the child fails to achieve these early motor milestones.

Atypical Motor Performance

The way in which a child moves when performing skilled motor acts is also affected. Depending on the type of cerebral palsy, the child may demonstrate a variety of motor abnormalities such as asymmetrical hand use, unusual crawling method or gait, uncoordinated reach, or difficulty sucking, chewing, and swallowing.

Types of Cerebral Palsy

Types of cerebral palsy are classified neurophysiologically into three major types: spastic; **athetoid** or dyskinetic; and **ataxia**.

1. Spastic is characterized by hypertonicity. This type is the most common and accounts for approximately 70% to 80% of the cases of cerebral palsy (8). The spasticity is a result of upper motor neuron involvement (18). Within this category, types are further subdivided anatomically according to the parts of the body that are affected.
2. Athetoid or dyskinetic is characterized by involuntary and uncontrolled movements. These movements are typically slow and writhing. This type accounts for approximately 10% to 20% of the cases of cerebral palsy (8). This type results from basal ganglia involvement (18).

3. Ataxia is characterized by unsteadiness and difficulties with balance, particularly when ambulating. It results from involvement of the cerebellum or its pathways (18). It is much less common than the other two types, occurring in only about 5% to 10% of the cases of cerebral palsy (8).

It is common for there to be mixed forms where two of the types occur together as a result of diffuse brain damage. The most common is spastic with athetoid. Persons with this type have signs of athetosis, and fluctuating postural tone fluctuates from hypertonicity to hypotonia. Athetoid combined with ataxia is less common (18).

Spastic

Spastic cerebral palsy is characterized by hypertonicity, retained primitive reflexes in affected areas of the body, and slow, restricted movement. The impact on motor function can range from a mild impairment that does not interfere with functional skills, such as not having isolated finger movement, to a severe impairment, where there is an inability to reach and grasp. **Contractures** and deformities are common. It is categorized anatomically by the area of the body that is affected. Spastic hemiplegia, spastic **diplegia**, and spastic **quadriplegia** are the most common types.

Spastic Hemiplegia. Spastic hemiplegia involves one entire side of the body, including the head, neck, and trunk. Usually the upper extremity is most affected. Early signs include asymmetrical hand use during the first year or dragging one side of the body when crawling or walking. The initial hypotonic stage is short-lived, with spasticity developing gradually (4). Most children begin walking after 18 months of age, with nearly all children walking by their third birthday (4). When walking, the child typically hyperextends the knee and the ankle in equinovarus or equinovalgus position on the involved side. The child often lacks righting and equilibrium reactions on the involved side and will avoid bearing weight on this side. The shoulder is held in adduction, internal rotation; the elbow is flexed; the forearm is pronated; the wrist is flexed and ulnar deviated; and the fingers are flexed. Spasticity increases during physical activities and emotional excitement. Arm and hand use is limited on the involved side, depending on the severity. The child may use more primitive patterns of grasping and lacks precise and coordinated movement. In more severe cases, the child may totally neglect the involved side or use it only as an assist during bilateral activities. Parietal lobe damage occurs in about 50% of cases and results in impaired sensation, including **astereognosis**, loss or lack of **kinesthesia**, diminished two-point discrimination, decreased **graphesthesia**, and **topagnosia** (4).

Spastic Diplegia. Spastic diplegia involves both lower extremities, with mild incoordination, tremors, or less severe spasticity in the upper extremities. It is most often attributed to premature birth and low birth weight and is, therefore, on the rise as more infants born prematurely survive as a result of medical advances. The ability to sit independently can be delayed up to 3 years of age or older because of inadequate hip flexion and extensor and adductor hypertonicity in the legs (19). Frequently the child will rely on the arms for support. The young child will move forward on the floor by pulling along with flexed arms while the legs are stiffly extended. Getting up to a creeping position is difficult because of spasticity in the lower extremities. Similarly, standing posture and gait are affected to varying degrees, depending on severity. Because of a lack of lower extremity equilibrium reactions, excessive trunk and upper extremity compensatory movements are used when walking. Lumbar **lordosis**, hip flexion and internal rotation (scissoring), plantar flexion of the ankles, and difficulty shifting weight when walking are common. Many of these problems result in contractures and deformities, including dorsal spine **kyphosis**, lumbar spine lordosis, hip subluxation or dislocation, flexor deformities of hips and knees, and equinovarus or equinovalgus **deformity** of the feet (19).

Approximately 85% of children with diplegia will walk independently. Another 10% to 15% will be able to walk in the community with the assistance of crutches or a walker (19). Independent walking occurs typically between 3 and 5 years of age in spastic diplegia (20).

Spastic Quadriplegia. With spastic quadriplegia, the entire body is involved. The arms typically demonstrate spasticity in the flexor muscles, with spasticity in the extensor muscles in the lower extremities. Because of the influence of the tonic labyrinthine reflex (TLR), shoulder retraction and neck hyperextension are common, particularly in the supine position. This results in difficulty with transitional movements such as rolling or coming up to sitting. In the prone position there is increased flexor tone, also a result of TLR influence, causing difficulty with head raising and weight-bearing on the arms. Independent sitting and standing are difficult for the child because of hypertonicity, the presence of primitive reflex involvement, and a lack of righting and equilibrium reactions. Only a small percentage of children with quadriplegia are able to walk independently, and less than 10% ever walk in the community after adolescence (21,22). Oral musculature is usually affected, with resulting **dysarthria**, eating difficulties, and drooling. Individuals are susceptible to contractures and deformities, particularly hip dislocation and **scoliosis**, and must be closely monitored.

Athetosis

Athetosis is the most common type of dyskinesia or dystonia, characterized by slow, writhing involuntary movements of the face and extremities or the proximal parts of the limbs and trunk. Abrupt, jerky distal movements (choreiform) may also appear. The movements increase with emotional tension and are not present during sleep. Head and trunk control is often affected as is the oral musculature, resulting in drooling, dysarthria, and eating difficulties. Whereas spasticity is characterized by hypertonicity in the affected muscle groups and restricted movement, athetosis is characterized by fluctuating tone and excessive movement. Contractures are rare, but hypermobility may be present because of fluctuating hypotonicity.

Associated Disorders

There are a number of disorders associated with cerebral palsy, in addition to the motor impairment that can significantly affect functional abilities.

Mental Retardation

Estimates of the incidence of mental retardation with cerebral palsy range from 40% to 70% (3,14,18). It occurs most often and most severely in spastic quadriplegia and mixed types. Individuals with spastic diplegia and hemiplegia often have normal intelligence (18). If it does occur, it is usually less severe (3,15).

Seizure Disorder

Reports of the incidence of seizures in people with cerebral palsy range from 25% to 60% (14,18). The incidence varies across the diagnostic categories. It is most common in spastic hemiplegia and quadriplegia, and rare with spastic diplegia and dyskinesia (15,19). A recent population-based study of children with cerebral palsy, found that the frequency of epilepsy was 38%. Partial seizures were the most common type and children with a cognitive impairment had a higher frequency of epilepsy (23).

Visual and Hearing Impairments

Visual and hearing impairments occur at a higher rate with cerebral palsy than in the general population. **Strabismus** is the most common visual defect, occurring in 20% to 60% of children with cerebral palsy, with the highest rates in spastic diplegia and quadriplegia (3,24). Other visual and ocular abnormalities include **nystagmus, homonymous hemianopsia** associated with spastic hemiplegia, and difficulties with visual fixation and tracking (3). Some children with athetosis have paralysis of upward gaze, which is a clinical manifestation of **kernicterus** (18). Hearing impairments include sensorineural hearing loss, present in approximately 12% of individuals with cerebral palsy. There is a four times greater prevalence in athetosis than in spasticity (3). Conductive hearing losses, caused by persistent fluid in the ears and middle ear infections, occur when there is severe motor involvement in children who spend a lot of time lying down (14).

Course and Prognosis

The course of cerebral palsy varies depending on type, severity, and the presence of associated problems. With mild motor involvement, the child will continue to make motor gains and compensate for motor difficulties. With more severe forms, little progress may be made in attaining developmental milestones and performing functional tasks. As the child grows older, secondary problems such as contractures and deformities will become more common, especially with spasticity. The life span for most persons with cerebral palsy is within the average range (14).

Medical/Surgical Management

No definitive test will diagnose cerebral palsy. Several factors must be considered. Physical evidence includes a history of delayed achievement of motor milestones. Delayed motor development can occur with mental retardation and other developmental disabilities. The quality of movement is the factor that helps provide a differential diagnosis. The findings of atypical or stereotypical movement patterns and the presence of infantile reflexes and abnormal muscle tone point toward a diagnosis of cerebral palsy. However, other causes must be ruled out, such as progressive neurological disorders, mucopolysaccharidosis, muscular dystrophy, and a spinal cord tumor. Many of these disorders can be ruled out by laboratory tests, although some must be differentiated by clinical or pathological criteria. A magnetic resonance imaging (MRI) or computed tomography (CT) scan may provide evidence of hydrocephalus, help determine the location and extent of structural lesions, and help to rule out other conditions. However, these scans are not definitive as far as making a diagnosis of cerebral palsy and are not predictive as far as the child's functioning (25). The yield of finding an abnormal CT scan in a child with cerebral palsy is 77% and for MRIs it is about 89% (26). An electroencephalogram (EEG) should not be used to determine the cause of cerebral palsy but should be obtained if there is an indication that the child may be having seizures. Because of the high occurrence of associated conditions, children with cerebral palsy should be screened for mental retardation, visual and hearing impairments, and speech and language disorders.

Cerebral palsy often is not evident during the first few months of life and is rarely diagnosed that early. Most cases, however, are detected by 12 months and nearly all by 18 months (14). In some cases early postural and tonal abnormalities in premature infants can resemble cerebral palsy, but the signs are transient with normal subsequent development.

Because of the complexity and diversity of difficulties affecting the individual with cerebral palsy, medical management requires a team approach using the skills of many professionals. Depending on the type of cerebral palsy and the presence of associated problems, team members typically include an occupational therapist, physical therapist, speech pathologist, educational psychologist, nurse, and social worker. The emphasis of intervention is usually on helping the child gain as much motor control as possible, positioning the child to minimize the effects of abnormal muscle tone, instructing the parents and caregivers on handling techniques and ways to accomplish various activities of daily living, recommending adaptive equipment and assistive technology to increase the child's ability to perform desired activities, providing methods to improve feeding and speech if difficulties are present, and helping parents manage behavioral concerns and family stresses.

The primary physician treats the usual childhood disorders and helps with prevention of many health problems. Physicians with various medical specialties may also be involved. The usual specialists include a neurologist to assess neurological status and help control seizures, if present; an orthopaedist to prescribe orthotic devices and any necessary surgeries; and an ophthalmologist to assess and treat any visual difficulties.

Medical management includes both surgical and nonsurgical approaches, with much of the focus on techniques to decrease spasticity. Oral medications such as diazepam (Valium), dantrolene (Dantrium), and baclofen have long been used to reduce spasticity with limited clinical success (26). More recently, the Food and Drug Administration (FDA) has approved the use of baclofen administered through a pump implanted in the abdominal wall to the spinal cord fluid to reduce spasticity in cerebral palsy. There have been few reported side affects. However, the spasticity returns after this treatment is stopped. Complications can occur, such as, overdose or infection, and long term consequences are not yet known (26,27). Another treatment more widely used in recent years is the injection of botulinum toxin into muscles. Spasticity is reduced for a period of 3 to 4 months after injection. Minimal side effects have been reported (26).

Orthotics and splinting are used to improve function and prevent contractures and deformities. Resting or night splints are used to maintain range of motion. Soft splints, dynamic splints, and those allowing movement of the fingers and thumb are used during waking hours and functional activities to reduce tone and promote more typical patterns of movement.

Orthoses prescribed include the ankle-foot orthosis (AFO) for children with hemiplegia to reduce spastic equinus positioning with supination or, occasionally, pronation of the foot. Children with bilateral spasticity who are ambulatory generally do not require or benefit from extensive bracing. However, AFOs are often used to improve abnormal alignment of the feet when the child pulls to a stand and begins walking (3). Supramalleolar orthoses (SMOs) are used when plantar flexor spasticity is mild and mediolateral malalignment is the main concern (3).

Inhibitory and progressive casting has gained acceptance as an alternative to bracing in recent years (28,29). A molded footplate is constructed that inhibits the primitive reflexes, thus reducing spasticity. The footplate is surrounded by a snug, bivalve below the knee cast. Inhibitory and progressive casting also is used with the upper extremities.

Surgical approaches are used to improve the function and appearance of affected areas of the body and to prevent or correct deformities. Tendon lengthening to increase range of motion and tendon transfers to decrease spastic muscle imbalances are done. These procedures, commonly used on the lower extremities, are performed more selectively in the upper extremities. Selective posterior rhizotomy is a neurosurgical technique that is used to reduce spasticity and improve function in carefully selected individuals (30–33). The procedure involves dividing the lumbosacral posterior nerve root into four to seven rootlets. Each rootlet is stimulated electrically. The dorsal rootlets causing spasticity are cut, leaving the normal rootlets intact. This approach is highly successful for individuals who meet the selection criteria (31–33). The most likely candidates are children with either quadriplegia or diplegia (30). An essential part of this treatment approach includes intensive postsurgical physical and occupational therapy for a period of several weeks.

Other surgical procedures include hip reconstruction for hip dislocation and spinal fusion to correct severe scoliosis. These surgeries are most often performed on children with severe quadriplegia. Although there are proponents of surgical intervention, some parents and physicians question whether the results are significant enough to warrant subjecting individuals to the risks of a surgery (28).

Impact on Client Factors

Virtually all of the body function categories and related body structures can be affected in the individual that has cerebral palsy. Which of the categories are affected depends on the type of cerebral palsy, the severity of the condition, and the presence of associated disorders. The one body function category that is always affected in all individuals with cerebral palsy is neuromusculoskeletal and movement-related function. Abnormal muscle tone and motor reflex functions affect joint stability and mobility, and muscle power functions are often diminished. Sensory functions may be involved if there is an associated vision or hearing impairment, or if there are difficulties with sensitivity or discrimination of sensory input. Mental functions, both global and specific, can be affected, particularly if there is an associated learning disability or mental retardation. Voice and speech functions can be affected if the oral motor and respiratory muscles have tonal abnormalities. Functions of the cardiovascular and respiratory system can be affected in a variety of ways, such as associated spinal deformities that can compromise respiration or decreased physical endurance or stamina as a result of the amount of effort that it takes to move.

CASE STUDY

Case Illustrations

■ CASE 1

L.N. is a 64-year-old woman with cerebral palsy, spastic quadriplegic type. She has lived alone in an apartment complex for the elderly and disabled for the past 15 years. Before then, she was in a nursing home. She supports herself on supplemental security income (SSI) and disability payments from the state. A personal-care attendant provided by the Department of Social Services comes in each morning and evening to assist her with activities of daily living, such as meal preparation, bathing, and dressing. L.N. has never been employed but has done volunteer work. She writes articles for a newsletter on her computer and has worked in her church's Sunday school. She has no family support but has many friends. She enjoys learning and taking classes through continuing education.

Spasticity, fluctuating tone, and retained primitive reflexes severely restrict L.N.'s purposeful movement. She has limited range of motion in her left upper extremity and both lower extremities. When reaching with the left arm, she cannot bring it to shoulder height or behind her back. She has a gross grasp in her right upper extremity and can grasp a joystick to operate her electric wheelchair. She cannot write or perform other activities requiring fine motor dexterity. Her left upper extremity is used as an assist for bilateral activities, with no grasping ability present. She can maintain an upright position in sitting, but her weight is shifted to the left (with resulting scoliosis). She can bring her head to an upright position, but neck flexion increases with activities requiring effort. Oral motor muscles are affected, resulting in severe dysarthria, drooling, and difficulty eating. Endurance is a problem, and L.N. becomes easily fatigued.

Communication/interaction skills are also affected. Articulation and modulation when speaking is affected by L.N.'s oral motor control. Limited dexterity and restrictions in movement limit her ability to use gestures and to orient her body in relation to others when engaged in social interactions.

All areas of occupation are affected. In activities of daily living, L.N. needs assistance with bathing, personal hygiene and grooming, toilet hygiene, and dressing. She brushes her teeth and performs light hygiene, such as washing her face, independently. She can transfer herself between her wheelchair and her bed. She needs assistance transferring to the shower seat she uses for bathing. She can transfer on and off the toilet in her apartment with grab bars and the toilet seat at the proper height and position, although it takes her a while to do this. In eating, L.N. can feed herself with her fingers if the food is set up for her, but the process is slow and messy. She drinks from a straw. She takes her own medications if they are set out for her.

In instrumental activities of daily living, L.N. needs assistance in clothing care, cleaning her apartment, household maintenance, and meal preparation. She can use a hand-held portable vacuum cleaner for small cleanups. She has a cat that she cares for. She shops independently but needs assistance getting money out of her wallet at the cash register. All areas of activities of daily living are affected except socialization. L.N. uses a computer for written communication. She uses a speaker phone for telephone communication and can use a tape machine if it is set up for her. If she falls or is in danger at home, she has an emergency alert system that she can activate. Because her speech is difficult to understand, she has an augmented output device for communication but uses it infrequently. She uses a motorized wheelchair for mobility. In the community, L.N. uses public transportation with no difficulty. She has some difficulty transferring herself to and from the toilet when using public restrooms, which sometimes results in incontinence.

In work activities, L.N. has never been employed but has worked as a volunteer for the past several years in the religious education program at her church. She enjoys the interaction with the children that are in the classes.

In leisure activities, L.N. has varied interests. She is an avid reader and enjoys computer games. Social activities include getting together with friends frequently and going out into the community, either alone or with friends. L.N. participates in church retreats as well as community-based trips through an independent living center.

■ CASE 2

A.K. is a 2-year-old girl who lives with her parents and older brother. She was born at 37 weeks gestation at a birth weight of 5 pounds 10 ounces. Pregnancy and birth were unremarkable. She was healthy at birth but her parents gradually became concerned when she did not attain the developmental milestones of sitting and rolling. Her family doctor had assured the family at her 6-month well-baby visit that there was no reason for concern. At 9 months of age, when she returned for another well-baby visit and still had not attained these milestones, she was referred by her family doctor to a behavioral-developmental pediatrician. This specialist diagnosed her with spastic quadriplegia type of cerebral palsy at 11 months of age. She was also seen by a rehabilitation physician who has recommended AFO to assist with ambulation. He has also recommended botulinum toxin (Botox) injections and selective posterior rhizotomy for consideration as future treatments. She was referred to her local school district for early intervention services. A multidisciplinary team assessment was completed by the physical, occupational, and speech therapist. Delays were noted in gross motor, fine motor, and self-help skills. Speech and language, social, and cognitive skills were all determined to be at age level. Weekly occupational and physical therapy home-based services were recommended.

Affected performance skills are in the motor area, which includes posture, mobility, coordination, and strength/effort. She demonstrates spasticity in all four extremities and her trunk. Her movement patterns reflect significant spasticity in her legs. Her joint range of motion is significantly limited in her hamstrings and hip adductors with mild limitations in her heel cords bilaterally. A.K. can sit independently, however it is difficult for her to sit on the floor with her legs extended in front of her as a result of hamstring and hip adductor tightness. She requires assistance moving in and out of sitting. In prone, she can push up to hands and knees and can crawl for short distances. She bears weight on her legs in supported standing with knees in a slightly flexed position, hips adducted, and feet plantar flexed and pronated. She has begun ambulating with a walker for short distances.

In her upper extremities, there is very slightly increased muscle tone in her right upper extremity and moderate hypertonicity in her left upper extremity. A.K. has a refined pincer grasp and active release in her right hand. On the left, she can grasp pegs and small blocks, but the grasp is not refined and release is difficult. She is able to hold an object in her left hand as she manipulates it with her right hand. She is able to use her left hand as an assist for activities requiring two hands such as looking at a book. More refined bilateral coordination tasks are more difficult such as stringing beads and holding paper as she snips with scissors, however she is able to perform these tasks. Strength is adequate for most tasks in her right upper extremity but strength is decreased in her left extremity.

Areas of occupation that are affected include activities of daily living (ADLs) and play. Because she is only 2 years old, instrumental activities of daily living, student, work, and leisure areas of occupational are not yet relevant areas for her. In ADL, because of her age she would not yet be expected to be independent. Given this, A.K.'s affected activities of daily living include bathing, dressing, feeding, and functional mobility. A.K. needs assistance with dressing skills such as undressing and removing shoes and socks. She is independent in feeding but needs some adaptations, such as a Dycem mat to prevent sliding of dishes and an adapted cup with handles that enables her to raise the cup up to drink from. She requires assistance with maintaining a stable sitting position in the bathtub and requires assistance getting in and out of the bath tub. She needs assistance with functional mobility, such as getting in and out of chairs and moving from one place to another.

Exploratory play skills are affected by A.K.'s difficulty with moving about her environment to obtain toys she wants to play with. Participation is affected by the need for a stable position in which to free up her upper extremities to manipulate toys. She uses a bench with a pelvis stabilizer and tray for refined fine motor tasks.

References

1. Freud S. Infantile Cerebral Paralysis. Coral Gables: University of Miami Press, 1968.
2. Hitzfelder N. Static encephalopathy: a basic explanation for parents. 1999. Easter Seals. Available at: http://dallas.easterseals.com/site/DocServer/StaticEncephalopathy.pdf? docID=1486. Accessed November 5, 2004.
3. Molnar G, ed. Pediatric Rehabilitation. 2nd Ed. Baltimore, MD: Williams & Wilkins, 1992.
4. UCP Research and Educational Foundation. Factsheet: Cerebral Palsy: Contributing Risk Factors and Causes. September 1995.
5. Little W. On the influence of abnormal parturition, difficult labor, premature birth and physical condition of the child, especially in relation to deformities. Trans Obstet Soc 1862;3:293.
6. Freeman J, Nelson K. Intrapartum asphyxia and cerebral palsy. Pediatrics 1988;82:240–249.
7. Illingsworth R. A pediatrician asks—why is it called a birth injury? Br J Med Obstet Gynecol 1985;92: 122–130.
8. Cerebral Palsy: Hope Through Research. National Institute of Neurological Disorders and Stroke. July 1, 2001. Available at:http://www.ninds.nih.gov/health_and_medical/pubs/cerebral_palsyhtr.htm. Accessed October 31, 2004.
9. Blickstein, A. Cerebral palsy: A look at etiology and new task force conclusions. OBG Management 2003;15:5.
10. UCP Research and Education Foundation Factsheet: Cerebral Palsy Facts and Figures. October 2001.
11. Lawson RD, Badawi N. Etiology of cerebral palsy. Hand Clin 2003;19(4):547–556.
12. Grether J, Nelson K. Maternal infection and cerebral palsy in infants of normal birth weight. JAMA 1997;278:3.
13. Marmer L. ACDC tracks disability in kids aged 3 to 10. In: Advance for Occupational Therapists. King of Prussia, PA: Merion Publications, Inc., 1997.
14. Blackman J. Medical aspects of developmental disabilities in children birth to three. 3rd Ed. Iowa City: The University of Iowa, 1997.
15. Metropolitan Atlanta Developmental Disabilities Surveillance Program. Center for Disease Control. August 4, 2004. Available at: http://www.cdc.gov/ncbddd/dd/ddsurv.htm. Accessed November 2, 2004.
16. Cerebral Palsy-Facts and Figures. United Cerebral Palsy. October 2001. Available at: http://www.ucp.org/ucp_generalddoc.cfm/1/9/37/37-37/447. Accessed November 1, 2004.
17. Multiple Births and Developmental Brain Damage. UCP Research and Educational Foundation. May 1997.
18 Berkow R, Fletcher A, eds. The Merck Manual of Diagnosis and Therapy. 16th Ed. Rahway, NJ: Merck Sharp & Dohme Research Laboratories, 1999.
19. Bobath K. A Neurological Basis for the Treatment of Cerebral Palsy. Philadelphia: JB Lippincott, 1980.
20. Koop S. Orthopedic aspects of static encephalopathies. In: Miller G, Ramer J, eds. Static Encephalopathies of Infancy and Childhood. New York: Raven Press, Ltd., 1992.
21. Bleck E. Locomotor prognosis in cerebral palsy. Dev Med Child Neurol 1975;17:18–25.
22. Russman B, Gage J. Cerebral palsy. Curr Probl Pediatr 1989;19:65–111.
23. Carlsson, M. et al. Clinical and aetiological aspects of epilepsy in children with cerebral palsy. Dev Med Child Neurol 2003;45:371–376.
24. Hiles D, Wallar P, McFarlane F. Current concepts in the management of strabismus in children with cerebral palsy. Ann Ophthalmol 1975;7:789.
25. Miller, F. Bachrach, S. Cerebral Palsy: A Guide For Care. Hopkins Press. 1998.
26. Ashwal S, Russman B, Blasco A, et al. Practice Parameter: Diagnostic assessment of the child with cerebral palsy. Neurology 2004;62:851–863.
27. United Cerebral Palsy Research and Educational Foundation. Factsheet: Baclofen and the Baclofen Pump: Update. October 2001.
28. Cusick B. Progressive Casting and Splinting for Lower Extremity Deformities in Children with Neuromuscular Dysfunction. Tucson: Therapy Skill Builders, 1990.
29. Hanson C, Jones L. Gait abnormalities and inhibitive casts in cerebral palsy: literature review. J Pediatr Med Assoc 1989;79:53–59.
30. Peacock W, Staudt L. Functional outcomes following selective posterior rhizotomy in children with cerebral palsy. J Neurosurg, 1991;74:380–385.

31. Berman B, Vaughan C, Peacock C, et al. The effect of rhizotomy on movement in patients with cerebral palsy. Am J Occup Ther 1990;44:6.
32. Kinghorn J. Upper extremity functional changes following selective posterior rhizotomy in children with cerebral palsy. Am J Occup Ther 1992;46:6.
33. Selective Dorsal Rhizotomy. The Cleveland Clinic Health Information Center. March 20, 2002. Available at: http://www.clevelandclinic.org/health/health-info/docs/0300/0368.asp? index=4591. Accessed November 4, 2004.

Recommended Learning Resources

Domans J, Pellegrano L. Caring for Children with Cerebral Palsy: A Team-based Approach. Baltimore, MD: Brooks Publishing, 1998. An interdisciplinary reference for team-based, collaborative care of children with cerebral palsy.

Fraser B, Hensinger R, Phelps J. Physical Management of Multiple Handicaps. A Professional's Guide. 2nd Ed. Baltimore, MD: Brooks Publishing, 1990. Valuable reference for those working with children and adults with severe physical or multiple impairments. Contains chapters on physical management and treatment, seating systems, therapeutic positioning and adaptive equipment, and activities of daily living.

Geralis, Elaine. Children With Cerebral Palsy—A Parent's Guide. 2nd Ed. Bethesda, MD: Woodbine House, 1997. Good reference for therapists and parents for young children with cerebral palsy. Contains comprehensive information on cerebral palsy including medical treatment information, and the effects of cerebral palsy on the child's development and education

Levitt S. Treatment of Cerebral Palsy and Motor Delay. 4th Ed. Oxford, England: Blackwell Science LTP, 2003. Book was written for occupational and physical therapists working with children with cerebral palsy. Good discussion of treatment approaches, principles of treatment, and description of procedures.

Morris S, Klein M. Pre-Feeding Skills. Tucson, AZ: Therapy Skill Builders, 1987. Excellent reference for oral-motor and feeding therapy for children. Very thorough and good overall approach to feeding issues.

United Cerebral Palsy National Office
1660 L Street, NW Suite 700
Washington, DC 20036
Tel: (202) 776–0406; toll free: (800) 872–5827
www.ucp.org
Leading source of information on cerebral palsy and national advocacy group.

Children's Hemiplegia and Stroke Association (CHASA)
4101 West Green Oaks Blvd.
PMB #149
Arlington, TX 76016
Tel: (817) 492–4325
www.hemikids.org
Comprehensive, practical resource related to children with hemiplegia type cerebral palsy.

National Institute of Neurological Disorders and Stroke (NINDS). Cerebral Palsy Information Page. Available at: www.ninds.nih.gov/disorders/cerebral_palsy. Lists resources including organizations, publications, links, and general information about cerebral palsy.

Autism Spectrum Disorders

Kathryn Shangraw

Key Terms

Ambiguous hand preference
Amygdala
Auditory processing
Autistic disorder
Asperger's disorder
Casein
Cerebellum
Childhood disintegrative disorder
Echolalia
Frontal lobes
Gastrointestinal (GI) disorder
Gene
Gluten
Hippocampus
Hyperlexia
Inferior olive
Joint attention
Limbic system
Neurobiological
Neuron
Purkinje cells
Rett's disorder
Rote memory
Tactile defensiveness
Theory of mind

Rachel was the beautiful first-born daughter to her parents, and during her first year of life, she appeared to be a typically developing child. She responded to people and objects in her environment with interest and enjoyment. Though slightly delayed in learning to walk, she mastered this skill between 14 to 16 months of age. In contrast, many of her language skills developed strongly during her first year. Rachel was exposed to three different languages in her home and learned several vocabulary words in each language by the time she was 14 months old.

When Rachel was approximately 14 months old, her parents noticed a startling change in her behavior. Eye contact became rare and she no longer turned in response when her mother called her name. As a result of this decreased responsiveness, her parents worried she was losing her hearing. However, an audiologic test indicated normal hearing abilities. Dressing this little girl became a challenge. Suddenly, she did not easily tolerate the sensation of clothes against her skin. She became intensely distressed when her mother tried to brush her hair or clip her nails. The vocabulary of approximately 30 words that she had previously developed was replaced by silence or babbling. Upon reflection, her mother realized Rachel had never used specific communicative gestures such as waving to greet others or pointing. Engaging Rachel in daily activities became increasingly difficult for she appeared frustrated, unable to express her needs and wants, and unable to leave familiar, preferred activities without becoming highly agitated. During these episodes of tantrums, Rachel would hit herself or bang her head repeatedly against a wall while crying. Her mother described that overall, "she no longer seemed happy." When Rachel was 2 years and 6 months old, her parents brought their concerns to the attention of early intervention specialists. As a result, Rachel began receiving occupational therapy, speech-language therapy, and special education services. During her preschool class, these specialists observed the same concerning characteristics her parents had described. Additionally, they noted she did not appear interested in the other children in her preschool class. Transitioning from room to room consistently distressed her, causing "meltdowns" during which she flung herself on the floor and cried inconsolably. She used only a few real words or echoed words of others but did not appear to understand what they meant. Many times, the classroom environment seemed to provide her with far too much sensory input. As a result, she would close her eyes or seek out places away from others. Yet Rachel still showed moments of attachment and joy, such as a strong, loving connection toward her parents and grandparents. Additionally, she smiled, laughed, and shared eye contact during specific activities, such as swinging, playing peek-a-boo, or singing.

Despite these moments of engagement, the changes and gaps in her development caused her parents and therapists to seek further neurodevelopmental testing. Rachel was therefore assessed by a local neurologist, who confirmed the suspicions of her family and therapists: Rachel presented with **autistic disorder,** one of the disorders on the autism spectrum.

Autism is a developmental disorder with significant life-long effects because it disrupts a child's ability to socially interact and communicate with others. Though the precise cause of the disorder is unknown, autism is of a **neurobiological** origin (1). In other words, undetermined abnormalities in the structure and/or function of a child's brain cause the atypical behaviors seen in autism (2). Autism is not seen as one disorder; rather, it describes a spectrum of disorders that range in severity of symptoms, onset and course of development, and presence of features such as cognitive impairment or language delay (1). *The Diagnostic and Statistical Manual, Fourth Edition, Text Revision (DSM IV-TR)* (3) lists five disorders under the synonymous term Pervasive Developmental Disorders: autistic disorder, **Asperger's disorder, childhood disintegrative disorder (CDD), Rett's disorder,** and **pervasive developmental disorder-not otherwise specified (PDD-NOS).**

The autism spectrum disorders (ASDs) share the following characteristics:

1. Impairment in social interaction
2. Impairment in communication
3. Restricted behavior (the child does not show new ideas) or repetitive/stereotyped behavior (a behavior is repeated to an extreme degree) (Fig. 3.1).

A child with ASD is deviant from, as well as delayed in, typical patterns of development. Some children evidence problems from birth, such as making far less eye contact than other infants. However, in most cases the characteristics of autism noticeably emerge between 12 to 36 months of age because of the following observations:

1. Because children with autism progress more slowly in several areas of development than

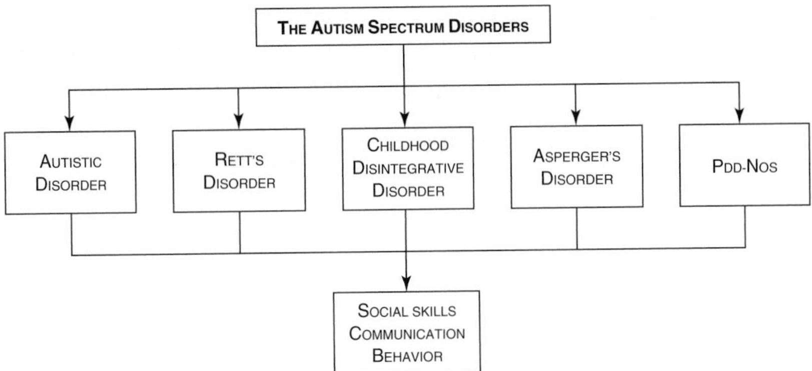

Figure 3.1 Autism spectrum disorders. Five disorders comprise the autism spectrum, with each disorder allowing for a range of skill sets and severity. All ASDs impact an individual's social, communication, and behavioral skills.

typical children, a gap in skills becomes clear at this age when children normally expand their language and social skills rapidly.

Children may have been typically developing before 12 to 36 months of age, with a sudden loss of previously acquired skills presenting in some cases of children with ASD (4).

2. Autism cannot be "cured." Intervention is available for individuals with autism that targets behavioral, language, cognitive, social, and sensory concerns. Though these individuals may improve their skills as a result of intervention, they usually struggle with the challenges of their disorder throughout their lives.

The Many Names of Autism

The terms used in the autism field are confusing for many people, since some terms are used interchangeably or inconsistently in literature and by professionals. The most accurate and generally agreed upon definitions are summarized as follows.

- The terms autism, ASDs, and PDDs are synonymous. Many professionals prefer using the term ASDs rather than PDDs, believing it more accurately reflects the variability that occurs both among the disorders and within an individual diagnostic category.
- This chapter will use autism and ASDs interchangeably, noting the term PDDs only when quoting another source that uses this phrase.
- Note that the similar term autistic disorder actually refers to one specific diagnostic category on the autism spectrum.

Etiology

Though researchers believe that certain factors (e.g., genetics) are more likely than others to cause autism, no one etiologic factor has clearly emerged. Therefore, autism is diagnosed based on observed behaviors, not by its cause. It was first described in literature in 1943 by Dr. Leo Kanner (5), and initial hypotheses that autism was caused by "cold" or unresponsive parents were dismissed (6). Rather, while not attributed to mental disorders, autism is a neurologic disability (1).

Abnormalities in Brain Structure/Function

Children with autism develop, process, and react differently to their world than typically developing children. This diversion from normal development means that children with autism begin life with brains that are physically different from nonautistic brains. Additionally, the way in which life experiences are mapped onto the brain is altered as a result of the physical differences (7). The precise distinctions are not yet entirely clear, since autism is not caused by a single obvious lesion in the brain. In fact, studies have indicated subtle differences in several areas of the brain with researchers unsure which area, or combination of areas, results in the manifestation of autism (8).

Through the study of postmortem brain tissue and imaging studies such as positron emission tomography (PET) scan and magnetic resonance imaging (MRI), consistencies have emerged in the research of brain abnormalities.

1. The brain is made up of about 100 billion **neurons**, or single cells, that interconnect and communicate information among the various brain regions and from other areas of the body. The behaviors of autism may result from abnormalities in the neural networking between the multiple areas of the brain, rather than in one area, as the brain processes complex information (9).
2. Though children with autism are born with normal head circumferences, increased brain volume and head circumference become evident in autistic children when they are 3 to 4 years old (8). However, individuals with Rett's disorder evidence smaller-than-usual brains (10).
3. There is a growing body of research that suggests that dysfunction of the **cerebellum** is a likely contributor to autism. This area of the brain has been traditionally known for its role in the coordination of movement. But the cerebellum, which sits over the brainstem, may also play a role in sensory discrimination, attention, emotions, mental imagery, problem solving, and some aspects of language processing; the speed, consistency, and appropriateness of mental and cognitive processes; and visual spatial orientation, spatial orientation, and visuomotor function (11,12). Neurons in the cerebellum known as **Purkinje cells** form a layer near the surface of the cerebellum and convey signals away from the cerebellum. In autistic individuals, an important deviation consistently noted is a decrease in the Purkinje cell number.
4. In the brainstem, the neurons in the **inferior olive** of individuals with autism also showed deviations depending on age. Cells were initially larger than normal but typical in appearance in young children; in adulthood, these cells were unusually small and pale (8,12).
5. Inferior olives are connected to Purkinje cells by climbing fibers, and this bond from the inferior olive to the Purkinje cell is made at 28 to 30 weeks gestation. Once this union occurs, if a Purkinje cell dies, then the inferior olive will also deplete. As previously noted, Purkinje cells are reduced in number in children with autism but the cells of the inferior olive are normal in quantity. The implication is that damage to the Purkinje cells in children with autism would have likely occurred in utero before the bond was established, prior to 30 weeks gestation (11,12).
6. Imaging studies have indicated reduced activation of the **frontal lobe** in individuals diagnosed with autism (8). Additionally, some areas of the frontal lobe appear markedly larger in children with autism compared with typically developing children (13). The frontal lobe's function is voluntary control of the body's movements. Specific regions of this lobe are also responsible for social behavior, spontaneous production of language, initiation of motor

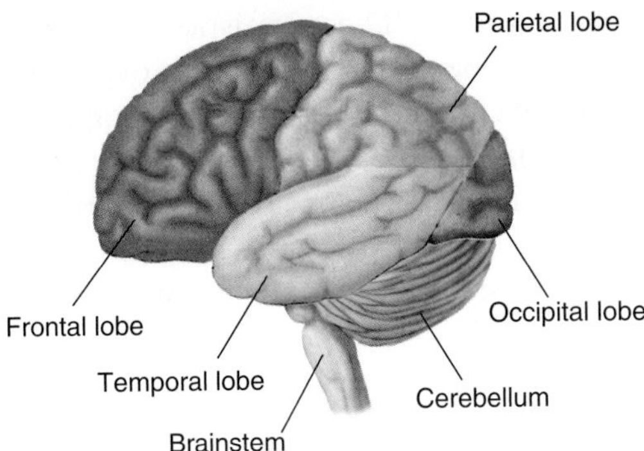

Figure 3.2 Cerebral cortex. Left lateral view of the brain, including the four lobes of the cerebrum and the cerebellum. (From Bickley LS, Szilagyi P. Bates' Guide to Physical Examination and History Taking. 8th Ed. Philadelphia: Lippincott, Williams & Wilkins, 2003.)

activity, processing sensory stimuli, and then planning reaction as a result of the input, abstract thinking, problem solving, and judgment (12). How the abnormalities affect the frontal lobe's ability to conduct these roles remains unclear, though many symptoms of autism appear related to problems in frontal lobe functioning (Fig. 3.2).

7. Within the **limbic system**, a network of structures that regulates emotion, structures known as the **amygdala** and **hippocampus** appear abnormal in the brains of individuals with autism.

"Memories, the desire to produce language, feelings, and the emotional coloring of thought are all mediated by the limbic system. Anatomical systems necessary for cognitive functions, such as language, spatial concepts, understanding of meaning in life, and so forth are all intimately linked to the limbic system" (14, p. 15). Since the functioning of these abilities is impacted in individuals with autism, it has been a logical step to focus research in this area. Thus far, anomalies include decreased size of the neurons that make up the structures of the limbic system, with a higher number of these neuronal cells packed into their respective spaces (12) (Fig. 3.3).

Scientists are persistently closing in on the differences in the brain structure and function of this population. In the meantime, the

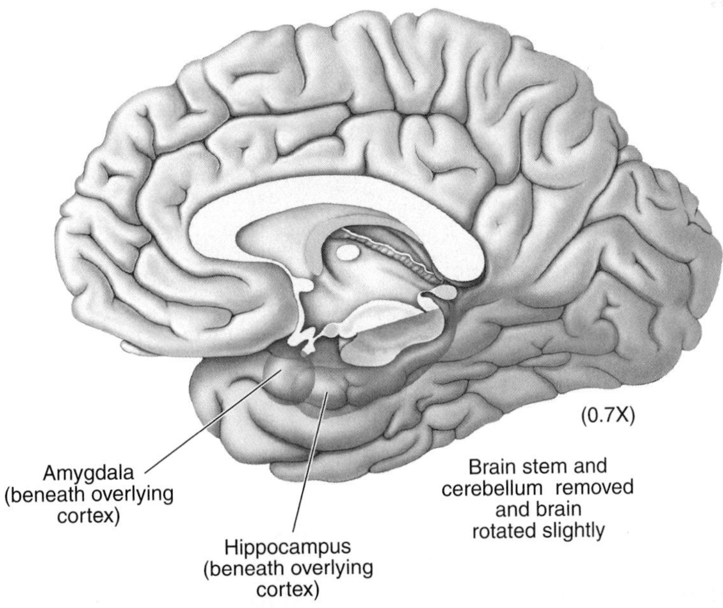

Figure 3.3 Amygdala and hippocampus. The limbic system is a group of subcortical structures in the brain that are responsible for learning, memory, and emotion. Deviations in the hippocampus and amygdala may contribute to autistic behaviors. (From Bear MF, Connors BW, Parasido MA. Neuroscience: Exploring the Brain. 2nd ed. Philadelphia: Lippincott, Williams & Wilkins, 2001).

question arises: What has happened in a child's system to cause these deviations in the brain to occur?

Hypothesized Causes of Autism

Parents of children with autism, upon hearing their child's diagnosis, typically search for reasons why this condition occurred in their child. The professionals who work with these parents must act as guides to discuss the most recent and accurate information in the autism field. Parents are likely to question professionals about many of the factors that will be discussed in the following sections. It is important to share with parents those theories that are likely and those that seem implausible based on current research.

Genetics. The differences in the neurobiology of children with autism are most likely accounted for by genetics. **Genes** are composed of DNA, and through heredity, determine the particular characteristics that distinguish one human from another. Genes are responsible for carrying the instructions for the brain. If these instructions are wrong, the brain deviates from a course of typical development (7). No single gene has been found to cause these disorders, therefore, current research is focused on finding a combination of genes that may be responsible for an individual's susceptibility to autism (8,15). Rett's disorder is the only one on the spectrum that has a confirmed genetic mutation as its cause, occurring on the methyl-CpG-binding protein 2 (MECP2) gene (16).

Support for Genetic Etiology.

- In sibling studies, where one monozygotic twin was diagnosed with autism, the other was also diagnosed somewhere on the spectrum in 90% to 95% of cases. For dizygotic (fraternal) twins, both children received an ASD diagnosis in only 10% of cases studied. These statistics imply that shared genetic codes significantly increase the likelihood of autism occurrence (15,17).
- In the general population, an individual has a 0.2% chance of having autism (15). Siblings of children with autism, however, are at a higher risk for presenting somewhere on the autism spectrum. For parents, the probability of having a second child with autism is 3% to 7% if the first child is male and autistic. If the first child is female with autism, the likelihood of a second child with autism increases to approximately 7% to 14% (17). A higher rate of speech-language disorders has also been found among these families (18), suggesting that these siblings received some, but not all, of the genes responsible for autism (7).
- Relatives of these children more commonly displayed traits of autism (e.g., anxiety, aloofness) than relatives of other children. The presence of these traits in family members may be genetically linked to the manifestation of autism. (19).
- Additional weight is given to the genetic link since a disproportionately higher number of males are diagnosed with autism (with the exception of Rett's disorder), with three to four males diagnosed for every one female (17).

Because specific genes have not yet been identified as the cause of autism, current research is exploring other factors as possible etiologies or covariables. Researchers are also considering that autism may be caused by a different set of variables for each child on the spectrum.

Environmental Factors. Environmental factors are external influences that may cause damage to people's systems if they are overexposed or exposed during a period of critical development. The United Kingdom Medical Research Council (8) reviewed the following environmental risk factors as possible causes of autism: prenatal or postnatal exposure to viruses, infections, drugs/alcohol, endocrine factors, and carbon monoxide. However, these factors are thus far not significantly linked to ASDs. In terms of obstetric complications, most mothers reported entirely normal prenatal or perinatal experiences. Researchers have paid particular attention to the measles-mumps-rubella (MMR) vaccination (which protects against those diseases) in recent years, with some researchers speculating that the mercury in this vaccination is responsible for causing changes in a person's system that lead to the symptoms of autism. When further investigated, a valid association between the MMR vaccine and autism was not found. Though exposure to mercury may lead to impairments that look similar to those found in autism, children with autism have not consistently evidenced elevated levels of mercury in their systems. In contrast, children with behavioral and/or developmental difficulties were discovered to have a higher level of lead in their systems, though it is unclear if exposure to lead results in autism (8).

Physiologic Abnormalities. Children with autism need to be closely monitored for additional medical concerns, since many of these children are not able to clearly express a medical problem. For those children who are nonverbal, acting out with inappropriate behaviors may be their only form of expressing discomfort. If a child demonstrates sudden aggressive, severe, or unusual behaviors, or awakens frequently from sleep, then medical attention by an experienced physician is necessary (20).

One medical condition an autistic child may experience is a **gastrointestinal (GI) disorder**, which is a disorder of the digestive tract. Unusually high rates of GI disorders in children with autism have been documented in recent years, including gastrointestinal reflux, gastritis, persistent gas, diarrhea, and constipation (20–22). These problems should be treated by a gastroenterologist, a physician who specializes in GI disorders. A common, though unproven, theory hypothesizes that children with autism experience abnormal digestion of **gluten**, a mixture of proteins that may be found in wheat and other products (e.g., some snack foods or delicatessen meats), and **casein**, a protein found in cow's milk. This theory suggests that children with autism children lack an enzyme that efficiently digests these substances; as a result, opioid or morphine-like substances accumulate and may be the reason these children socially withdraw or engage in repetitive behaviors (23,24).

The idea of a vulnerability to immune system disorders in children with autism has gathered interest and has been widely debated, but similar to theories of food allergies, there is currently a lack of research to prove or disprove this as a factor.

Combination of Factors. It is plausible that the interaction of gene susceptibility and environmental factors gives rise to autism. In other words, an individual may be genetically at risk for this disorder, but in order for characteristics to appear, an individual would also need to be exposed to a yet-to-be-identified environmental factor (8).

Prevalence and Incidence

Autism is the third most common developmental disorder, occurring more frequently in the population than congenital malformations (physical body or organ malformations that are present at birth) and Down syndrome (25). In children younger than 8 years, about 60 children per 10,000 present with some type of ASD. Approximately 10 to 30 children per 10,000 have autistic disorder, with Asperger's disorder occurring more infrequently at 2.5 per 10,000 children. Childhood disintegrative disorder and Rett's disorder are less common, with CDD occurring in 0.1 to 0.6 children per

10,000 and Rett's disorder occurring in 1 in 10,000 to 1 in 15,000 children (8,16). Prevalence information for the adult population on the autism spectrum is not known.

Prevalence of autism has been on the rise since the early 1990s. Though this increase has raised speculation of a possible "epidemic," the rise in prevalence likely results from better identification and availability of services, along with changes in diagnostic criteria that allow more children to fit the diagnosis of autism (19,26,27).

Incidence, or the measure of new cases per year, is best studied in disorders that have a clear onset. Because the age of onset in autism is usually unclear, accurate incident rates are difficult to measure. Estimates range from 2.1 to 8.3 per 10,000 for all children diagnosed with an autism spectrum disorder (8).

Signs and Symptoms

Each ASD is related to the other disorders in social, language, and behavioral deviations, and each differs in terms of age of onset, severity of symptoms, and presence of other features such as cognitive impairment (1). However, these core behaviors do not nearly encompass the entire picture of these complex human beings. Motor abnormalities, sensory integration disorders, and co-occurring medical disorders (e.g., seizures, sleep disturbances, GI problems) are only some of the additional concerns that arise in this population. Every child with autism displays a separate matrix of strengths and challenges; even two children who fall into the same diagnostic category on the spectrum (e.g., Asperger's disorder) will exhibit individual differences resulting from personality and experiences (8).

The first of the core symptoms, difficulty in social interaction, includes limited use of eye contact, facial expressions, social gestures (e.g., pointing, shrugging, reaching arms up to be lifted by parent), and body postures. Additionally, children on the autism spectrum are usually challenged to accurately interpret the body language and facial expressions of other people. A child with ASD may not seek out others to share enjoyment, share interest in the same objects, or look for approval or reassurance from parents. Moreover, individuals experience challenges in developing friendships with same-age peers. These obstacles range from showing a lack of interest in others to desiring friends but having difficulty understanding how to relate appropriately to peers. Problems with interaction may exist because children with autism are hypothesized to have limitations in **theory of mind**, which is the ability to understand another person's thoughts, feelings, or intentions. It is how an individual "reads" someone's thoughts, understands another person's perspective on an issue, and predicts another's feelings (28). Without this ability, a person is not able to predict or understand the actions of others (4). Other social disturbances that manifest in children with autism include a preference for playing alone, limited or repetitive play routines, and limited or absent pretend play skills (1,3,29).

Language impairments in the autism population include delays in language development as well as abnormalities in language use. Typically developing children progress through several communication milestones in their first few years (4). During a child's first year of life, a toddler gazes at others with interest, begins babbling, and reacts to sounds and voices. By 12 months, gestures and first words emerge and the child shows recognition of his name and some words and phrases. By 2 years of age, the child has built a substantial vocabulary and combines words into two- to three-word phrases. However, children with autism frequently show delays in learning to speak, with some children unable to use words until their school-age years (3,4). In severe cases of autism, spoken language may not be acquired at all. A child's ability to respond to voices or comprehend verbal language (**auditory processing**) may also be impacted. Many parents report that their child with autism does not respond when spoken to or called by name. Social impairments further affect these children's communication because they may not be motivated to communicate with others, are typically challenged to use or understand social cues such as intonation and facial expressions to interpret meaning, and have difficulty maintaining the "give and take" of conversations (e.g., a child may discuss only his topic of interest without allowing others to take a turn).

The language of verbal children appears even more peculiar because of the presence of **echolalia**, pronoun reversal, and out of context words. Echolalia is speech in which the child echoes back what he has previously heard. Though all young children use echolalia as they are learning language, children with autism retain this characteristic and often apply it in abnormal ways. It results from poor auditory processing while auditory memory remains intact (30). Echolalia may be immediate, meaning that it occurs just after another speaker's utterance, or delayed, occurring significantly after hearing a speaker (e.g., reciting an entire children's book from memory an hour or day later) (30). Though it may appear unusual in conversation, children with autism frequently use this inappropriate device in meaningful ways (e.g., reciting lines from his favorite movie as a self-calming strategy when he feels anxious). Because children with autism often fail to understand language, pronouns (e.g., "you" and "me") are also often used incorrectly. Other times, these individuals may use language in a context that seems out of place; for instance, saying "ball" when he is actually requesting juice.

In the area of repetitive behaviors, individuals with ASD may exhibit an abnormal or intense preoccupation with routines or patterns. For instance, a child may line up blocks or toy cars for hours without playing with others or using these toys in pretend play. Additionally, the child may scream or cry in reaction to someone joining his play or moving the lined-up toys. Obsessions with specific topics are common, such as showing an unusual interest in elevators or numbers and letters (4). Additional common characteristics include rigidity in daily routines; abnormal, stereotyped behaviors such as repetitive hand-flapping or body rocking; and unusual, nonfunctional preoccupation with parts of an object (e.g., spinning the wheels of a toy car without showing interest in any other type of play with this toy) (3,4).

All children with autism demonstrate some combination of these social, language, and behavioral symptoms. Additionally, specific characteristics are associated with each disorder on the autism spectrum and are discussed in the following sections.

Autistic Disorder

Autistic disorder is diagnosed when severe challenges occur in each area of social, language, and behavioral characteristics. Marked delays and deviations are noted in language development, which are the most common initial concerns of parents and pediatricians. Approximately half of children with autistic disorder remain nonverbal or struggle with severely impaired speech as adults (26). Because both the comprehension and the use of language are affected, these individuals are additionally challenged to compensate for lack of verbal language with another mode of communication, such as meaningful social gestures (pointing or acting out what they want/need) or sign language (1). Even those who develop verbal language may struggle in the initiation, maintenance, or relevance of conversation. Cognitive deficits are evident in the majority of children with autistic disorder, though these children often demonstrate a scattered pattern of skills (26). For instance, a child may be exceptional at puzzles and matching colors but poorly comprehends time concepts. A child does not need to evidence

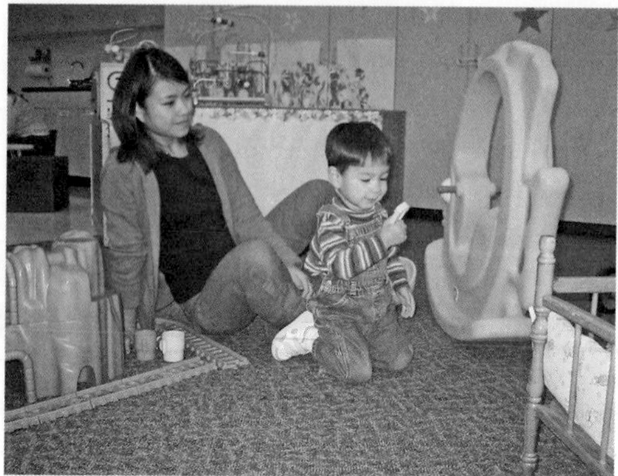

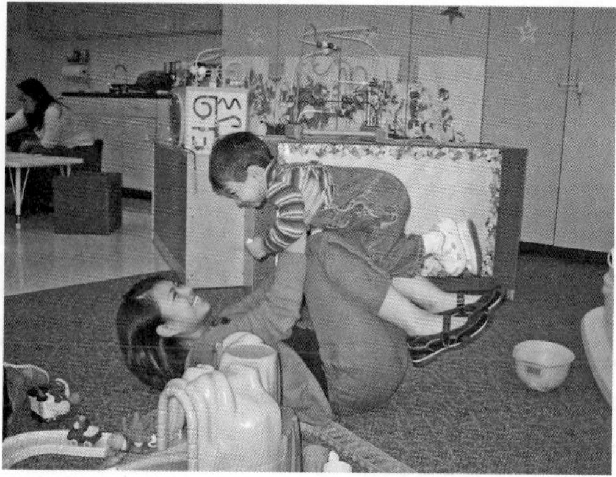

Figure 3.4 Young child with autistic disorder. **A,** Children with autism bear no obvious physical features that distinguish them from other children; rather, it is their behaviors set them apart from their peers. Here, though a familiar adult approaches this little boy to play, he prefers gazing at an object for an unusual length of time. **B,** Initially, children with autism were thought to be incapable of any social interaction with others. This generalization no longer holds true. Though it requires more effort to engage this child in social interaction than it takes with typically developing children, he is clearly capable of sharing moments of joy with other people.

cognitive challenges to receive a diagnosis of autistic disorder (Fig. 3.4).

Rett's Disorder

Rett's disorder primarily affects females who evidence a significantly deviant pattern of development. Individuals with Rett's disorder show an unusual progression of development. These children's prenatal and perinatal experiences are normal, and following birth, typical development progresses for several months. However, unusual onset of characteristics begins after this period of normal growth, as head growth decelerates between 5 and 30 months of age and hypotonia appears (3,31). Use of previously acquired functional hand skills diminishes between 5 to 48 months of age and is replaced by frequent, stereotyped hand movements, such as hand wringing (3). At the same time, dementia, autistic features, and possible onset of seizures appear (31). Poor coordination may be noted in gait or trunk movements. The pattern of social development is quite unusual. These children lose their previous ability to socially engage with others; however, social interaction is often later reacquired in a child's development. Expressive language, receptive language, and psychomotor skills are significantly impaired in this population (3,31). Rett's disorder stands alone as the only ASD with a known etiology caused by a single gene disorder (16).

Childhood Disintegrative Disorder

In this rare disorder, children with CDD develop normally for a minimum of 2 years following birth. Prior to ten years of age, a loss of skills is noted in at least two areas of development, including receptive/expressive language, social/adaptive functioning, bowel/bladder control, play abilities, and motor skills (3). Skills disintegrate until the child exhibits features consistent with those in autism. However, before the loss of skills has occurred, children with CDD have usually acquired far more words, phrases, and even sentences than children with autistic disorder or PDD-NOS (30), meaning that the loss of language is more obvious in CDD than in autistic disorder.

Asperger's Disorder

The hallmarks of this disorder include the social and behavioral challenges observed in other ASDs; however, children with Asperger's disorder do not exhibit delays in cognitive, language, or adaptive functions. Though early language milestones are met, children with Asperger's have difficulty using language appropriately in reciprocal interactions. Problems occur in the interpretation of others' gestures and nonverbal signals. Therefore, they may discuss a topic of interest while using impressive vocabulary words, but not observe their partner's signals of disinterest in a conversation (e.g., bored expression, fingers drumming on a table in exasperation). Unfortunately, because these children do develop language at a typical age, their symptoms may not be apparent until a later age, resulting in a diagnosis at a later age than children with autistic disorder (3). Though the term "high-functioning autism" is at times used synonymously with Asperger's disorder, these two terms actually refer to two different diagnostic categories.

Pervasive Developmental Disorder-Not Otherwise Specified

This category is used when children demonstrate a significant impairment in social interaction, as well as impairment either in the use of language or with the presence of stereotypical behaviors (3). Children given the diagnosis of PDD-NOS display less severe forms of ASD behaviors, with fewer of the symptoms of autism present (30) (Table 3.1).

Table 3.1 THE AUTISM SPECTRUM DISORDERS

Disorder	Characteristics
Autistic disorder (classic autism)	Presence of ≥6 of 12 potential deficits involving all three behavioral domains that define the autistic spectrum: ≥2 deficits in sociability, empathy, and insight into other persons' feelings and agendas ≥1 deficit in communicative language and imagination ≥1 deficit in behavioral and cognitive flexibility Detectable before the age of 3 years Diagnosis not excluded by the level of cognitive competence or the existence of other handicaps
Asperger's disorder	Troublesome social ineptness Behavioral inflexibility with a narrow range of interests IQ ≥ 70 (affected children may be normally intelligent or gifted) No delay in the emergence of speech Often clumsiness
Pervasive developmental disorder not otherwise specified	Applies to less severely affected children who do not meet criteria for either autistic disorder or Asperger's disorder
Childhood disintegrative disorder	Early development entirely normal, including speech Severe regression between the ages of 2 and 10 years, affecting language, sociability, cognition, and competence in skills of daily life
Rett's disorder	Severe global regression in infant girls (rarely in boys), resulting in lifelong severe mental retardation, lack of language and purposeful hand use, and other neurologic deficits

Co-Occurring Conditions

Autism has been associated with medical or genetic conditions in approximately 10% of its population. These conditions include fragile X syndrome, tuberous sclerosis, metabolic disorders, rubella syndrome, haemophilus influenza meningitis, and structural brain abnormalities (27).

Seizure disorders are not specific to autism, but occur more frequently than in the general population. An estimated one third of children are reported to have experienced at least two seizures before reaching adulthood. The probability of experiencing seizures is highest during adolescence and has been linked to causing or worsening cognitive and motor impairment (32).

Course and Prognosis

Because each category in the autism spectrum presents with a range of abilities, the course of the disorder during one's lifetime depends on the child's diagnosis and individual differences (1). In addition, a diagnosis can change for an individual. For instance, a child with autistic disorder may show improvement in his symptoms, thereby displaying characteristics more similar to PDD-NOS (30). Most individuals with autism tracked by longitudinal studies have retained ASD symptoms to some degree throughout their lives (1).

Autistic Disorder

A child displays traits of autism before the age of 3 years, and these symptoms are generally most apparent following the child's second birthday. In some cases, deviations in a child's developmental and interaction skills are noted shortly following birth (e.g., hypersensitivities and limited eye contact), while other infants appear to develop normally and seem to lose skills between 12 to 36 months of age. Though gains may be made in developmental and social skills, these children are typically not able to catch up with their peers and remain autistic once the loss has occurred (29). In some cases, behavioral challenges increase as a child reaches school age, while these challenges may decrease in other children. Longitudinal studies have found that few individuals with autistic disorder reach full independence as adults; many are not able to live on their own or find employment. Even those who evidence higher skills in this category (known as high-functioning autism) frequently struggle with social interactions throughout their lives. In fact, it is older children with higher-functioning autistic disorders who often make more attempts to socialize, and may feel greater distress and loneliness than younger or lower-functioning children with ASD when they are unsuccessful in reciprocal interactions (29). For the many individuals who do not reach independence in adulthood, families must continue to provide support or these adults may enter residential programs. These programs offer special education, developmental, and behavioral techniques to teach adults new skills and to generalize these skills into functional community activities (33).

Rett's Disorder

Rett's disorder is evident before a child reaches four years of age, and most frequently presents in the first or second year of life following a period of typical development. Challenges in communication and behaviors are typically continuous throughout the individual's life. Gains in developmental skills are usually not significant in later childhood or adolescence, though the child may show a heightened desire to socially interact with others (3).

Childhood Disintegrative Disorder

Symptoms appear in this disorder following the age of 2 years but prior to the age of 10 years, and children progress through typical developmental milestones before the onset of this disorder. Following the onset, a significant loss of skills is noted. If this disorder occurs in isolation, the loss of skills ceases and minimal improvement is observed later in life. This disorder may co-occur with a progressive neurological condition, in which case, the child will continue to lose skills (3).

Asperger's Disorder

A child with Asperger's disorder typically exhibits strong verbal skills in the school-age years; however, professionals and peers should not let these skills be misleading in terms of the child's social impairments. These children may show a strong interest in having friends but lack the understanding of the social rules that apply to these interactions. As a result, these individuals may appear more comfortable with others either older or younger than themselves. Longitudinal studies suggest that prognosis is better for Asperger's disorder than autistic disorder because more individuals are able to function independently in employment and self-sufficient living (3).

General Prognostic Indicators

Overall, children's language levels and IQ scores are the strongest indicators related to prognosis in independence and appropriate functioning in adulthood, particularly in the area of verbal IQ (1,3).

In terms of communication skills, a child's ability to spontaneously, meaningfully, and consistently combine words into phrases or sentences before 5 years of age is a good prognostic indicator of cognitive, language, adaptive, and academic achievement measures (1). It is important to observe that the child is able to spontaneously construct sentences rather than echo others' utterances (echolalia) or use memorized chunks of language to communicate. A child's use of **joint attention** has been found to be a predictor of language outcome. Joint attention is the ability to use eye contact and gestures in order to share experiences with others. Children who fail to use early gestural joint attention (e.g., failing to point at an object and to turn to his mother to determine if his mother shares his interest) seem to struggle in the development of meaningful language (1). In Lord and McGee's review of autism research (1), one longitudinal research finding implied that early joint attention, symbolic play, and receptive language were strong predictors of a child's future outcomes. Another study in this review examined severity of repetitive, stereotyped behaviors and social symptoms, and found that the severity later predicted adaptive functioning (1).

Early success in hand-eye coordination may predict vocational abilities later in life. Fine motor skills also predicted later leisure pursuits (1). Children with autism who displayed a definite hand preference performed significantly better on motor, language, and cognitive tasks (34). The ability to imitate body movements has been linked to expressive language development, and imitation of actions with objects predicted later levels of play abilities (1). The more established behavioral challenges become without intervention, the more these problems persist and worsen (1).

Surgical/Medical Management

Diagnosis

Autism is now diagnosed at a younger age than ever before since characteristics of autism have become more defined and better recognized in recent years. Receiving a diagnosis at an early age is optimal because the sooner the disorder is recognized, the more likely the child can make dramatic reductions in symptoms and gains in learning (1,4). One study examined children diagnosed with autism. A specialized review of home videotapes from their first birthdays revealed interaction and behavioral differences clearly at 12 months of age. Consistent signs among these children who were later diagnosed with autism included lack of the following skills: pointing, showing objects to others, looking to others, and responding to their names (35). In fact, researchers are now wondering if these initial characteristics may show that not as many children as originally thought have a sudden onset of autism but rather show these early subtle signs.

A child is usually referred for an assessment because those who interact closely with him (e.g., family members, pediatrician, teachers) may observe warning signs either specific to autism or to a development delay in one or more areas. When these concerns become apparent, the child is initially screened, usually by primary care providers or early child care professionals, to look for the "red flags" that may indicate autistic behaviors. Published screening instruments for children with autism include:

- The Checklist for Autism in Toddlers (CHAT) (36)
- The Autism Screening Questionnaire (ASQ) (37)
- The Screening Tool for Autism in Two-Year-Olds (38)
- Australian Scale for Asperger's Syndrome (39)
- Pervasive Developmental Disorders Screening Test-Stage 1 (PDDST-I) (40)
- The Modified Checklist for Autism in Toddlers (M-CHAT) (41)

If the child does not pass the screening, this indicates that enough warning signs of autism are present to warrant a thorough assessment for autism. Since each child on the autism spectrum disorder displays a unique matrix of strengths and weaknesses, no two children on the autism spectrum will look the same. Therefore, critical to an accurate diagnosis is an assessment with clinicians who are experienced in identifying the characteristics of autism. Additionally, a thorough diagnosis with a team of professionals can gather insight into each child's skills across several areas of development, which, in turn, helps with intervention planning. The following elements should be included in every sensitive, comprehensive evaluation of a child with autism:

1. History: Though autism is not known to result from complications during pregnancy, it is important to discuss any unusual pre- or perinatal events to rule out other disorders. Because of autism's genetic implications, it is important to determine if other family members have been diagnosed with autism, psychiatric concerns, or developmental disorders. The history portion should also include questioning about autism-specific behaviors in the areas of social, language, behavioral, play, cognitive, and sensory processing abilities (32).
2. Medical History: During this portion of the assessment, parents report when their child's developmental milestones were reached (e.g., what age their child said his first word, learned to walk), if regression of developmental skills occurred at any point, or if any other medical problems are occurring (e.g., psychiatric, sleeping, or eating problems) (42).
3. Physical/Neurological Examination: Other illnesses such as fragile X syndrome, tuberous sclerosis, or congenital rubella need to be ruled out, since these disorders may look similar to autism (32). The physician also checks for other medical illnesses (e.g., GI disorders, ear infections), measures head circumference, gives a general physical examination, examines mental status, verifies that cranial nerves function normally, and performs a motor examination (42).

4. Parent Interviewing: Many diagnostic tools are available to gain parents' insight into their child's autism-specific behaviors. A clinician should also ask parents about their overall impression of their child, since more general questions may reveal further insight beyond the scope of these tools (1,42).
   Parent Interview Tools:

   The Autism Diagnostic Interview: Revised (43)
   Autism Diagnostic Observation Schedule-General (ADOS-G) (44)
   Functional Emotional Assessment Scale (FEAS) (45)
   The Gilliam Autism Rating Scale (GARS) (46)
   The Pervasive Developmental Disorders Screening Test-Stage 2 (PDDST-II) (47)
5. Tests in developmental areas, including language, social, motor, cognitive, and adaptive skills.
6. Informal observation of the child interacting with others. This is considered one of the most valuable pieces of the evaluation process, since it typically reveals the qualitative impairments of the child (such as lack of eye contact, limited initiation of interaction, or difficulty transitioning between tasks).
7. Audiological testing: An audiologic evaluation is necessary to rule out hearing disorders. Children with autism are often unresponsive to verbal auditory stimuli, and it is important to determine that this behavior is not caused by a hearing impairment. If hearing loss co-occurs with autism, language comprehension may be further impacted than with a diagnosis of autism alone (42).
8. Other testing: Certain tests may prove beneficial to specific circumstances. For instance, an electroencephalograph (EEG) may be needed if the child is suspected of having seizures (42). Some children are assessed through university studies, and MRIs are typically included in these autism assessments (11,42). Genetics testing may be appropriate for parents who are considering having another child (42). Some parents are also concerned about heavy metal contamination and wish to pursue a lead screening for their child.

During the comprehensive assessment, a diagnostic instrument should be used that examines autistic behaviors while the clinician observes the child's interests and interactions with others.

The instruments that are currently available include:

1. The Autism Diagnostic Observation Schedule-Generic (ADOS-G) (44).
2. The Childhood Autism Rating Scale (CARS) (48).
3. The Screening Tool for Autism in Two-Year-Olds (STAT) (38).

Medical/Surgical Treatment

Overall, treatment for autism does not heavily rely on medical intervention, and surgical interventions are not practiced for this disorder. Intensive early intervention is most effective in reducing problem behaviors while increasing language, social, sensory, motor, and cognitive skills (1,32,49). A variety of approaches are available, ranging from highly structured to naturalistic. Because no two children with autism present with the same set of symptoms, no one treatment plan is successful for all children with autism. Effective intervention must account for the child's individual strengths and challenges, and must consider functional skills to be generalized across a variety of settings in the child's life. Substantial literature supports early intervention for children 0 to 3 years as the most beneficial time to connect new pathways for more appropriate functioning and behavior, though an individual may continue to make substantial gains following this period of development (1,32,49). Because it is beyond the scope of this book to discuss these approaches, this chapter focuses on current knowledge of medical interventions meant to accompany intervention techniques.

Pharmacologic Therapies. Use of medication does not cure the core social, language, and repetitive behavioral deficits of autism because "in most cases, the brain has undergone atypical cellular development dating from the earliest embryonic stages" (26, p. 303). Research in this area is presently limited or inconclusive. In addition, many parents and clinicians are cautious because use of pharmacotherapy with children presents the risk of harmful side effects. Lindsay and Aman (50) reviewed existing literature on pharmacologic intervention, and found that when certain medications are used appropriately, behavioral dysregulations such as hyperactivity, irritability, anxiety, and perseveration may be reduced. For instance, risperidone, an atypical antipsychotic agent, shows promising results in emerging research for reducing tantrums, irritability, aggression, and self-injurious and repetitive behaviors (50–52). Because autism is likely a genetic disorder determined before the child is born, pharmacologic treatments could probably not "undo" this disorder. Therefore, these treatments are not investigated to replace educational services but rather to supplement them. For those children who respond successfully to medication, behavioral and educational intervention may be even more beneficial since they do not struggle as greatly with challenging behaviors.

Medical Conditions. Medical intervention is necessary for any co-occurring medical conditions, such as seizures or gastrointestinal disorders. Children with autism need to be monitored closely for behaviors that may reflect a medical condition, and should receive a complete medical work up and treatment through a physician who specializes in the child's medical condition.

Complementary and Alternative Medicine. Complementary and alternative medicine has gained popularity in the past decade as a supplementary treatment to educational services. Complementary and alternative medicine is defined as "a broad domain of healing resources that encompasses all health systems modalities and practices and their accompanying theories and beliefs, other than those intrinsic to the politically dominant health system" (53, as cited in 22, p. 418). Those who support complementary and alternative medicine believe the methods target underlying medical difficulties, such as GI and sleep disorders, which are not addressed through educational intervention. The goal of many of the complementary and alternative medicine treatments is to aid in the associated problems of autism, rather than claim to cure the disorder. Statistics reveal that 30% to 50% of children with autism in the United States are using complementary and alternative medicine; however, approximately 9% are using potentially harmful treatments and 11% are using multiple complementary and alternative medicine treatments (22). Several studies are currently underway to examine the effectiveness and the risks of these treatments since many parents have reported a decrease in associated problems (e.g., GI problems) and an increase in developmental skills. Table 3.2 summarizes the potentially harmful side effects of these methods. The following sections describe commonly used complementary and alternative medicine treatments.

Supplements. The use of vitamins and minerals to address ASD concerns purports that because children with autism experience GI inflammation and intestinal disorders, their ability to absorb nutrients is thereby reduced. As a result, development that relies on nutrients such as vitamins A, B1, B3, B5, biotin, selenium, zinc, and magnesium is altered. Frequently used supplements

Table 3.2 POTENTIAL SIDE EFFECTS OF COMPLEMENTARY AND ALTERNATIVE MEDICINE

Proposed Mechanisms	Example	Potential Adverse Side Effects
Neurotransmitter production or release	DMG B6/magnesium Vitamin C Omega 3 Fatty acids Secretin	No reported side effects (Excessive doses) B6: peripheral neuropathy; Mg: arrhythmia Renal stones No reports of side effects from excessive administration Unknown impact of long-term administration of secretin
Change in gastrointestinal function	Gluten-free/casein-free diet Secretin Pepcid Antibiotics	If nutritional state not monitored by clinicians, at risk for inadequate calcium, vitamin D, protein intake Unknown impact of long-term administration Hepatotoxicity in high doses Superinfection or antibiotic resistance with long-term use, implications for population at large with resistance
Putative immune mechanism or modulators	Antifungal agents Intravenous Immunoglobulin Vitamin A/Cod liver oil	Possible superinfections or resistance with long-term use Aseptic meningitis, renal failure, or infection Hypervitaminosis A or pseudo-tumor cerebri
Agents that might remove toxins	Chelation – DMSA, DMPA Other detox agents or protocols	Renal and hepatotoxicity of oral agents Possible magnesium intoxication from Epsom salts ingestion

Levy SE, Hyman SL. Use of complementary and alternative medicine for children with autistic spectrum disorders is increasing. Pediatr Ann 2003;32(10):687. Reprinted with permission.

include vitamin C, cod liver oil (for vitamins A and D), and the combination of vitamin B6 with magnesium (2).

Gluten-Free, Casein-Free Diet. Parents and professionals who support the theory that gluten and casein negatively impact a child's development recommend a diet that completely eliminates these products (23). Parent reports of improvement have been inconsistent, as some parents claim to see significant improvements in their child's behavior and/or developmental skills (e.g., improved eye contact), while others report that no change occurs by implementing this diet. Data are currently limited and inconclusive. Anecdotal information comprises the majority of reports rather than controlled studies.

Other Common Complementary and Alternative Medicine Treatments for Autism.

- Secretin: The human body naturally produces secretin, which is a hormone produced in the small intestine that stimulates secretion by the pancreas and liver. The use of extra secretin through injections became a popular complementary and alternative medicine treatment before it was scientifically analyzed, and studies now show few changes for children with ASDs who have used the extra hormone injection (24).
- Chelation: Because mercury poisoning produces symptoms similar to those seen in autism, mercury and other heavy metals have been suggested as causes of autism. Though research has not found a link between mercury and autism, those who believe their children have experienced metal poisoning may choose chelation, a process to remove toxins from a child's system (24).
- Antibiotic treatment: Immune system dysfunctions and antibiotic treatments have been targeted as possible causes of autism, and those who believe in these theories use further antibiotic treatment to alter the course of the symptoms in autism (24).
- Antifungal treatment: Yeast overgrowth in the colon is hypothesized to cause many medical disorders, including autism, with a low-sugar diet and the use of probiotic agents (which encourage helpful intestinal bacteria) used as treatments (24).

Conclusion of Complementary and Alternative Medicine Treatments. The effectiveness of complementary and alternative medicine stands largely unproven and highly controversial, though attempts are underway for further studies since many parents report positive results by using these methods. Complementary and alternative medicine treatments are intended to supplement educational services rather than to replace them. Clinicians are currently encouraged to use an empathetic stance with families providing complementary and alternative medicine to their children, though no alternative method should be administered without the guidance of an experienced physician.

Impact of Conditions on Client Factors

Global Impairment

Autism is considered a global impairment, meaning that it does not reflect damage as a result of one specific lesion in the brain. Since autism likely affects several regions of the brain, this global impact means that autism impairs multiple areas of a child's development. As a result, even a child's ability to regulate basic functions is impaired, such as consistent sleep patterns or emotional stability.

Irregular sleeping patterns are common in children with autism, particularly in the quality rather than the quantity of their sleep (54–56). Disturbances include problems falling asleep, disoriented awakening, difficulty sleeping in an unfamiliar place, and nightmare-type disturbances such as screaming (54,56). Children may exhibit sleep disturbances as early as 2 years of age, and higher occurrence of sleep disorders seem to exist in children with more severe forms of autism (54).

Children with autism often have difficulty regulating their own emotions and interpreting the emotions of others. These children often experience depression, a sense of loneliness, and a limited range of emotions that results in a flattened affect. For example, they may show they are happy or angry, but more subtle emotions such as worry, jealousy, or disappointment are less commonly seen in these children. Additionally, difficulty in reading facial expressions, body postures, and intonation of voices to infer another's feelings are common challenges. An unusual characteristic of autism is emotional lability, which is a child's use of laughing or crying for unclear reasons or during inappropriate situations. Some parents may describe their children as "laid back" or less reactive to emotional stimuli, while other parents note a tendency to frequently cry inconsolably. Heightened anxiety is evident in many children, as are temper tantrums that often result from disrupted routines (29). Other children show a lack of fear during dangerous situations (1). Aggressive behaviors such as hitting, biting, self-mutilation (head banging, hitting self), or self-stimulatory behaviors (e.g., body rocking) may occur when the child does not get his way or his routine is disturbed.

Specific Mental Functions

As previously mentioned, each child with autism presents with different areas of strengths and weaknesses; therefore, children with an ASD show various combinations of concerns in their mental skills. Attention deficits, however, are nearly universal in this population. Unique patterns of attention include distractibility, disorganization, intense preoccupation for preferred, self-initiated activities for unusual lengths of time, and lack of boredom for repeating same action or play schema (29). The ability to focus jointly on an activity with another person is significantly impaired.

A child with autism often shows a scattered pattern of memory functions (57). Overall, "memory performance of individuals with autism becomes increasingly impaired as the complexity of the material increases" (58, p. 1099). Children with autism also use fewer organizational strategies, relying on stereotyped rules regardless of the task's complexity (58). Therefore, a child with autism performs more poorly on tasks with higher complexity. Word recall is more significantly impacted than digit recall, and these children often have difficulty recalling activities in which they have recently participated (59). However, certain areas of memory remain intact, particularly in the areas of visual and **rote memory**. Rote memory describes the memorization and use of previously heard chunks of language rather than the spontaneous generation of language.

In the area of perceptual functioning, individuals with ASDs perceive sensory stimuli, but often process and react abnormally to it. Integration of perceptual and sensorimotor information allows individuals to respond appropriately with physical and emotional responses. In autism, this integration does not occur in the same efficient way; therefore, this population of individuals has difficulty responding with typical emotional and physical responses to the sensory stimuli around them. Between 30% and 100% of individuals with autism demonstrate deviant sensory-perceptual abilities (60).

Cognitive impairments are common in, though not universal to, the autism population. Approximately 75% of these individuals have IQ scores below 70 (3), indicating mental retardation. Those with Asperger's disorder, however, show IQ scores within the normal range. Individuals with cognitive deficits typically demonstrate scattered skills; in other words, they may present with strong skills in some areas with significant concerns in other areas. These children often have difficulty sequencing a series of items, imitating the actions and words of others meaningfully, generalizing concepts across a variety of situations, demonstrating theory of mind, and playing with toys appropriately and symbolically (1). In her 1991 literature review of autistic features (29), Rapin described that children with autism tend to have better visual-spatial skills than auditory verbal skills on IQ tests. Children in this population may show above-average skills in very specific areas, such as calculating numbers, completing puzzles, or demonstrating rote verbal memory, while demonstrating overall cognitive impairment. Some children with autism are able to read at a young age with minimal instruction, but they have little or no understanding of what they read. This unusual occurrence is known as **hyperlexia** (29).

Studies examining higher level cognitive functions have revealed that executive functioning skills such as forward planning, cognitive flexibility, and the use of assistive strategies (e.g., creating a mnemonic such as a rhyme to assist in remembering information) in learning are impacted for those who have autism (51).

As previously described, children with autism typically show language delay, with the exception of those with Asperger's disorder. Deviations from typical language are noted across all diagnostic categories. Children on the autism spectrum typically have limitations in using language in appropriate contexts and for social purposes. Some children may be highly verbal and articulate though literal, echolalic, and repetitive; other children may remain nonverbal or use very little speech (32). Additionally, comprehension of language is affected and exacerbated by a decreased motivation to use language for interacting with others. Often these children are challenged to understand what topics interest others and have difficulty interpreting nonverbal language such as gestures and facial expressions, as well as abstract language such as jokes or idioms. For those who are verbal, intonation of their voices may sound unnatural as a result of a singsong or monotone pattern. Speaking at unusually loud volumes is another unusual characteristic of children with autism. Though the words may be clear, content may be memorized chunks of language or may focus on topics that are not relevant to a conversation partner's. Echolalia is also common for verbal children (29). Some children do not master fluent speech and their sounds in words are difficult to understand. Decoding the sounds that they hear may be severely compromised; therefore, these children may not understand what they hear and, in turn, are unable to produce the sound accurately (32).

Sensory Functions and Pain

"The experience of being human is imbedded in the sensory events of everyday life. When we observe how people live their lives, we discover they characterize their experiences from a sensory point of view" (61, p. 608). If a child's sensory system does not interpret stimuli in a typical way, it is easy to understand why this individual may react to the world differently. These sensory disturbances appear to occur more commonly in children than adults, and since the severity of sensory impairment seems to be related to the severity of stereotypic and behavioral abnormalities, sensory processing problems should be addressed through early intervention to reduce these abnormal behaviors (1,60).

The prevalence of sensory impairments in children with autism is significantly higher than in the population of typically developing children, though each child with autism shows a different profile of hyper- and hyposensitivity to sensory stimulation. Despite the variability in sensory thresholds from child to child, some general patterns have emerged in research.

Visual perception is usually an area of relative strength, and may be used to compensate for challenging areas. For instance, the integration of vestibular, visual, and somatosensory afferent systems is needed to maintain upright postural stability. Molloy, Dietrich, and Bhattacharya (62) measured the postural stability in children with autism, and found that these children relied on visual cues to help them maintain stability. When these visual cues were omitted, children had difficulty maintaining their upright balance and reducing their sway. One area of visual processing that is consistently impaired is integrating details of a figure into a whole (63). For instance, if given a line drawing of a house made up of geometric shapes, these children focus on the shapes rather than seeing the image of a house.

Auditory processing is often a significantly challenging area for children with autism. Frequently, children with ASDs are unresponsive to some auditory stimuli while being oversensitive to others. For instance, a child may not respond when her name is called, but screams in response to hearing a vacuum cleaner running. Furthermore, children with autism may be distracted, irritable, or have difficulty functioning in activities in noisy environments (64).

These children also show mixed patterns of craving and/or avoiding vestibular sensations. Some children appear to seek out, others withdraw from, and some show mixed preferences for certain types of these sensations. Common vestibular movements include swinging, spinning on a sit-and-spin or merry-go-round, and playing with spinning toys (64).

Food tastes and textures are difficult for many children on the autism spectrum. Many parents note their child with autism has unusual taste preferences. Due to sensory issues, this population are frequently picky eaters" and may have a limited repertoire of food preferences (65). They may be sensitive to certain textures, such as avoiding wet (e.g., oranges in fruit syrup), "goopy" (e.g., macaroni and cheese), and/or mixed textured foods (e.g., a casserole). Though nutritional intake generally appears adequate (8), it is often stressful for families to meet nutritional needs of these children who have very specific food preferences. Parents and clinicians typically observe these individuals to crave strong tastes, such as spicy or salty foods, and crunchy foods that give the child significant sensory input.

As with taste, many individuals with autism have abnormal smell interests. Unusual behaviors are observed in the person's inappropriate smelling of objects or unusual attachment to or aversiveness from certain smells (29,65).

Reports of clumsiness are common for children who are higher functioning on the autism spectrum (e.g., children with milder cognitive impairment, such as those with Asperger's disorder) (66). Weimer et al. (67) suggest that in children with Asperger, this observed clumsiness may result from a deficit in proprioception, not from a motor disturbance.

Tactile defensiveness is a hypersensitivity to certain touch situations that most people find nonthreatening. Children with this symptom frequently exhibit an avoidance-withdrawal response (e.g., rubbing/scratching, avoiding certain textures, or crying when exposed to a specific texture) (68). The presence of tactile defensiveness appears to co-occur with stereotyped behaviors such as rocking of the body, hand flapping, unusual interest or focus on objects (69). A significant relationship also appears between tactile defensiveness and rigid behaviors (e.g., child has difficulty breaking out of own agenda), repetitive verbalizations, visual stereotypes, and abnormaly focused affections. Though these children experience significant tactile hypersensitivities, many also appear to have a reduced response to pain (29).

Functions Related to the Digestive System

Children with autism may be at a higher risk for experiencing gastrointestinal problems such as reflux or gastritis, with persistent gas, diarrhea, and constipation also frequently reported (20–22). Additionally, hypotheses exist regarding functioning of the digestive system, such as increased intestinal permeability that allows absorption of morphine-like compounds from gluten and casein. The buildup of these substances theoretically results in the social withdrawal and stereotypical behaviors seen in autism, but as previously described, this theory has not been proven (24).

Urinary and Reproductive Functions

In children with autism, the urinary tract is usually typical in its structure and function. However, for those children with cognitive and sensory impairments, toilet training is often complicated. Children with autism often learn to toilet train at a later age than typically developing children; evidence problems such as fear, pain, confusion, frustration, and constipation when learning to train; urinate or defecate in inappropriate places; and experience difficulty when a change of routine occurs or when entering an unfamiliar bathroom (70).

Because individuals with autism have difficulty interacting, inappropriate sexual behavior is also a concern. Close relationships with others are challenging for these individuals; therefore, few person-oriented behaviors are noted. Additionally, discouraging inappropriate sexual behaviors may be difficult. The most frequently reported inappropriate sexual behaviors include public masturbation or public touching of one's own private parts (71,72).

Gross and Fine Motor Skills

Though individuals with ASDs often show relative strengths in movement functions, some abnormalities in motor skills have been observed, including overall motor joint laxity, hypotonia, clumsiness, apraxia, and chronic toe walking (32). Females with Rett's disorder frequently demonstrate poor coordination in gait or trunk movements. In children with Asperger's disorder, "clumsiness" has been more specifically defined as poor performance on tests of apraxia, tandem gait, one-leg balance with eyes closed, and repetitive finger-thumb apposition (67).

Further fine and gross motor impairments include problems in skilled movement, hand-eye coordination, speed, praxis and imitation, posture, and balance (60). A particularly debilitating abnormality in individuals with autism includes deficits in motor imitation skills despite intact perceptual and motor capacities, which is most apparent in younger groups of children (73). Furthermore, these children perform poorly on tasks of executing a sequence of movements, such as a sequence of hand or facial actions in imitation (74). Reduced stride lengths, increased stance times, increased hip flexion at toe-off, reduced knee extension at initial ground contact, abnormal heel strikes, and decreased knee extension and ankle dorsiflexion at ground contact were noted in an earlier study of children with autism (75).

In addition, a disproportionate number of children with autism display **ambiguous hand preference** (approximately 40%) long past the age that dominant hand preference typically develops. A person who is ambidextrous will usually choose one hand for a specific task (e.g., left hand for writing, right hand for throwing a football). An ambiguous hand preference, however, refers to switching hands within the same activity (34). When this behavior persists into the school-age years, it may indicate abnormal functioning of the brain.

Motor stereotypes are common in those on the autism spectrum and often manifest through hand flapping, pacing, spinning, running in circles, and flipping light switches. More severe, self-injurious forms include biting, hitting oneself, or head banging (32).

Brain Structure

The most significant abnormalities in a child's body structure include the anomalies of the brain that are currently under investigation. Likely caused by genetic abnormalities, these deviations in the brains of individuals with autism are not yet clearly defined, nor is it clear precisely how the differences cause the characteristics of autism. Studies have found consistent abnormalities in the cerebellum, frontal lobes, brainstem, limbic system, and brainstem (8–14). Research is also examining potential deviations in the way different regions of the brain communicate (9).

CASE STUDY

Case Illustrations

■ CASE 1

At 1 year of age, Jacob was brought to an early intervention clinic because of delays in motor and cognitive skills. An initial evaluation conducted by an occupational therapist, educator, and speech-language pathologist confirmed these concerns. In the area of gross motor skills, Jacob was delayed in learning to walk and demonstrated moderate hypotonia in his trunk. Fine motor concerns included tactile defensiveness of wet or sticky substances, and delays in grasping and manipulating objects appropriately. Cognitively, Jacob showed little interest in playing with toys or imitating the words and actions of others. Language impairments were not yet observed since Jacob frequently vocalized, babbled, and expressed his feelings through behaviors such as smiling or crying. At this young age, ASD was not initially suspected. Jacob was clearly a delightful little boy who showed a strong attachment to his parents and was interested in watching children and other adults in his environment.

Jacob was placed in a playgroup at the clinic where his occupational therapist and educator worked directly with him, while a speech-language pathologist monitored his language. As time passed, further concerns became evident. His language skills failed to further develop; as a result, first words did not emerge. Nor was he using gestures to indicate what he wanted. At the age of fourteen months, he evidenced limitations in language comprehension and speech production, and his use of eye contact decreased. As the months progressed, he showed frustration more frequently through crying, banging his head, throwing himself on the ground, and arching his back to pull away from a person trying to hold him. His feeding skills were limited since he was not able to bring his hand to his mouth, and he demonstrated extreme sensitivities to many tastes and textures. He did not show an interest in other self-help skills such as learning to bathe or dress himself. While other children his age learned to imitate motor movements in songs, Jacob seemed to content to only listen to the songs. He did not demonstrate typical play skills for his age such as exploring how toys worked, taking toys in or out of a container, or taking turns with others. However, musical or flashing toys captured his attention for long periods of time. While he was engrossed with these toys, he evidenced unusual, repetitive behaviors such as rocking his body back and forth.

Through early intervention by his therapists and parents, Jacob's gross motor skills improved during the following months and he successfully learned to walk at 18 months. He delighted in walking through his home, through the early intervention center, and outside. His eye contact improved, becoming more spontaneous and consistent. His repertoire of sounds increased and he vocalized to take a turn in songs or games; in addition, he began signing "more" to request something desirable to happen again. He learned to play with toys in a more functional manner, including stacking rings and blocks and taking toys in and out of containers. Yet other skills continued to be challenging. When he was left to play on his own, he repetitively turned the pages of books or walked aimlessly around a room. He showed hypersensitivities to touching or mouthing certain textures, limited motor or imitation skills, difficulty understanding others, a lack of verbal words, and repetitive behaviors during play.

Currently, at slightly older than 2 years of age, Jacob continues to struggle in several areas of development. However, he has made steady progress in these developmental skills, and his family and team are encouraged that he will continue to make significant gains. More importantly, despite being faced with more challenges than typically developing children, Jacob is a young boy who is often able to share and express joy with others.

References

1. National Research Council. Educating children with autism. Committee on Educational Interventions for Children with Autism. Lord C, McGee, JP, eds. Division of Behavioral and Social Sciences and Education. Washington, DC: National Academy Press, 2001.
2. Autism Society of America. Autism Info [Fact Sheets], 2004. Bethesda, MD: Autism Society of America. Available at: http://www.autism-society.org. Accessed April 11, 2004.
3. American Psychiatric Association. The Diagnostic and Statistical Manual. 4th Ed, text revision. Washington, DC: American Psychiatric Association, 2000.
4. Strock M. Autism spectrum disorders. NIH Publication No. NIH-04-5511, National Institute of Mental Health, National Institutes of Health, U.S. Department of Health and Human Services, 1996. Available at: http://www.nimh.nih.gov/publicat/autism.cfm. Accessed June 19, 2005.
5. Kanner L. Autistic disturbances of affective contact. Nervous Child 1943;2:17–250.
6. Bettelheim B. The Empty Fortress: Infantile Autism and the Birth of the Self. New York: Free Press, 1967.
7. Siegel B. Helping Children with Autism to Learn. Oxford: Oxford University Press, 2003.
8. United Kingdom Medical Research Council. MRC review of autism research: epidemiology and causes. December 2001. Available at: http://www.mrc.ac.uk/pdf-autism-report.pdf. Accessed July 25, 2004.
9. Piven J, Saliba K, Bailey J, et al. An MRI study of autism: the cerebellum revisited. Neurology 1997;49(2):546–551.
10. Bauman ML, Kemper TL. Brief report: neuroanatomic observations of the brain in pervasive developmental disorders. J Autism Dev Disord 1996;26(2):199–203.
11. Bauman M. Innovative interventions in autism/nonverbal learning disabilities. Conference presentation, December 3–4, 2004; Seattle, WA.
12. Kemper TL, Bauman M. Neuropathology of infantile autism. J Neuropathol Exp Neurol 1998;57(7): 645–652.
13. Carper RA, Courchesne E. Localized enlargement of the frontal cortex in early autism. Biol Psychiatry 2005;57(2):126–133.
14. Helm-Estabrooks N, Albert ML. Manual of Aphasia Therapy. Austin, Texas: Pro-Ed, 1991.
15. Veenstra-VanDerWeele J, Cook E, Lombroso PJ. Genetics of childhood disorders: XLVI. Autism, Part 5: genetics of autism. J Am Acad Child Adolesc Psychiatr 2003;42:116–118.
16. Webb T, Latif F. Rett syndrome and the MECP2 gene. J Med Gen 2001;38:217–223.
17. Rapin I, Katzman R. Neurobiology of autism. Ann Neurol 1998;43:7–14.
18. Rutter M, Silberg J, O'Connor T, et al. Genetics and child psychiatry: II Empirical research findings. J Child Psychol Psychiatr 1999;40(1):19–55.
19. Jick H, Kaye JA. Epidemiology and possible causes of autism. Pharmacotherapy 2003;23(12): 1525–1530.
20. Horvath K, Papadimitriou JC, Rabsztyn A, et al. Gastrointestinal abnormalities in children with autistic disorder. J Pediatr 1999;135(5):559–563.
21. McQueen JM, Heck AM. Secretin for the treatment of autism. Ann Pharmacother 2002;36:305–311.
22. Levy SE, Mandell DS, Merhar S, et al. Use of complementary and alternative medicine among children recently diagnosed autistic spectrum disorder. J Dev Behav Pediatr 2003;24(6):418–423.
23. McCandless J. Children with Starving Brains: A Medical Treatment Guide for Autism Spectrum Disorder. 2nd Ed. Paterson, NJ: Bramble Books, 2003.
24. Levy SE, Hyman, SL. Use of complementary and alternative medicine for children with autistic spectrum disorders is increasing. Pediatr Ann 2003;32(10):685–691.
25. Gadia CA, Tuchman R, Rotta NT. Autism and pervasive developmental disorders. Journal of Pediatrics (Rio J) 2004;80(2 Suppl):S83–S94.
26. Rapin I. The autistic spectrum disorders. N Engl J Med 2002;347(5):302–303.
27. Fombonne E. The epidemiology of autism: a review. Psych Med 1999;29:769–786.
28. Leslie AM, Frith U. Metarepresentation and autism: how not to lose one's marbles. Cognition 1987;27(3): 291–294.

29. Rapin I. Autistic children: diagnosis and clinical features. Pediatrics 1991;87:751–760.
30. Siegel B. The World of the Autistic Child. Oxford: Oxford University Press, 1996.
31. Dunn HG, MacLeod PM. Rett syndrome: review of biological abnormalities. C J Neurol Sci 2001;28(1): 16–29.
32. Rapin I. Autism. N Engl J Med 1997;337:97–104.
33. Holmes, DL. Community-based services for children and adults with autism: the Eden family programs. J Autism Dev Disord 1990;20:339–351.
34. Hauck JA, Dewey D. Hand preference and motor functioning in children with autism. J Autism Dev Disord 2001;31(3):265–277.
35. Osterling J, Dawson G. Early recognition of children with autism: a study of first birthday home videotapes. J Autism Dev Disord 1994;24(3):247–257.
36. Baron-Cohen S, Allen J, Gillberg C. Can autism be detected at 18 months? The needle, the haystack, and the CHAT. Br J Psychiatr 1992;161: 839–843.
37. Berument SK, Rutter M, Lord C, et al. Autism screening questionnaire: diagnostic validity. Br J Psychiatr 1999;175:444–451.
38. Stone WL, Coonrod EE, Ousley OY. Brief report: screening tool for autism in two-year-olds (STAT): development and preliminary data. J Autism Dev Disord 2000;30:607–612.
39. Garnett MS and Attwood AJ (1998). Australian scale for Asperger's syndrome. In: Attwood, T. Asperger's syndrome: a guide for parents and professionals. London: Jessica Kingsley. 1998.
40. Siegel, B., Early screening and diagnosis in autism spectrum disorders: The Pervasive Developmental Disorders Screening Test (PDDST). Paper presented at the NIH State of the Science in Autism Screening and Diagnosis Working Conference, Bethesda, MD, June 15–17. 1998.
41. Robins DL, Fein D, Barton ML, et al. The modified checklist for autism in toddlers: an initial study investigating the early detection of autism and pervasive developmental disorders. J Autism Dev Disord 2001;21:131–144.
42. Filipek PA, Accardo PJ, Baranek GT, et al. The screening and diagnosis of autistic spectrum disorders. J Autism Dev Disord 1999;29(6):439–484.
43. Lord C, Rutter M, LeCouteur A. Autism diagnostic interview-revised: a revised version of a diagnostic interview for caregivers of individuals with possible pervasive developmental disorders. J Autism Dev Disord 1994;24:659–685.
44. Lord C, Rutter M, Goode S, Heemsbergen J, Jordan H. Autism diagnostic observation schedule: a standardized observation of communicative and social behavior. J Autism Dev Disord 1989;19: 185–212.
45. Greenspan SI, DeGangi G, Wieder S. The Functional Emotional Assessment Scale for Infancy and Early Childhood: A Manual. Madison: International Universities Press, 1999.
46. Gilliam GE. Gilliam Autism Rating Scale. Austin, TX: Pro-Ed, 1995.
47. Siegel B. Pervasive developmental disorders screening test-Stage 2, 1998.
48. Schopler E, Reichler RJ, Renner BR. The Childhood Autism Rating Scale. Los Angeles: Western Psychological Services, 1988.
49. Rogers SJ. Brief report: early intervention in autism. J Autism Dev Disord 1996;26(2):243–246.
50. Lindsay RL, Aman MG. Pharmacologic therapies aid treatment for autism. Pediatr Ann 2003;32(10): 671–676.
51. Gordon B. Autism and autistic spectrum disorders. In: Asbury AK, McKhann GM, McDonald WI, et al., eds. Diseases of the nervous system. 3rd Ed. Volume I. Cambridge: University Press, 2002: 406–418.
52. Pediatric Psychopharmacology Autism Network. Risperidone in children with autism and serious behavioral problems. N Engl J Med 2002;347(5): 314–321.
53. Panel of Definition and Description. Defining and describing complementary and alternative medicine. Paper presented at CAM Research Methodology conference, April 7–9, Washington, DC.
54. Hoshino Y, Watanabe H, Yashima Y, et al. An investigation on sleep disturbance of autistic children. Folia Psychiatr Neurol Jpn 1984;38(1):45–51.
55. Hering E, Epstein R, Elroy S, et al. Sleep patterns in autistic children. J Autism Dev Disord 1999;29(2): 143–147.
56. Schreck KA, Mulick J. Parental report of sleep problems in children with autism. J Autism Dev Disord 2000;30(2):127–135.
57. Hill E, Berthoz S, Frith U. Cognitive processing of own emotions in individuals with autistic spectrum disorder and in their relatives. J Autism Dev Disord 2004;34(2):229–235.
58. Minshew NJ, Goldstein G. The pattern of intact and impaired memory functions in autism. J Child Psychol Psychiatry 2001;42(8):1095–1101.
59. Boucher J. Memory for recent events in autistic children. J Autism Dev Disord 1981;11:293–302.
60. Dawson G, Watling R. Interventions to facilitate auditory, visual, and motor integration in autism: a review of the evidence. J Autism Dev Disord 2000;30(5):415–421.
61. Dunn W. The sensations of everyday life: empirical, theoretical, and pragmatic considerations. Am J Occup Ther 2001;55(6):608–620.
62. Molloy CA, Dietrich K, Bhattacharya A. Postural stability in children with autism spectrum disorder. J Autism Dev Disord 2003;33(6):643–652.
63. Deruelle C, Rondan C, Gepner B, et al. Spatial frequency and face processing in children with autism and Asperger Syndrome. J Autism Dev Disord 2004;34(2):199–210.
64. Kientz MA, Dunn W. A comparison of the performance of children with and without autism on the sensory profile. Am J Occup Ther 1997;51(7): 530–537.

65. Williams PG, Dalrymple N, Neal J. Eating habits of children with autism. Pediatr Nurs 2000;26(3): 259–264.
66. Ghaziuddin M, Butler E. Clumsiness in autism and Asperger syndrome: a further report. J Intellect Disabil Res 1998;42:43–48.
67. Weimer AK, Schatz AM, Lincoln A, et al. "Motor" impairment in Asperger syndrome: evidence for a deficit in proprioception. J Dev Behav Pediatr 2001;22(2):92–101.
68. Baranek GT, Berkson G. Tactile defensiveness in children with developmental disabilities: responsiveness and habituation. J Autism Dev Disord 1994;24(4):457–471.
69. Baranek GT, Foster LG, Berkson G. Tactile defensiveness and stereotyped behaviors. Am J Occup Ther 1997;51(2):91–95.
70. Dalrymple NJ, Ruble L. Toilet training and behaviors of people with autism: parent views. J Autism Dev Disord 1992;22(2):265–275.
71. Ruble LA, Dalrymple NJ. Social/sexual awareness of persons with autism: a parental perspective. Archiv Sex Behav 1993;22:229–240.
72. Van Bourgondien ME, Reichle NC, Palmer A. Sexual behavior in adults with autism. J Autism Dev Disord 1997;27(2):113–125.
73. Williams JHG, Whiten A, Singh T. A systematic review of action imitation in autistic spectrum disorder. J Autism Dev Disord 2004;34(3):285–299.
74. Hughes C. Brief report: planning problems in autism at the level of motor control. J Autism Dev Disord 1996;26(1):99–107.
75. Vilensky JA, Damasio AR, Maurer RG. Gait disturbances in patients with autistic behavior: a preliminary study. Arch Neurol 1981;38(10): 646–649.

Recommended Learning Resources

Organizations

Autism Society of America
7910 Woodmont Ave., Suite 300
Bethesda, MD 20814–3067
www.autism-society.org/site/PageServer

National Alliance of Autism Research
99 Wall Street, Research Park
Princeton, NJ 08540
www.naar.org

National Institute of Mental Health
Office of Communications
6001 Executive Blvd
Room 8184, MSC 9663
Bethesda, MD 20892–9663
www.nimh.nih.gov/publicat/autism.cfm

Autism

Cohen DJ, Volkmar FR. Handbook of autism and pervasive developmental disorders. 2nd Ed. New York: John Wiley & Sons, 1997

Ozonoff S, Dawson G, McPartland, J. A parent's guide to Asperger syndrome and high functioning autism. New York: Guilford Press, 2002.

National Research Council. Educating children with autism. Committee on Educational Interventions for Children with Autism. Lord C, McGee, JP, eds. Division of Behavioral and Social Sciences and Education. Washington, DC: National Academy Press.

Quill KA. Do-Watch-Listen-Say: Social and Communication Intervention for Children with Autism. Baltimore, MD: Paul H. Brookes Publishing, 2000.

Siegel B. Helping Children with Autism Learn: Treatment Approaches for Parents and Professionals. New York: Oxford University Press, 2003.

Siegel B. The World of the Autistic Child: Understanding and Treating Autism Spectrum Disorders. New York: Oxford University Press, 1996.

Wing L. The Autistic Spectrum: A Guide for Parents and Professionals. London: Constable and Company Limited, 1996.

Sensory Integration Disorder

Ayres AJ. Sensory Integration and the Child. Los Angeles: Western Psychological Services, 1998.

Kranowitz CS. The Out-of-Sync Child: Recognizing and Coping with Sensory Integration Dysfunction. NY: Perigree, 1998.

Developmental Challenges

Greenspan SI. Wieder, S. The Child with Special Needs: Encouraging Intellectual and Emotional Growth. Reading, MA: Perseus Books, 1998.

Diagnostic Guidelines Online

Filipek, P. Autism diagnostic guidelines. Screening and Diagnosis of Autism http://www.neurology.org/cgi/reprint/55/4/468.pdf. Accessed June 8, 2006.

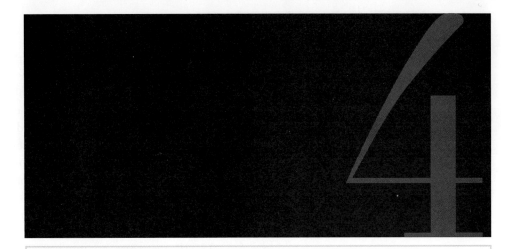

Mental Retardation

Ben J. Atchison

Key Terms

- Cortical atrophy
- Craniostenosis
- Cytomegalovirus
- Down syndrome
- Fragile X syndrome
- Hydrocephaly
- Hyperphenylalaninemia
- Hypoxia
- Muscular dystrophy
- PICA
- Spina bifida
- Tay-Sachs disease
- Teratogenic
- Toxemia

Joanna, aged 4 years, 6 months, was interviewed by the director of a preschool when her parents applied to have her enrolled. Joanna smiled a great deal and was interested in the toys in the office. The director, however, was concerned about Joanna's inability to say her own name and address, to communicate basic information about her family, and to express herself verbally. After an evaluation, Joanna was diagnosed as mildly mentally retarded, and she is now enrolled in a special school where she receives individual help in language development and academics. Her teachers feel that she is benefiting from the program and will be ready to enter a mainstream kindergarten.

Michael, now 5, was diagnosed by his pediatrician shortly after his birth as having Down syndrome, because of certain physical characteristics such as his round face, flattened nose bridge, abnormally small head, low-set ears, short limbs, and abnormally shaped fingers. Mental retardation (MR) is inevitable in children with Down syndrome. Michael's parents were helped to locate an appropriate early intervention program that also provides parent education.

Eddie, now in fifth grade, was always considered a little slower than his peers, but he was a likeable child who got along well with family members and friends. When academic work became demanding and he fell behind in second grade, the school conducted an evaluation. He was diagnosed as having moderate MR and was placed in a special education class where the material is appropriate for his cognitive ability and learning pace.

Definition

The official definition of the disability is as follows and includes three specific criteria:

> "*Mental retardation is characterized by significant limitations both in* intellectual functioning *and in* adaptive behavior *as expressed in conceptual, social, and practical adaptive skills. This disability* originates before the age of 18" *(1)*.

Intellectual Functioning

The first component of this definition, intellectual functioning (or intelligence), is considered to the general mental capability of an individual. This capability includes the ability to reason, plan, solve problems, think abstractly, comprehend complex ideas, learn quickly, and learn from experience. While it has its limitations, the accepted measure of intelligence is that which is determined by an intelligence quotient (IQ) score, which involves administration of standardized tests given by a trained professional. In the 1992 publication of the AAMR, a significant limitation of intellectual functioning was defined as being equivalent to an IQ score of approximately 70 or 75 and below (2, p. 5). The rationale for this range was logical in that an obtained IQ score must always be considered in light of its standard error of measurement, appropriateness, and consistency with administration guidelines. Since the standard error of measurement for most IQ tests is approximately 5, the ceiling may go up to 75. However, this range of 5 points, while seemingly small, was highly controversial for the reason that the difference between an "IQ of 75 and below" and an "IQ of 70 and below" resulted in an inexact cutoff for determining those eligible for diagnosis of MR. Twice as many people are eligible for the diagnosis when the cutoff was 75 or below (4). In an effort to address this issue, the most recent diagnostic classification published by the AAMR describes an intellectual deficit as being at two or more standard deviations from the mean (3).

The term MR may also be referred to in the literature as "intellectual disability or cognitive impairment." The Arc, a national advocacy group. does not use the term MR in their mission statement as it is felt to be offensive to many people:

> "*The term should not be thought of as guaranteeing individual access to needed supports. Rather, access to supports under federal programs such as IDEA, SSI and Medicaid is usually based on a combination of functional assessments and state and local administrative plans. In most programs other than IDEA, financial eligibility is required. People still need to use the term "mental retardation" to be eligible for some services in a few states, but in no case does having the label guarantee that supports will be available" (1).*

The Arc recognizes that the term is used in the public mainstream, especially among policy makers and legislators. It is most likely that the general public, including families, individuals, funders, administrators, and public policy makers at the local, state, and federal level are not aware of the negative feelings about the term and use the term with positive intentions:

> "*We find it necessary to use the term from time to time, as in this Q&A, to help people understand our issues. We try to use newer, more acceptable language as much as possible.*

We hope one day everyone will be known by their name, not by a label" (1).

Nevertheless, the term MR continues to be used in the mainstream literature as well as by the principal organizations, which historically and currently establish official definitions and classifications. In particular, the American Association on Mental Retardation (AAMR) was founded in 1876 and is an international multidisciplinary association of professionals dedicated to the development of services for persons with MR. Since 1921, the Association has published an official definition of MR with its most recent publication in 2002.

Adaptive Behavior

Adaptive behavior is most related to the domain of concern among occupational therapists. Thus, it is our focus of assessment and intervention for persons with MR. As defined by the AAMR, "adaptive behavior is the collection of conceptual, social, and practical skills that people have learned so they can function in their everyday lives" (3). Significant limitations in adaptive behavior impact a person's daily life and affect the ability to respond to a particular situation or to the environment. Table 4.1 describes specific examples of these three areas, which are provided by AAMR.

Limitations in adaptive behavior can be determined by using standardized tests referenced to the general population, including people with disabilities and people without disabilities. On these standardized measures, significant limitations in adaptive behavior are operationally defined as performance that is at least two standard deviations below the mean.

Onset Before the Age of 18

The final component of the definition of MR is that it begins early in life and therefore, a diagnosis of MR is usually made at or near birth. A diagnosis of MR is not considered in adult-onset degenerative diseases such as dementia or those associated with adult onset traumatic brain injury.

In considering this definition, the AAMR notes that there are five assumptions that need to be considered in the diagnostic process (2):

1. Limitations in present functioning must be considered within the context of community environments typical of the individual's age peers and culture.
2. Valid assessment considers cultural and linguistic diversity as well as differences

Table 4.1 ADAPTIVE SKILLS

Conceptual Skills	Social Skills	Practical Skills
Receptive and expressive language Reading and writing Money concepts Self-directions	Interpersonal Responsibility Self-esteem Gullibility (likelihood of being tricked or manipulated) Naiveté Following rules Obeying laws Avoiding victimization	Personal activities of daily living such as eating, dressing, mobility and toileting. Instrumental activities of daily living such as, preparing meals, taking medication, using the telephone, managing money, using transportation, and doing housekeeping activities. Occupational skills Maintaining a safe environment

in communication, sensory, motor, and behavioral factors.

3. Within an individual, limitations often coexist with strengths.
4. An important purpose of describing limitations is to develop a profile of needed supports.
5. With appropriate personalized supports over a sustained period, the life functioning of the person with MR generally will improve.

Etiology

The causes of MR may be classified according to when they occurred in the developmental cycle (prenatally, perinatally, or postnatally) or by their origin (biomedical vs. environmental) (2,4). There are hundreds of causes of MR (5).

Despite knowing the many factors that can cause MR, in a large proportion of cases the cause remains unknown. The ability to determine cause is highly correlated with the level of the retardation. The etiology of MR is much less likely to be known with individuals who are mildly retarded (IQs of 50 to 70) than with those who are severely retarded (IQs of <50) (2,4,6).

In a large United States population-based study describing probable causes of MR in school-aged children, the following results were obtained (5):

- No defined cause 78.0%
- Prenatal conditions 12.4%
- Genetic 7.1%
- Perinatal conditions 5.9%
- Intrauterine/intrapartum 5.2%
- Postneonatal events 3.6%
- **Teratogenic** 2.9%
- Central nervous system (CNS) birth defects 1.5%
- Other birth defects 0.8%
- Neonatal 0.7%

Prenatal factors that can cause MR include genetic aberrations, birth defects that are not genetic in origin, environmental influences, or a combination of factors (5). Up to 50% of the individuals diagnosed with MR may have more than one causal factor (2). With genetic aberrations, the problem is either with the genes, which are the basic unit of heredity, or the chromosomes, which carry the genes. Each nongerm cell (cells other than the ovum and spermatozoa) contains 23 pairs of chromosomes, including one pair of sex chromosomes that determine the sex of the person. Males have an X and a Y chromosome, and females have two X chromosomes.

In many cases of MR, the gene or chromosome that has caused the condition can be identified specifically. In fact, more than 350 inborn errors of metabolism that result from genetic changes have been identified. Many of these metabolic errors lead to MR (7). The two most common genetic causes of MR are Down syndrome and **fragile X syndrome**. (8) Down syndrome is generally caused by an extra 21st chromosome, and fragile X syndrome is the result of a mutation at what is known as the fragile site on the X chromosome (9). In other cases, the specific genetic aberration has not been identified. Factors such as higher incidences of a condition in specific families or increased recurrence rates among siblings suggest that the defect is genetic (6).

Birth defects that are not considered genetic in origin also can contribute to or cause MR. These could include such things as malformation of parts of the CNS **(cortical atrophy, hydrocephaly, spina bifida, craniostenosis)** (4), congenital cardiac anomalies (10), or metabolic disorders not associated with a genetic defect (hypothyroidism) (11).

Environmental factors may also be involved in prenatal development of MR. They may include exposure to chemical agents, such as alcohol or nonprescription drugs ingested by the mother during the pregnancy, maternal conditions such as **hyperphenylalaninemia**, (12)

toxemia, hypertension, and diabetes, or to congenital infections such as **cytomegalovirus**, rubella, and syphilis (4).

Genetic Causes

Genetic causes can be divided into two types: single gene disorders and chromosomal abnormalities. In single gene disorders, there is a problem with the quality of the genetic material; a specific gene is defective. In chromosomal abnormalities, the problem is with the quantity of material. There is either too much or too little genetic material in a specific chromosome (13).

Single Gene Disorders

Single gene disorders follow specific patterns of transmission: autosomal dominant, autosomal recessive, or sex-linked. Table 4.2 presents the transmission patterns and risk factors associated with each type.

The autosomal dominant type is caused by a single altered gene. Either parent may be a carrier or there may have been a spontaneous mutation of the gene. Dominant inheritance occurs when one parent passes on the defective gene. This occurs even if the other parent passes a healthy gene. Because the defective gene can be passed by either parent, there is a 50% risk of the child being affected in each pregnancy (8). An example of this type of inherited disorder is tuberous sclerosis.

In the autosomal recessive type, both parents are carriers but show no outward signs or symptoms of having the disorder. Inheritance occurs when both parents pass the defective gene to their offspring. Each pregnancy has a 25% risk of the child being affected (8). Examples of this type of disorder are phenylketonuria (PKU) and **Tay-Sachs disease**.

With X-linked disorders, the affected gene is on the sex chromosomes, specifically the X chromosome, and can occur in either parent. Because males have only one X chromosome, if the father has an affected gene, he will always

Table 4.2 SINGLE GENE DISORDERS

Type	Autosomal Dominant	Autosomal Recessive	Sex Linked
Transmission Pattern	Either parent carries gene or spontaneous transmission	Both parents are carriers	Either parent can transmit gene: mother usually a carrier, father cannot be a carrier but can have the disorder
Risk Factors	50% risk of child being affected with each pregnancy	25% risk of child being affected with each pregnancy	If mother has affected gene, 25% risk of having affected son or carrier daughter; if father has affected gene, all his daughters will be carriers and his sons will be normal
Sex Distribution	Male and female children equally at risk	Male and female children equally at risk	Primarily male children at risk for having disorder, female children at risk for becoming carriers

have the disorder and cannot be a carrier. Because the female has two X chromosomes, she can either be a carrier of the disorder (if only one X chromosome is affected) or have the disease herself (if both X chromosomes are affected). A carrier mother has a 25% risk of having an affected son. If the father has the affected gene, all his daughters will be carriers, but his sons will not be affected (8). Examples of X-linked disorders are Duchenne **muscular dystrophy**, fragile X syndrome, Lesch-Nyhan syndrome, and Hunter's syndrome.

Chromosomal Aberrations

Chromosomal aberrations include missing or extra chromosomes, either in part, such as a short arm, or the total chromosome, as is found in the trisomal types. Either the autosomes or sex chromosomes can be affected, with the autosomal type resulting in more serious neuromotor impairments (14). The most common are trisomy 21, 18, and 13. The patterns of transmission are not as readily identified as those of specific gene defects.

Environmental Influences

Prenatal Factors

There are numerous environmental causes of MR in the prenatal period, including maternal infections such as rubella, cytomegalovirus, toxoplasmosis, and syphilis. Low birth weight that results from prematurity or intrauterine growth retardation can also be a contributing factor. Maternal factors associated with low birth weight include smoking, lack of prenatal care, infections, poor nutrition, toxemia, and placental insufficiency. Exposure to industrial chemicals or drugs, including certain over-the-counter (OTC) prescriptions and illegal substances, also can affect birth weight, particularly during the first trimester of pregnancy.

Perinatal Factors

Two major causative factors of MR in the perinatal period are mechanical injuries at birth and perinatal **hypoxia**. Mechanical injuries are caused by difficulties of labor because of malposition, malpresentation, disproportion, or other labor complications that result in tears of the meninges, blood vessels, or other substances of the brain. Factors that cause perinatal hypoxia or anoxia include premature placental separation, massive hemorrhage from placenta previa, umbilical cord wrapped around the baby's neck, and meconium aspiration. Very premature infants also may have impaired respiration or an intracranial hemorrhage that can result in brain damage.

If a mother has an active case of herpes simplex II and is shedding the virus at the time of delivery, the baby can acquire the infection in the birth canal, which can cause severe developmental disability. This can be avoided by testing to determine whether the mother has an active case and, if so, delivering by cesarean section.

Postnatal Factors

Traumas or infections that result in injury or a lack of oxygen to the brain are a major cause of MR during the postnatal period. Traumas include near-drowning or strangulation, child abuse, and closed head injuries. Infections include encephalitis and meningitis. MR that results from meningitis caused by *Haemophilus influenzae* is now preventable, however, with the introduction of the *Haemophilus influenzae* type b (HiB) vaccine (15).

Another major postnatal factor is sociodemographic characteristics or environmental influences. When an analysis of the relationship of sociodemographic characteristics and MR was completed for a large population of children with MR, it was found that boys, children with two or more older siblings, African-American children, children whose mothers had not completed high school, and children of older mothers (with Down syndrome factored out) were more likely to experience MR (2).

Incidence and Prevalence

MR is the most frequently occurring developmental disability. Estimates of the prevalence of MR in this country range from 1% to 3%. Most professionals associated with the AAMR accept a prevalence of 2.5% and they recognize that the prevalence varies with chronologic age (1). A recent review of prevalence studies found that 2.5% to 3% is probably an accurate estimate of distribution in the general population (16). Boys are 1.5 times more likely to experience MR than girls (17), which may be related to the sex-linked genetic disorders that result in MR (2).

Signs and Symptoms

MR often occurs in tandem with, or as a secondary manifestation of, another diagnosis. One study's results found that two thirds of the children with severe MR (IQ <50) had an additional neurological diagnosis; less than 20% of children with mild MR were found to have an additional neurological diagnosis. These diagnoses included conditions such as cerebral palsy, epilepsy, and hearing and visual impairments (1). With certain genetic conditions, such as Down syndrome, MR is one of the clinical signs of the condition.

MR is defined by the AAMR as a condition that is present from childhood (age 18 or younger), with an IQ below 70 to 75 as measured on a standardized test, and significant limitations in two or more adaptive skills areas (3). As previously stated, adaptive skill areas include communication, self-care, home living, social/interpersonal skills, leisure, health and safety, self-direction, functional academics, use of community resources, and work. Adaptive skills should be assessed in all of the individual's performance contexts. Someone with limited intellectual function who does not have adaptive skill deficits is not considered mentally retarded (3).

There are currently two major systems of classification for MR. The American Psychiatric Association (APA) uses the older, more traditional system of classifying MR based on performance on standardized intelligence tests using somewhat arbitrary cutoffs to assign levels of function. It is essentially used for diagnostic purposes (2). In 1992, the AAMR introduced a system of classification based on adaptive skills levels and supports needed to function (3). The AAMR system, because it focuses on function and supports needed in adaptive skills across performance contexts, is more useful to the practice of occupational therapy.

In the traditional system, MR is classified according to the severity of the impairment in intellectual functioning. This is determined through standardized intelligence testing. To be considered mentally retarded, the person's performance on these tests must be two standard deviation units or more below the mean. The levels of MR as identified by IQ tests are mild, moderate, severe, and profound. Approximately 85% of individuals with MR are in the mild range, 10% are in the moderate range, 3.5% are in the severe range, and 1.5% are in the profound range of function (17,18). Table 4.3 presents the classifications, IQ levels, and general level of functioning as an adult. This information is adapted from the *Diagnostic and Statistical Manual of Mental Disorders*, *Fourth Edition (DSM-IV)* which is the diagnostic standard for mental healthcare professionals in the United States. The *DSM-IV* classifies four different degrees of MR: *mild*, *moderate*, *severe*, and *profound*. These categories are

Table 4.3 LEVELS OF RETARDATION

Classification	IQ Range	When Identified	Adaptive Behavior As Adult
Profound	Less than 20/25	Infancy	Independent functioning ■ Requires total supervision ■ Dependent upon others for personal care Communication ■ Very minimal language ■ Occupation ■ Minimal participation
Severe	20/25–35/40	Early childhood	Independent functioning ■ Can contribute partially to self-care with total supervision ■ Communication ■ Care engage in simple conversation ■ Recognizes signs and selected words Occupation ■ May prepare simple foods, can help with simple household tasks, e.g., bed making, vacuuming, setting and clearing table Requires much supervision
Moderate	35/40–50/55	Early childhood	Independent functioning ■ Feeds, bathes, and dresses self; prepares simple foods for self and others; able to care for own hair (wash and comb) ■ May function semi-independently in supervised living situation Communication ■ Carries on simple conversation, uses complex sentences; recognizes words, reads sentences, ads, and signs with comprehension Occupation ■ May do simple routine household chores (dusting, garbage, dishwashing); prepares food requiring mixing ■ May function in supported employment or sheltered workshop setting ■ Can learn some functional living skills: shopping, using post office, laundry
Mild	50/55–70/75	Elementary school	Independent functioning ■ Exercises care for personal grooming, feeding, bathing and toileting; may need health or personal care reminders; may need guidance and assistance when under unusual social or economic stress Occupation ■ Prepares meals, perform everyday household tasks ■ Can hold semi/skilled or simple skilled job

based on the functioning level of the individual. (2,3,9,19). It is important to remember that not all individuals in a particular classification will function at exactly that level.

The classification system developed by the AAMR involves a three-step process. The first step is to have a qualified person administer standardized intelligence and adaptive skills assessments that are appropriate for the individual's age, communication abilities, and cultural experience. The second step is to describe the individual's strengths and weaknesses across the dimensions of (a) intellectual and adaptive behavior skills, (b) psychological/emotional considerations, (c) physical/health/etiological considerations, and (d) environmental considerations. The third step is to have the interdisciplinary team determine needed supports across these four dimensions. Supports are classified based on level of intensity and include intermittent, limited, extensive, and pervasive. Intermittent support is provided on an "as-needed" basis. Limited support occurs over a limited time span. Extensive support is assistance provided on a daily basis in a life area. Pervasive support refers to the need for support in all life areas across all environments on a daily basis (3).

In addition to the performance deficits produced by MR and the associated conditions already mentioned, a high proportion of individuals with MR also have some form of mental illness. Estimates of prevalence of mental illness among people with MR range from 10% to 20% (19) to 40% to 70% (18). Some of the common types of mental illness seen in people with MR include personality disorders, affective disorders, psychotic disorders, avoidant disorder, paranoid personality disorder, severe behavior problems that may include self-injurious behavior (20) and dementia associated with Down syndrome (21). Several misconceptions about people with MR may complicate or prevent appropriate care for their mental illness, including the beliefs that people who are mentally retarded cannot also be mentally ill, do not experience normal feelings and emotions, and are not affected by changes in their environment. Substance abuse problems, especially with alcohol, may be overlooked and there is controversy about the benefit of using antipsychotic drugs with individuals who are mentally retarded (17). Because of limitations in communication skills and abstract thinking caused by the MR, the diagnosis of mental illness and mental health problems can be a very difficult process and is frequently inexact. Good communication with caregivers and significant others in the life of the individual with MR is essential.

Course and Prognosis

MR is generally considered a lifelong condition, but the course and prognosis will vary depending upon the cause(s) of the retardation (21,22). Most cases of MR are nonprogressive, that is, once the initial insult to the brain occurs, there is no further damage. The emphasis is on managing the medical aspects of the condition and helping individuals to achieve their highest potential. However, certain genetic conditions (e.g., muscular dystrophy and Tay-Sachs disease) are progressive, with incremental loss of function and, in some cases, associated early death. The goal for these individuals is to help them achieve the highest level of independence and maintain it as long as possible. Those with Down syndrome experience degenerative changes in the brain, beginning at about age 40 years, that eventually result in progressive dementia similar to Alzheimer's disease (20). On a positive note, it is possible for individuals with mild MR to gain adaptive behavior skills through remedial programs to the extent that they no longer meet the diagnostic criteria for being mentally retarded, although their intellectual function has probably not changed significantly (2).

Diagnosis

An evaluation must be performed to determine whether a person meets the criteria for being mentally retarded. Besides ascertaining that the onset of the condition occurred before age 18, there are two main aspects to this process. The first part involves administration of appropriate standardized intelligence tests by a qualified individual. "The choice of testing instruments and the interpretation of results should take into account factors that may limit test performance (e.g., the individual's sociocultural background, native language, and associated communicative, motor, and sensory handicaps)" (2).

The second aspect of the process is the evaluation of adaptive behavior as it relates to the targeted adaptive life skill areas. "Adaptive functioning refers to how effectively individuals cope with common life demands and how well they meet the standards of personal independence expected of someone in their particular age group, sociocultural background, and community setting" (2). The skills needed for adaptive behavior become more complex and varied as the person ages. For instance, eating and dressing independently are major skills for the young child, but the child does not need to be able to use a telephone or manage money. Evidence for deficits and strengths in adaptive function should be gained from one or more independent, reliable sources who are familiar with the individual's abilities in different performance contexts. This information should be used to complete a standardized scale designed to provide a composite "picture" of the individual's adaptive function. As with the selection of an intelligence test, care should be taken that the adaptive behavior scale chosen is appropriate for the individual's sociocultural background, education, associated handicaps, motivation, and cooperation level (2). There are more than 200 adaptive behavior measures and scales. The most common scale is the Vineland Adaptive Behavior Scales (23), which purports to assess the social competence of individuals with and without disabilities from birth to age 19 years. It is an indirect assessment in that the respondent is not the individual in question but someone familiar with the individual's behavior. The VABS measures four domains: Communication, Daily Living Skills, Socialization, and Motor Skills. An Adaptive Behavior Composite is a combination of the scores from the four domains. The AMMR Adaptive Behavior Scale (ABS): The ABS has two forms which address survival skills and maladaptive behaviors in individuals living in residential and community settings or school-age children (24). It is limited in scope and should be used with caution. A new scoring method has recently been devised that can generate scores consistent with the ten adaptive behavior areas suggested in the 1992 definition of MR (24). The results of this assessment can be readily translated into objectives for intervention.

Medical/Surgical Management

There is no drug treatment for the condition of MR; however, medications may be needed for some of the conditions that may occur in tandem. Concomitant mental health problems such as affective or psychotic disorders, and severe behavior problems would all benefit from appropriate medical intervention; seizure disorders would require drug therapy. Neuromuscular aberrations (spasticity, rigidity, etc.) seen in cerebral palsy may also be helped by medication.

Impact of Conditions on Client Factors and Occupational Performance

Virtually all areas of occupational performance and many client factors can be affected by MR, depending on the cause and severity of the retardation. As stated previously, the diagnostic criteria for individuals with MR identify ten adaptive behavior skill areas that may be affected in persons with MR, and at least two of these areas must be substantially limited to meet the criteria for being mentally retarded (2,3). If these areas are compared with the occupational performance areas, we see that all ten (communication, self-direction, self-care, home living, social/interpersonal skills, leisure, health and safety, functional academics, use of community resources, and work) fall into all occupational performance areas including (basic) activities of daily living, instrumental activities of daily living, work, play, leisure, and social participation.

Although all of the occupational performance areas and client factors can be influenced by MR, those that are affected will depend on factors such as the presence of additional medical diagnoses and the severity of the retardation. It is imperative that the clinician be informed about the specific diagnosis that accompanies the identification of MR to determine the specific associated client factors that are involved. For example, occupational therapists often work with persons who have Down syndrome. Babies with Down syndrome often have hypotonia, or poor muscle tone. Because they have a reduced muscle tone which results in oral motor dysfunction such as protruding tongue, feeding babies with Down syndrome is often difficult. Hypotonia may also affect the muscles of the digestive system, in which case constipation may be a problem. Atlantoaxial instability, a malformation of the upper part of the spine located under the base of the skull, is present in some individuals with Down syndrome. This condition can cause spinal cord compression as well as craniovertebral instability (25). Additionally, half of children with Down syndrome are diagnosed with a congenital heart. In addition to hearing disorders, visual problems also may be present early in life. Cataracts occur in approximately 3% of children with Down syndrome but can be surgically removed.

Approximately half of the children with Down syndrome have congenital heart disease and associated early onset of pulmonary hypertension, or high blood pressure in the lungs. Echocardiography may be indicated to identify any congenital heart disease. If the defects have been identified before the onset of pulmonary hypertension, surgery has provided favorable results. Seizure disorders, though less prevalent than some of the other associated medical conditions, still affect between 5% and 13% of individuals with Down syndrome, a 10-fold greater incidence than in the general population. Congenital hypothyroidism, characterized by a reduced basal metabolism, an enlargement of the thyroid gland, and disturbances in the autonomic nervous system, occurs slightly more frequently in babies with Down syndrome. Recent studies indicate that 66% to 89% of children with Down syndrome have a hearing loss of greater than 15 to 20 decibels in at least one ear, due to the fact that the external ear and the bones of the middle and inner ear may develop differently in children with Down syndrome (26). Given that 85% of all MR cases fall in the mild range of cognitive impairment, global and specific mental functions will be most affected with this population. The following case studies illustrate how MR affects an individuals' area of occupational performance in different stages of the life cycle.

CASE STUDY

Case Illustrations

■ CASE 1

K.R. is a 21-year-old young woman with Down syndrome. Despite the fact that she has reached the legal age of adulthood, she is still in the process of transitioning from the developmental stage of adolescence to young adulthood. She still receives special education services but is also working on developing work and job skills through traditional vocational services. Her "disability" is expected to be lifelong.

K.R.'s condition was identified at birth. She has received continuous support and direct services to facilitate development of her abilities since then. She has always lived at home with her parents and still does so. She has her own room and bathroom at home and generally has exclusive use of the family room for her leisure pursuits. Her parents are professionals who are actively involved in their professions and the community. They are very realistic about her abilities and extremely supportive, allowing her to make most of her life choices. K.R. has a younger sister who is now away at college. K.R. has always been exposed to and involved in many social and cultural opportunities in the community, both with her family and on her own. Her social circle includes friends with and without disabilities, and she has several close friends as well as many social acquaintances.

K.R. has recently declared her life goals to be getting a job, getting an apartment of her own, and spending leisure time at the local community drop-in/recreational center for individuals with disabilities. Her mother feels that, with appropriate supports, all of these goals are attainable.

K.R. is independent in most areas of personal care. As a result of limited fine motor coordination that seems to be complicated by visual perceptual deficits, she needs assistance with regulating the water temperature for her bath, fastening zippers and buttons, and tying her shoes. She also occasionally needs reminders to straighten her clothing and brush the back of her hair. She has a speech impediment that makes it difficult for individuals who are unfamiliar with her to initially understand her. K.R. has learned to adapt to this limitation and works very hard to make people understand what she is trying to communicate. When cued, she will slow down and work on enunciating her words. She is independent in functional mobility, but because of problems with depth perception, she is very cautious when climbing steps and negotiating between different surface levels. She is able to travel independently in community areas she is familiar with and can ride the community "Dial-a-Ride" bus if the ride is arranged for her. Her mother feels that K.R. would be aware of danger in her home, such as a fire, and would get out of the house. She does not consistently answer the phone when it rings, although she is capable of doing so. For this reason, she is generally not allowed to be at home alone because her parents have no way of checking in with her if she does not answer the phone.

K.R. is able to perform many home management tasks and has recently become motivated to attempt more activities given her desire to have an apartment of her own. She generally dislikes "housework" but knows it is necessary in order to be a good roommate. She folds laundry and puts it away, and is learning to sort light and dark clothing and operate the washing machine. Her mother questions her ability to make judgments about what should or should not go into the dryer, however. She is able to sweep, vacuum, and dust but is not thorough and this may be a result of her lack of interest and/or her visual-perceptual impairment. She keeps her bathroom clean and makes her bed. She is currently dependent in meal preparation and this is the area that will probably require the most support for her to live in her own apartment. She cannot safely regulate stove and oven temperatures because of her fine motor problems. At the current time, K.R. attends school in a self-contained special education classroom in the local high school for half a day, focusing on vocational and prevocational skills, and spends the other half-day at Goodwill Industries in a work adjustment trial placement. K.R. has told her mother that she no longer enjoys going to school and would rather go to Goodwill. In addition to school and vocational activities, K.R. volunteers at the local community theater and at her church office doing clerical tasks. She is very interested in obtaining employment and would prefer to work at a video store, a music store, at the mall, or Pizza Hut. She is very interested in clerical tasks and has been working at her father's medical practice putting monthly billings in envelopes to be mailed. K.R. has many leisure interests and activities. She enjoys music and videos, likes to eat out, participates in Special Olympics, goes to a community center for structured activities, and socializes with her friends. She prefers not to do strenuous physical activities, probably because of the difficulty she has as a result of generalized hypotonia. She has participated in team sports at the center but does so mostly for the social interaction. K.R. is very aware of her limitations and takes herself out of situations that she knows will be difficult or where she might not succeed.

■ CASE 2

F.B. is a 60-year-old man who is mentally retarded. He has a history of behavior problems, including **PICA** and obsessive-compulsive type behaviors of picking at his skin and clothing and stuffing toilets. He was retired from a sheltered workshop approximately 18 months ago when the emphasis of the program shifted to work readiness for community placement. It was determined that he would not be a good candidate for community work because of his age and lack of necessary supports (e.g., transportation). He currently attends a day program for social/leisure activities. F.B. has no known family and has spent most of his life in public residential institutions or in adult foster care (AFC) homes. He currently has a court-appointed guardian who makes most significant life decisions for him, including those regarding medical care and living arrangements. His guardian supports and encourages F.B. to make his wishes known about how he would like to spend his leisure time and allowed him input into his last housing change. In addition to his intellectual limitations, F.B. also experiences fairly frequent medical problems related to his obsessive-compulsive behaviors (e.g., skin infections). Medical problems, which may be age related, are emphysema and frequent fractures of bones in his lower extremities. F.B. currently lives in an AFC with 11 other adults who are developmentally disabled. His home is only required by law to provide basic care and so it does not offer training in or support for participation in many home management tasks. His social groups generally consist of other adults with developmental disabilities or paid paraprofessional staff, either at home or the day program. His cultural experiences have been very limited and because of his background, it would be fair to say that he has been encultured as a "mentally retarded person."

F.B. is independent in most self-care tasks but needs supervision when using the bathroom because of his history of stuffing the toilet. He needs assistance and supports for taking medication owing to his cognitive limitations. He also needs very close monitoring of health status because he has a very high pain tolerance. He tends to prefer solitary activities but has become more verbal, social, and outgoing since going to the day program. He generally seeks out staff to interact with, and this usually takes the form of teasing. He will share activities with day program peers if prompted and has shown protective behaviors toward clients who are more limited and vulnerable than he is. Although he is verbal, he has a speech impediment that makes it difficult for people who are unfamiliar with him to understand what he is saying. He is independently ambulatory; however, he has reduced endurance as a result of an old hip fracture and neuropathy of the right lower extremity caused by a degenerative disease in the lumbar spine. He is dependent for all community mobility as a result of cognitive limitations and lack of experience and training. It is not clear whether he understands emergency situations, but he is cooperative with emergency drill procedures at the day program. It is likely that he would need ongoing supervision to maintain his personal safety.

Because of a lack of experience and opportunity, F.B. is dependent in all home management tasks. He has no responsibility for caring for others but seems to be very aware when one of his peers needs assistance or protection and alerts staff to these needs. He has been retired from the vocational arena for 18 months and now attends a day program that emphasizes social and leisure activities.

F.B. is generally not open to exploring new activities and has to be coaxed and teased by staff to try them. He generally prefers solitary activities and appears to enjoy assembly activities that result in a finished product like picture puzzles and building with Erector-Set components. He does not seem to be very interested in watching television or listening to music but does enjoying going on automobile rides with his guardian, especially when she drives her convertible with the top down.

References

1. Introduction to Mental Retardation. Arlington, TX: The Arc, May, 2005. Available at: http://www.thearc.org. Accessed February 16, 2006.
2. American Association on Mental Retardation. Mental retardation: Definition, classification, and systems of supports. 10th Ed. Washington, DC: 1992.
3. American Association on Mental Retardation. Mental retardation: Definition, classification, and systems of supports. 10th Ed. Washington, DC: 2002.
4. Yeargin-Allsopp M, Murphy C, Cordero J, et al. Reported biomedical causes and associated medical conditions for mental retardation among 10-year-old children, metropolitan Atlanta, 1985 to 1987. Dev Med Child Neurol 1997;39:142–147.
5. Introduction to Mental Retardation. Arlington, TX: The Arc, 1993. http://www.thearc.org. Accessed January 10, 2006.
6. Matilainen R, Airaksinen E, Monomen T, et al. A population-based study on the causes of mild and severe mental retardation. Acta Paediatr 1995;84:261–266.
7. Scriver C. The Metabolic and Molecular Bases of Inherited Disease. 7th Ed. New York: McGraw-Hill, 1995.
8. Genetic Causes of Mental Retardation. Arlington, TX: The Arc, 1996. http://www.thearc.org. Accessed December 19, 2005.
9 Kaplan H, Sadock B, Grebb J. Synopsis of Psychiatry. 7th Ed. Baltimore: Williams & Wilkins, 1994.
10. Rogers B, et al. Neurodevelopmental outcome of infants with hypoplastic left heart syndrome. J Pediatr 1995;126:496–498.
11. Reuss M, Paneth M, Pinto-Martin J, et al. The relation of transient hypothyroxinemia in preterm infants to neurologic development at two years of age. N Engl J Med 1996;334:821–827.

12. Jardim L, Palma-Dias R, Silva L, et al. Maternal hyperphenylalaninemia as a cause of microcephaly and mental retardation. Acta Paediatr 1996;85: 943–946.
13. Gror M, Shekleton M. Basic Pathophysiology, A Conceptual Approach. St. Louis: CV Mosby, 1979.
14. Harris S, Tada W. Genetic disorders. In: Umphred D, ed. Neurological Rehabilitation. St. Louis: CV Mosby, 1990.
15. Baraff L, Lee S, Schriger D. Outcomes of bacterial meningitis in children: a meta-analysis. Pediatr Infect Dis J 1993;12:389–394.
16. Frayers T. Epidemiological thinking in mental retardation: issues in taxonomy and population frequency. Int Rev Res Ment Retard 1993;19: 97–133.
17. Hauser M, Ratey J. The patient with mental retardation. In: Hyman S, Tesar G, eds. The Manual of Psychiatric Emergencies. Boston: Little Brown & Co, 1994:104–109. Available at: http://www.psychiatry. com. Accessed December 27, 2005.
18. Silka V, Hauser M. Psychiatric assessment of the person with mental retardation. Psychiatr Ann 1997;27:3. Available at: http://www.psychiatry.com. Accessed January 16, 2006.
19. Reiss S, Goldberg B, Ryan R. Mental illness in persons with mental retardation. Arlington, TX: The Arc, 1993. Available at: http://www.psychiatry.com. Accessed January 16, 2006.
20. Zigman W, Schupf N, Zigman A, et al. Aging and Alzheimer disease in people with mental retardation. Int Rev Res Ment Retard 1993;19:41–70.
21. Behrman R, Kliegman R, Nelson W, et al, eds. Nelson's Textbook of Pediatrics. 14th Ed. Philadelphia: WB Saunders, 1992.
22. Beers M, Berkow R, eds. The Merck Manual of Diagnosis and Therapy. 17th Ed. Rahway, NJ: Merck Sharp & Dohme Research Laboratories, 1997.
23. Sparrow S, Balla D, Cicchetti D. Vineland Adaptive Behavior Scales. Circle Pines, MN: American Guidance Service, 1984.
24. Nihira K, Leland H, Lambert NM. Adaptive Behavior Scale–Residential and Community. 2nd Ed. (ABS-RC:2). Austin, TX: Pro-Ed, 1993.
25. Brockmeyer D. Down syndrome and craniovertebral instability: Topic review and treatment recommendations. Pediatr Neurosurg 1999;31(2):71–77.
26. National Institutes of Health: Facts about Down Syndrome. Available at: http://www.nichd.nih.gov/publications/pubs/downsyndrome/down. Accessed February 12, 2006.

Recommended Learning Resources

American Association on Mental Retardation. Mental Retardation: Definition, Classification, and Systems of Support. 10th Ed. Washington DC: American Association on Mental Retardation, 2002.

Baker B, Brightman A, Blacher J, et al. Steps to Independence: Teaching Everyday Skills to Children with Special Needs. 4th Ed. Baltimore, MD: Paul H. Brookes, 2004.

Behrman R, Kliegman R, eds. Nelson Essentials of Pediatrics. 4th Ed. Philadelphia: WB Saunders, 2002.

Case-Smith J. Occupational Therapy for Children. 5th Ed. St. Louis: Mosby, 2005.

American Journal on Mental Retardation
American Association on Mental Retardation
444 No. Capitol St., NW, Suite 846
Washington, DC 20001

Education and Training in Mental Retardation and Developmental Disabilities
Division on Mental Retardation & Developmental Disabilities
The Council for Exceptional Children
1920 Association Drive
Reston, VA 22091–1589

Journal of the Association for Persons with Severe Handicaps
Division on Mental Retardation & Developmental Disabilities
The Council for Exceptional Children
1920 Association Drive
Reston, VA 22091

Advocacy Resources

American Association on Mental Retardation (AAMR)
444 North Capitol St., NW, Suite 846
Washington, DC 20001
Tel: (202) 387–1968; toll free: (800) 424–3688;
Fax: (202) 387–2193

The Arc
500 E. Border St., Suite 300
Arlington, TX 76010
Tel: (817) 261–6003; TTY: (817) 277–0553;
Fax: (817) 277–3941

The Association for Persons with Severe Handicaps (TASH)
11201 Greenwood Ave. N.
Seattle, WA 98133
Tel: (206) 361–8870

Division on Mental Retardation & Developmental Disabilities
The Council for Exceptional Children
1920 Association Drive
Reston, VA 22091–1589
Tel: (703) 620–3660

National Down Syndrome Congress
1605 Chantilly Dr., Suite 250
Atlanta, GA 30324
Tel: (800) 232-NDSC

National Down Syndrome Society
666 Broadway
New York, NY 10012
Tel: (212) 460–9330; toll free: (800) 221–4602

President's Committee on Mental Retardation (PCMR)
U. S. Department of Health & Human Services
330 Independence Ave., SW
Washington, DC 20201
Tel: (202) 619–0634

People First International (self-advocacy group)
1340 Chemeketa St., NE
Salem, OR 97301
Tel: (503) 588–5288

Special Olympics International, Inc.
1350 New York Ave., NW, Suite 500
Washington, DC 20005
Tel: (202) 628–3630

Schizophrenia

Yvonne Russell Teske

Key Terms

Affect
Alogia
Anhedonia
Antipsychotic medications
Cogwheel rigidity
Delusions
Delusions of grandeur
Delusions of persecution
Fixed ideas
Flight of ideas
Genotype
Hallucinations
Ideas of reference
Negative symptoms
Neurotransmitters
Phenotype
Positive symptoms
Relapse
Tangential thinking

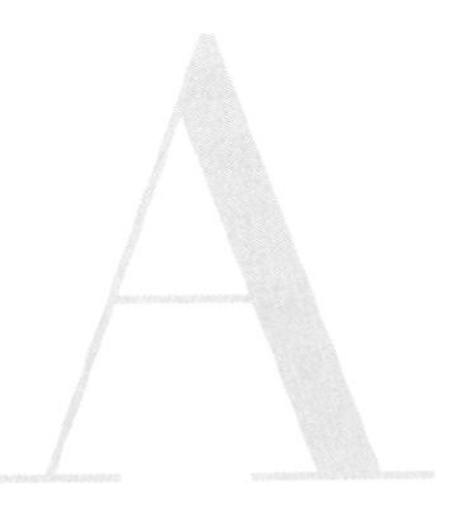

An occupational therapy professor and two occupational therapy students drove to a house where eight former mental patients lived. The local community mental health agency owned and operated the house as a supervised residence for individuals who were recently discharged from a state-run mental hospital. The students had prepared to administer a goal-setting, interview assessment to individuals who had a history of mental illness. In order to live in the house, residents had agreed to set goals for living in the community setting.

On the way to the house, the professor and students saw a man rapidly walking down the street, taking long strides. In spite of his hunched-over shoulders, he looked straight ahead without turning his head to look at the people or the physical environment as he passed. His face reflected a look of concentration, with a squint and wrinkled forehead. The man talked to himself as he walked. Even though the temperature that day was in the 60s, he wore a long wool coat. His long hair flowed behind him as he walked. He was smoking a cigarette, rapidly taking the cigarette in and out of his mouth as he puffed and talked.

At the house, the students met the residents and staff member supervisors who were seated in the dining room. The man who was walking down the street was one of the residents. When the students introduced themselves, he responded with an unstoppable stream of speech. No one could help him. He had been hospitalized 8 years and people tried to help him, it didn't work out and he had to help himself. Over and over, he repeated the same ideas. The professor replied, "Fine." He continued his thoughts about being helped, but the more he spoke the more unusual the phrases became with biblical references to the end of the world, pestilence, rape, and sex. The professor heard his disturbance about several issues including the presence of young women students, past failures, and fear about change and the future.

The students' faces showed surprise at his outburst but the man did not look at their faces. Once he stopped talking, he became quiet for a moment. Then he repeated over and over, "I'm sorry, I'm sorry." He expressed his concern with great emotion. The students could not respond to the emotional intensity of what they heard, so the professor spoke to validate the man's beliefs about people's ability to help themselves. As the professor continued speaking quietly the man calmed down and retreated to his room. The students interviewed other residents in the house, but the man did not re-appear. Later the students learned about the man's history of repeated, long hospitalizations, and his family's distress over his problems (class experience, Y. Teske, 2000).

Even though the interviews went smoothly, the professor and students felt stressed by their experience with the intensity of the man's speech, so after the session they stopped for ice cream before returning to the university. In a quiet corner in an empty restaurant, the students talked about the changes in society and culture over the period of 8 to 10 years of hospitalization for mental illness, changes in the technology of computers, telephones, television; changes in the landscape of communities; changes in local, state, national, and international policies and politics. In the past, a diagnosis of schizophrenia resulted in long and repeated periods of hospitalization. However, research into the etiology and treatment of schizophrenia leads to reduced periods of hospitalization and increased opportunities for living and participating in community life.

Schizophrenia is a brain disorder because of brain neuropathology. Even though schizophrenia is commonly labeled as a single disorder, individuals who have schizophrenia have a complex array of observable symptoms and more subtle cognitive deficits. In diagnosing schizophrenia, psychiatrists look for symptoms of psychosis. Psychosis consists of three major types of observable symptoms—**hallucinations**, **delusions**, and disorganized thinking. Individuals who have schizophrenia have an increase or excess of these symptoms beyond what typical individuals may have. Therefore these symptoms are called **positive symptoms** (1). Psychosis is present in other conditions such as Alzheimer's disease, substance abuse, and mood disorders. The psychiatrist also will look for decreases or deficits in typical behaviors. The deficit symptoms are called **negative symptoms** (1). The psychiatrist will try to identify a pattern of positive and/or negative symptoms.

Positive symptoms (1,2) include:

- Hallucinations—atypical auditory, visual, and/or olfactory sensory perceptions. Auditory hallucinations are the most common type. For example, an observation of a woman sitting on a chair in the lunchroom of a day program for individuals with mental illness shows her looking ahead intently listening to something not heard by others in the room. She has a slight smile on her face and occasionally nods her head. When asked if she is hearing voices, she says "yes" but is unwilling to share what the voices say to her. Individuals with visual hallucinations may see someone from their past enter the room or see a symbol of a religious nature.

The visualizations are not seen by others in the room. Olfactory hallucinations are the least common. Hallucinations are not unique to schizophrenia but can occur with other disorders such as Alzheimer's disease and substance abuse. Altered mental states such as hallucinations also can occur with other physiological changes such as those that come in the period before death.

- Delusions—atypical yet well-organized, systematic beliefs not explained by evidence or culture. Delusions, like hallucinations, are a result of the brain disorder in schizophrenia. To someone who does not have schizophrenia, the delusions sound unusual but in many cases the delusions reflect literature such as the Bible, poetry, and novels, as well as historical and political events. **Delusions of grandeur** consist of inflated self-views. Patients talk about the powerful and influential jobs and remarkable adventures they have had. A listener may find a challenge in figuring out what parts of the stories are true and what parts are not. Accurate reports may be threaded through the delusional stories, leading to confusion for the listener. The actual facts are not important; the listener hears what the individual with schizophrenia believes to be true. **Delusions of persecution** are consistent and organized beliefs that other people are demeaning, accusing, or spying on the individual who has schizophrenia. The individual can explain the who, what, when, where, and how of the delusion. The federal government is a common source of accusations and negative acts in delusional systems.

Ideas of reference are beliefs that people are talking about the individual with schizophrenia. The individual looks at a small group of people and assumes the group is talking about him or her. The logic of this type of delusion is that because the world view of the individual is focused on the self, therefore others must be talking about him or her.

Fixed ideas are part of delusions. An individual has an idea that resists change through logical arguments, evidence, or persuasion. An example seen by this author involved three men who believed they were Jesus Christ. Though all three men were in the same room, and the psychiatrist presented them with logical reasons against their beliefs, all three men remained fixed in their ideas (class experience, Y. Teske, 1972).

- Disordered thinking—thoughts are illogical, are not presented in sequence, and do not reflect cause and effect relationships.
- Unusual speech and behavior—complete dictionaries of psychological and psychiatric terms are important resources for mental health practice settings. Many terms define and describe atypical speech and behavior.

The man described in the introductory paragraph of this chapter shows **flight of ideas** because of his rapid rate of speech and changing ideas. One word led to another without logical links among the ideas. Because of the rapid speech and illogical ideas, the professor and students could not understand the man.

Negative symptoms (1,2) include:

- **Alogia**—absence of speech because of mental illness.
- **Anhedonia**—lack of pleasure or enjoyment in life activities.
- Avolition—lack of initiative and motivation to engage in tasks and relationships with other people.
- Flat, sometimes called blunt, **affect**—lack of facial expression during or in response to emotional expression.
- Movement reduced in amount or rate.

Etiology

The cause of schizophrenia remains unknown despite extensive research efforts through the National Institute of Mental Health (NIMH) and universities around the world. Researchers continue to identify small parts of the genetic, neurobiological, and environmental picture of schizophrenia. Biological vulnerability to schizophrenia determined at birth results from the interaction of genetic and prenatal environmental factors. Then, at critical periods in brain development such as adolescence, stressful events trigger the behavioral expression of the vulnerability. Family members observe symptoms of hallucinations, delusions, and disordered thinking in their adolescent child. Though other members of the family may have similar genetic characteristics and early environmental factors, each family member's brain responds to stressful events in a unique way. Environmental factors disrupt the neuronal circuits of the brain leading to schizophrenia in the adolescent or young adult family member.

Genetic Causes

No one gene is responsible for schizophrenia. Researchers conclude that the pattern of inheritance in schizophrenia involves multiple genes acting together or many single genes acting separately in heterogeneous patterns of genes (3). These heterogeneous patterns of genes leading to a brain disorder show how complex the cause of schizophrenia must be. Genetic patterns of dominant and recessive traits do not seem to answer the research questions about the causes of schizophrenia (3). Recognizing the genetic complexity, international efforts continue to identify genes that can predict a high risk or vulnerability for schizophrenia in families.

At least four genes have a role in schizophrenia: Neuregulin 1, Dysbindin, catechol-O-methyl transferase (COMT), G72 (3). Some regulate chemical substances such as dopamine and glutamate; others influence nerve myelination and plasticity at nerve synapses. Dopamine may interfere with short-term memory while glutamate is the primary activator for neuron function in the brain (3). Schizophrenia research efforts showed that the COMT gene on chromosome 22 q slightly increased the risk of the brain disorder by impairing the frontal cortex function in animals (4). Research in schizophrenia shows evidence that genes located on several different chromosomes affect each other through linkages among the chromosomes and together may lead to some of the brain abnormalities in the disorder.

In addition to the search for specific gene patterns, researchers also seek genetic markers that may be present in family members even though only one family member has the disorder. Genetic markers are actually **phenotypes**, which come from the **genotype** or genetic makeup of a living organism (5). The gene is a unit of heredity and the genotype describes the pattern of genes for each of us. Phenotypes are the observable physical characteristics for each of us. Unlike genotypes, phenotypes can be observed and studied directly in living organisms including human beings. Researchers who are interested in inherited characteristics regard phenotypes as observable markers for genotypes and study phenotypes for clues to the neurobiology of schizophrenia. To qualify for a marker of a specific disease, a phenotype must meet rigorous research criteria. For example the phenotype must be present in nonaffected family members at a rate higher than the general population. Occupational therapists can see some evidence of phenotypes when a patient is unable to focus on a task in the presence of a mild distraction. The patient is unable to screen out the irrelevant distraction.

The genotype may be present but is not seen in parents, siblings, or close relatives, whereas phenotypes are observable in the individual who has schizophrenia and in family members. The closer the family relationship to an individual who has schizophrenia, the more likely family members will also have the disorder. For example a child of someone who has schizophrenia is ten times more likely to have the disease than the average person. The fact that the disorder is not seen in predictable inherited patterns through each generation strengthens the evidence that many genes are involved in the cause. Although environmental factors may influence schizophrenia, the chance of environmental factors alone causing the disorder is slim.

Phenotypes for schizophrenia include several major cognitive deficits that are central to the brain disorder (6,7). These include deficits in perception, memory, and social interaction. Cognitive deficits are the major barriers to independent living, work and education, and social participation in community life and need to be the focus of interventions (7).

Perceptual Deficits

- Backward masking. Individuals who have schizophrenia and their family members view stimuli on a computer screen. Then testers briefly interrupt the stimuli with a grid followed by the original stimuli. The individuals and some family members do not recognize the original stimuli (6).
- Vigilance and sustained attention. Psychologists measure vigilance by presenting a series of stimuli on a computer screen including stimuli relevant to the task and irrelevant stimuli that represent distractions like noise. Individuals and their family members who have this phenotype remain vigilant to all stimuli. They have reduced resources for attention (6,7).
- Sensory gating. If a quiet stimulus precedes or acts as a gate for a startling stimulus, the eye blink response to the startling stimuli will be less. For individuals and family members with this phenotype, the quiet first stimulus does not reduce the startle response. They cannot attend to or ignore the first stimulus, even when asked. The sensory gating deficit, sometimes called P50 gating response, shows there is a genetic link to the hippocampus in the brain (6,8).

Memory, Problem-Solving, and Executive Functions

- Immediate memory. Individuals with schizophrenia and family members may mentally rehearse a telephone number, dial it, and immediately forget it (6).
- Secondary or explicit memory. After writing a grocery list of 15 items, a person goes to the store but forgets to take the list. The typical person will recall most if not all of the items, but individuals with schizophrenia will be unable to remember the items (6).
- Motor/procedural memory and speed. Information is retained but takes longer to learn and must be learned in the context of performance. Information from memory takes longer to recall and use, causing slow motor responses. The brain disorder causes the slow motor speed.
- Executive function. Schizophrenia affects problem-solving planning, and alternating between two or more tasks. These factors are related to prefrontal cortex function and affect mental process skills (6).
- Context. Context refers to the sense of overall goal for a series of activities. Schizophrenia reduces the ability to retain the intent or goal of activities. Even when not interrupted, individuals have difficulty pursuing goal-directed activity (6).

Social Interaction Deficits

- Verbal fluency. Much of social interaction depends on cognitive abilities to process information and respond quickly and appropriately. By the time an individual who has schizophrenia comprehends the words themselves, processes word meaning with a response, and then articulates a response, the social interaction no longer seems spontaneous. The rate of speech and quality of speech is deficient in schizophrenia because of deficits in semantic memory, executive function, and articulation (9).

- Perception of emotion. Individuals with schizophrenia and some of their family members are unable to recognize emotion on a face, in a voice, or on a video. The deficit results in decreased communication and social interaction skills (8).
- Social understanding. Typically, individuals can deduce what others are thinking and what others are thinking about them. Because they lack abstract reasoning, individuals with schizophrenia cannot put together a social understanding of others and of themselves in relation to others.

The phenotypes just described represent changes in brain structure and function starting in adolescence and young adulthood. Changes in mental processes can affect relatively simple tasks like dressing, and making a sandwich. Changes in perceptions and thoughts isolate individuals by giving them a view of the world not shared by family members and friends. Since social behavior depends on a world view, social interaction becomes limited.

Brain Abnormalities

Research using techniques such as computerized axial tomography (CAT), positron emission tomography (PET), and magnetic resonance imaging (MRI) show physical abnormalities in brain structure and function. While researchers report many abnormalities, no single abnormality is characteristic of all individuals with schizophrenia or applies to schizophrenia alone. Similar abnormalities appear in the brains of individuals who have disorders other than schizophrenia.

Changes in brain structure precede the observable symptoms of the disorder. Many researchers report shrunken areas in the brain implying a shortage of neurons in the gray matter and reduced myelin covering the connecting axons (8,10). Research shows reduced size and volume in the hippocampus and thalamus. The region of the hippocampus consistently emerges as the one area of the brain that distinguishes individuals who have schizophrenia from healthy individuals (11). Located in the medial temporal lobe, the hippocampus and the adjacent amygdala form memories, interpret the emotional importance of specific memories, and determine which memories will be retained. Memory deficits as a result of schizophrenia affect daily occupations. The physical and functional changes in the brain are important areas of research but do not address the cause of the schizophrenia.

Changes in brain function using MRI and PET show reduced activity in the frontal and temporal lobes while individuals who have schizophrenia perform cognitive tasks. Since more than one region of the brain shows atypical activity, scientists believe the primary deficits in schizophrenia are in the connections through neuronal networks and circuits in several regions. Functional imaging data indicate that the pathophysiology in schizophrenia is a result of abnormal, excitatory, and bizarre activity in neuronal circuits in and among the prefrontal cortex, hippocampus, and other subcortical structures. White matter inside the brain's gray matter consists of myelin-covered axons that connect neurons. According to research evidence, cells in the myelin sheath around the axons have a genetic predisposition to misfire leading to defects in neuronal circuits that connect all regions of the brain (8). However the defects in myelin sheaths around axons in the brain are not unique to schizophrenia.

Neurons secrete chemical substances called **neurotransmitters** that bind receptors on nearby cells. More than 25 neurotransmitters have been identified (5). Neurotransmitters are considered paracrine hormones because they influence nearby cells instead of influencing cells throughout the body, as other hormones do. Five neurotransmitters most commonly appear in schizophrenia research: dopamine, glutamate, γ-aminobutyric acid (GABA), serotonin, and noradrenalin (12). Dopamine is responsible for neurotransmission between the cortex and subcortical regions of the brain (13). Abnormalities in dopamine that are reported in research results for schizophrenia include excess production, increased number of dopamine receptors over those of normal individuals, and abnormal production and release (13). Glutamate connects the hippocampus, prefrontal cortex, and thalamus (7). Individuals with schizophrenia in some studies have shown reduced transmission of glutamate. Dopamine and glutamate work together in the frontal cortex region. Glutamate excites neuronal circuits, whereas GABA inhibits function. The two neurotransmitters work in concert and so it is likely that both would be affected in schizophrenia. Serotonin and noradrenalin have more limited evidence for their role in decreased brain function in schizophrenia (7). The neurocognitive deficits presented above and the brain abnormalities just described provide evidence that schizophrenia affects brain function but do not show that specific areas of the brain affect day-to-day performance for individuals who have schizophrenia.

Complications of Pregnancy and Birth

Because obstetrical complications can affect development of the fetal brain, conditions such as maternal preeclampsia and lack of oxygen (hypoxia) for the fetus can lead to schizophrenia. Preeclampsia is a condition in pregnancy characterized by maternal hypertension, edema, and excess protein in the urine (7). Usually the woman has high blood pressure before the pregnancy and the physiological stress of pregnancy leads to hypertension, a condition caused by very high arterial blood pressure. Individuals who have hypertension retain fluid in their bodies slowing down the elimination of fluids by the kidneys. Pregnant women with hypertension have excessive swelling, called edema, in their hands and legs. In addition to fetal brain changes in-utero, women with preeclampsia may deliver premature children who experience developmental problems like schizophrenia. During birth, hypoxia happens when oxygen to the fetus is reduced. According to data from the National Collaborative Perinatal Project, the chances of schizophrenia directly increased as the incidents of hypoxia at birth increased (14).

Many studies show that individuals born between December and March have higher that average rates of schizophrenia (15). Viral infections like influenza commonly occur in late fall and early winter. Mothers may have influenza or may carry viral infections during the second trimester of pregnancy when important brain development occurs.

Traumatic events that affect the mother during pregnancy like the death of a spouse can affect fetal development and increase the risk of schizophrenia. One explanation for the effects of maternal traumatic, stressful events has to do with the link between stress and release of high levels of the hormone cortisol into the adrenal glands affecting hypothalamus, pituitary and adrenal relationships (7).

Environmental Stress

Evidence from research results shows several relationships between stressful environments and events on the behavioral expression of schizophrenia in vulnerable individuals. The number of stressful events increases in the months before an individual who has schizophrenia experiences a **relapse**, the return of symptoms and readmission to treatment. Negative environments in which family members fight, argue, and are unable to give each other positive support increase the chances of relapse in schizophrenia. These studies provide direct evidence of the effects of stress on already-diagnosed patients.

Indirect evidence comes from studies that are retrospective, studies that look back on the lives of patients. Dysfunctional families, abuse by parents with mental illness, removal of children from mothers who have schizophrenia, and parental substance abuse are stress-producing conditions for individuals who are vulnerable to schizophrenia (7). Researchers conclude that these documented environments are significant in the behavioral expression of schizophrenia in vulnerable individuals but would not necessarily have the same effects on individuals who did not carry the genetic vulnerability. Recall how high levels of cortisol can affect the hypothalamus, pituitary, and adrenal glands and create hypersensitivity to stress situations.

Incidence and Prevalence

Figures for the incidence and prevalence of schizophrenia are collected every several years in large data-collection projects. The incidence of schizophrenia in the United States and around the world has remained stable for many years. In the United States, 1.1% of the population has schizophrenia at any given time (16). The United States has a population of 281,422,509 according to 2000 census data (17). In 1 year, over 2 million people will have schizophrenia. The population within the city limits of Houston, Texas is just above 2 million people (17). The prevalence of schizophrenia is 1 in 100 individuals. So in a small city of 30,000 people, about 300 will have schizophrenia. The average age of onset of schizophrenia for men is 18 years, and for women, 25 years. This is a time when men and women begin new developmental tasks of achieving a college education, starting new careers, marrying, and becoming parents. A diagnosis of schizophrenia affects the entire young adult milestones (18).

Signs and Symptoms

While schizophrenia can first appear with sudden onset, symptoms may be evident for some time. Parents with an adolescent or young adult child who is diagnosed with schizophrenia, say that they noticed changes in hygiene, dress, facial expression, speech, and interaction for a period before they realized what the behavioral change might indicate (NAMI-Virginia, March 2004, personal communication). They began to realize the child was no longer the one they previously knew. Subtle changes added up to a different person. Common problems in the premorbid or pre-illness stage of schizophrenia include learning problems in school; a change in activity level, either hypoactive or hyperactive; changes in mood, euphoric or depressed; disturbances in sexual behavior; complaints about the body; obsessiveness, guilt, unpredictable or odd behavior, suspicion, anxiety, and fearfulness (19).

One family reported that their generally well-groomed son no longer wanted to shower. He repeatedly wore the same clothes. No matter what the emotion, facial expression was flat or blunted with little genuine or spontaneous expression of feeling. At times he refused to come out of his room to join family members or friends. The event that finally alerted the parents to mental illness and led to hospitalization was his disappearance. When the parents called the police after the son was gone for 1 day, the police concluded that the behavior was common for teenagers. When the police did find the son, the parents insisted the police call the mental health agency for a psychiatric evaluation. The evaluation led to immediate hospitalization.

Symptoms appear gradually for children under the age of 12 years. Parents first notice developmental delays in language and motor skills and a lack of empathy for others. Children may accuse parents and teachers of reading their minds or plotting against them. Otherwise, their symptoms are like adult symptoms.

Positive Symptoms

Previously we discussed positive and negative symptoms. While in real-life cases distinctions between positive and negative symptoms are not clear cut, the categories facilitate understanding of symptoms. Mark, age 45 years, has positive symptoms even when in treatment. His conversation consisting of stories about his life at the time his family took him to the state mental hospital, his hospital stay, and his thoughts about mental illness is difficult to listen to without interrupting. One thought merges into another and the listener becomes unable to follow the story, but can hear the anger with which he expresses it. Mark recalls that he smoked marijuana and used other substances which made it difficult to study at the community college he attended. He mutters phrases about illegal drugs he took that made him crazy. He rambles as his continues to tell his story about working part-time to put himself through school, the motorcyclists cruising through the gas station where he worked to taunt him for being different. He says he became addicted to recreational drugs and alcohol, and addiction caused his schizophrenia. After one aggressive outburst, his mother took him to the hospital because she was afraid for his life. Once in the hospital acute admissions unit, the enforced security and limitations in his freedom made him feel like he was in "a Nazi prison camp" and was going to be tortured. Over the years of multiple hospitalizations, he believes his progress has been because of his caring mother and an effective psychiatrist who remained supportive of him over a long period of time.

Negative Symptoms

While Mark has the rambling speech, **tangential thinking**, and delusional ideas of positive symptoms, Tim, age 35 years, has the brief conversation, concrete thinking, social withdrawal, and reduced facial expression of someone with negative symptoms. Though he has been on medication treatment for several years, he still has blunt affect. Tim does not initiate or continue conversation without prompting. With periodic prompting, Mike relates how successful he felt when playing high school football. Tim is married to a woman with bipolar disorder who has helped him interact with friends, take pride in his part-time work at a maintenance job, and take care of his hygiene, grooming, and nutrition. With the help of medication and support, Tim manages to conquer his anhedonia to participate in weightlifting and tossing a football with a friend, activities he enjoyed before his illness. He now initiates activities instead of remaining passive, a symptom referred to as avolition. He no longer withdraws and becomes socially isolated from family and friends.

Insight

The lack of insight into their own behavior is one symptom Mark and Tim continue to have, though their symptoms have improved because of treatment. Both men learn best through concrete experiences of trial and error, but even with specific feedback they lack insight into the meaning of behaviors.

Before and even after treatment neither one wanted to take medication. They saw little relationship between medication and other treatments and their behaviors. They did not understand the reasons why the disruptive behavior or the withdrawal behavior occurred or that the behaviors were related to their mental illness. They just acted.

Course and Prognosis

The premorbid period of schizophrenia begins during childhood, several years before onset of schizophrenia. Premorbid refers to the period before an illness receives a diagnosis when symptoms are present but are not recognized as an illness (7). The period covers the initial vulnerability as a result of genetic and obstetrical complications up to diagnosis in late adolescence and young adulthood. While siblings may have a common vulnerability, children who later have schizophrenia show several differences from their siblings in lower scores on standardized test of intelligence and achievement, lower grades, less positive emotion, deficits in bilateral manipulation and walking (7). These behaviors are not unique to children who develop schizophrenia by adolescence but are signs of problems in their brain neuronal circuitry.

By adolescence, children who develop schizophrenia show marked adjustment problems of noncompliance in school and home, irritability, and withdrawal. The signs are similar to other mental illnesses. Some teenagers develop psychotic-like symptoms similar to schizophrenia but less severe than full-blown schizophrenia. They may be diagnosed with schizotypal personality disorders at first but later the diagnosis may change to schizophrenia as the symptoms such as unusual beliefs and sensory experiences persist. According to Walker, et al. several studies report the genetic links and transitions from a diagnosis of schizotypal personality disorder to schizophrenia (7). Children may have limited emotional expression in social interaction and prefer to be alone. They show little enjoyment in activities, are isolated and indifferent to others (2). Parents hesitate to have their children diagnosed with a mental illness in general and specifically with schizophrenia because of the stigma mental illness carries in the United States. However diagnosis leads to specific intervention to prevent continuing developmental interruptions, functional decline, and death from suicide.

Suicide is the leading cause of death among individuals with schizophrenia (20). One in 10 patients who have schizophrenia commits suicide. The highly personal themes in auditory hallucinations and delusions can provoke attempts at suicide. Patients hear voices telling them to take dangerous actions and calling them names until patients try to carry out the orders from the voices or try to harm themselves to get rid of the voices. Suicidal behavior also is the result of disordered thinking including cognitive deficits such as lack of insight. Altogether, symptoms create powerful disturbances in the daily lives of individuals who have schizophrenia and even though psychiatric and rehabilitation programs can improve their lives, symptoms often continue to create a rocky course to recovery.

Once diagnosed, the individual course of schizophrenia varies by the degree of symptoms, medical and environmental stability, and willingness to accept the illness and treatment. The idea of relapse is important in describing the course of schizophrenia over time. Patients may have long periods of having reduced symptoms and increased function. Then symptoms and dysfunctional behavior reappear leading to hospitalization. This process of illness, function, and return of illness describes a relapse.

Weiden et al. (21) divided patients into three groups to describe the course of schizophrenia—mild, moderate, and severe.

Some patients have a mild course which follows a pattern of mild symptoms, few if any relapses, and full compliance with treatment. Other patients have a moderate course with moderate symptoms, several relapses by middle, and partial compliance with treatment regimens. A severe course of schizophrenia often is complicated by medical illness in addition to schizophrenia. The symptoms and relapses of a severe course of illness interfere with activities of daily living that require cognition such as money management and cooking. Symptoms persist and increase during stress. Major relapses dominate the period through middle age, often because of problems coming from new symptoms, ineffectiveness of past medications to control symptoms, and patient refusal to continue on medications and other treatment regimens. Patients who have a severe course of schizophrenia are described as seriously and persistently mentally ill.

The American Psychiatric Association also describes the course of mental illnesses including schizophrenia in their diagnostic manual (22). Even though the patients may meet the full diagnostic criteria at the onset of illness, with re-admissions to treatment settings, the admitting psychiatrist may see a different pattern of symptoms. The course of schizophrenia is one of repeated episodes with varying symptoms. If during a relapse, the patient does not show full criteria for the illness, then the patient is in one of the following periods:

- In partial remission; patient met full criteria in the past, but only has some of the symptoms in the current admission.
- In full remission; patient does not have the symptoms or signs of schizophrenia because of medication and other treatments. The diagnosis of schizophrenia remains important to the patient's care.
- Prior history; no current signs or symptoms; no current disorder, but the diagnostic label may be important to the patient's future.

Prognosis depends on how soon and if patients can return to typical lives, meaning living independently and keeping a job. About 20% to 30% of individuals can live and work in the community, 20% to 30% have moderate and persistent symptoms; and more than half have significant disability throughout life (7). Factors associated with a poor course of schizophrenia also include male gender, gradual onset, early age of onset, poor functioning before onset of the disorder, family history of schizophrenia, and presence of other conditions such as substance abuse (7).

Many Americans depend on their jobs for health and retirement benefits. Schizophrenia prevents access to these benefits for those who have significant disabilities. Schizophrenia is one of the top ten causes of disability worldwide (23). Patients become dependent on family income and benefits, as well as state and federal disability income for routine physical and dental examinations and treatment. Since not all physicians and dentists are willing to accept patients who have disability benefits from governmental systems, families must search for care. If the individual lives alone without family members in the area, the problems become more severe without support.

Patients can recover from schizophrenia but most will need to remain on medication. Recovery means a return of performance in occupations. Performance in social activities in the community may be the greatest challenge in recovery because effective social relationships require perception and cognition. Several factors are keys to recovery. Early diagnosis and treatment reduce the permanent disability from the effects of cognitive deficits on education, social relationships and work, and improve function. Patients have shorter time-outs from the community during treatment because of fewer hospitalizations. Supportive families and friends make early diagnosis possible but beyond diagnosis, families may have limited access to quality care in areas where they live. Illegal substance use reduces recovery but prescribed use of treatment medications helps recovery. To recover, patients must follow the advice and prescriptions of their doctors just like in medical illnesses. In the United States, 50% of individuals who have chronic conditions do not take their medications (24). Support from family, physicians, teachers, friends, and therapists can help an individual recover from schizophrenia.

Medical Management

Diagnosis

In all medical research and treatment, standard categories improve the consistency of diagnosis. The American Psychiatric Association manual for standard diagnoses is the resource in the United States (22). The current edition, called the *DSM IV-TR* is a transitional edition between editions four and five. The *DSM* criterion A includes several characteristic, observable symptoms: delusions, hallucinations, disorganized speech, atypical or disorganized behavior, and negative symptoms (22). If a patient has delusions and auditory hallucinations, the individual fits into the paranoid subtype of schizophrenia. However, if the same patient also has a depressed mood, the diagnosis of paranoid schizophrenia no longer applies. Because of variety in presenting symptoms in schizophrenia, diagnosis using inclusion and exclusion criteria is a challenge. Patients may have symptoms of more than one subtype or may not neatly fit into one subtype, or their symptoms may overlap with other mental illnesses. Schizophrenia has five subtypes: paranoid, disorganized, catatonia, undifferentiated, and residual (22).

- Paranoid: Includes persistent delusions or auditory hallucinations. Excludes disorganized speech and behavior, flat affect, inappropriate affect.
- Disorganized: Includes disorganized speech and behavior, flat or inappropriate affect. Excludes catatonic signs and symptoms.
- Catatonic: Includes the signs and symptoms of: physical immobility, unusual postures.
- May show aimless wandering and agitation, repetitive movements, grimacing. Includes lack of awareness of the immediate environment; lack of reaction to stimulation; negativism and mutism.
- Undifferentiated: Meets Criterion A for Schizophrenia; does not meet the above criteria for a specific type.
- Residual: Includes continued negative symptoms, or two or more symptoms in Criterion A. May include odd beliefs, unusual perceptual experiences.

The psychiatrist like other medical specialists pays attention to differential diagnosis by comparing the observed symptoms with diagnostic criteria of schizophrenia with medical and psychiatric diagnoses that might have overlapping symptoms. During diagnosis, the psychiatrist analyzes the patient symptoms including the psychological, social, and mental characteristics; physical, social and cultural environment; and the overall function of the patient in the past and present. The DSM system organizes the client clinical picture along five Axes (22).

- Axis I—clinical disorders, such as schizophrenia and major depression.
- Axis II—personality disorders, such as personal make-up and behaviors such as emotional expression, social interaction, and beliefs that are longstanding and very different from the culture. Mental retardation, such as below average intellectual performance as measured by a standardized test.
- Axis III—mental disorders directly a result of general medical conditions such as

cerebrovascular accident (stroke), and Parkinson's disease (see Index).

- Axis IV—prominent psychosocial and environmental disorders such as family, work, and financial problems in the patient's life.
- Axis V—global assessment of functioning (GAF). On a scale of 1 (lowest) to 100 (highest) the psychiatrist reports the patient's function in work, leisure, social participation, and activities of daily living.

The GAF has 10 levels of function, one level for every 10 points. From 1 to 100 the categories move from many symptoms and low function to decreasing symptoms and increasing function. The lowest category from 1 to 10 includes the psychiatric definition of mental illness: danger to self or others, or the inability to meet the basic requirements of self care.

A patient who has schizophrenia may have a diagnostic assessment of:

Axis I: Schizophrenia, paranoid, chronic with acute worsening of symptoms.
Axis II: No diagnosis.
Axis III: Mild blockage in right carotid artery.
Axis IV: Lack of psychosocial support; serious mental illness.
Axis V: GAF-20. Some danger of hurting self or others, occasionally fails to maintain minimum hygiene, and gross impairment in communication (class experience, Y. Teske, 2004).

Assessment

Regardless of patient psychiatric symptoms, psychiatrists use two important psychiatric assessment methods, the history interview and the mental status examination (MSE) (25). The standard procedures help psychiatrists differentiate among the various mental illness diagnoses. All psychiatrists receive training and certification to use the two procedures. Because both assessments are unstructured interviews, psychiatrists must be skilled observers and interpreters of patients' verbal and physical behavior.

The psychiatric history interview moves from open questions to specific closed questions to gather detailed information about medical and psychiatric history, family health history, social history, and occupations such as education and work.

The MSE assesses appearance, mood such as happy or sad, affect as seen on the face, communication, rate and volume of speech, thought processes like problem solving and the subject matter of thoughts and speech. One method psychiatrists use to assess thought processes and speech is to ask a patient to interpret a saying such as "a rolling stone gathers no moss." Patients with schizophrenia may interpret the saying concretely: moss won't stick to a rolling stone; the moss will rub right off. Another person who is able to think abstractly will have a philosophical interpretation. Through the interview and MSE, psychiatrists determine if the patient is mentally ill, if the patient is suicidal or homicidal, and if the patient is oriented to time, place and date, spatial relationships, and other cognitive processes. Psychiatrists may use other tests in assessment and throughout treatment to determine patient status and progress.

After collecting information from assessment, the psychiatrist reviews patient data to determine the mental illness and the best least-restrictive, treatment setting to meet patient needs. In actual situations the legal system, health care system, and family may be involved before a psychiatrist sees the potential patient. A psychiatric evaluation may occur in a judicial center office, emergency room, mental health agency, or jail. Law enforcement officers, officers of the court such as judges or magistrates and mental health agency staff members, and family members all may be involved with an individual before psychiatric evaluation. If the individual is acutely ill, a complete psychiatrist evaluation is delayed until the individual is in a safe setting and is coherent (25,26).

The legal system with input from mental health professionals determines the setting for care. The laws defining mental illness, criteria for hospital admission and commitment for care differ among states. If an individual who has schizophrenia meets the criteria for mental illness, hospitalization occurs. At this point the psychiatrist can begin the diagnostic process and prescribe medication to reduce stress, agitation, and aggression the patient may be experiencing.

An individual who has the signs and symptoms of schizophrenia may not require hospitalization but hospitalization is likely. The process of complete diagnosis and stabilization on medications usually occurs in a hospital setting for individuals with schizophrenia.

By law, patient rights must be closely protected. The right to confidentiality refers to the privacy of medical records, including diagnosis, results of tests and treatment. Patients cannot be photographed. In many mental hospital settings, patients are considered too ill to understand the implications of giving their consent to release information. Another patient right is protected by a United States Supreme Court ruling. That is, patients must be treated and discharged to the least-restrictive environment possible considering their diagnoses (26). For example, parents who have been coping with the increasing agitation and decreasing self-care of their 18-year-old son, will not be asked to take part in the psychiatric evaluation. The judge or psychiatrist may ask the parents for information in a separate session but the ill son may have to give permission for the parents to give information and learn the results of the psychiatric evaluation.

To protect patient rights, federal and state laws dictate the procedures for psychiatric admissions to hospitals. States differ in definitions of mental illness, requirements for admission, and assessment (27). Patients can voluntarily admit themselves to a hospital but many admissions for schizophrenia are involuntary.

- Informal voluntary—patients enter the hospital under their own free will and may leave at any time, even against medical advice of the psychiatrist. Patients who are considered dangerous to themselves or others would not be admitted under this category.
- Formal voluntary—patients can be admitted but cannot leave against medical advice. Patients can request discharge in writing.
- Involuntary—patients are admitted against their will based on the results of psychiatric evaluations by two different psychiatrists. Both independent evaluations must recommend hospitalization for reasons of safety and disability. Patients can make a written request for case review of the legal procedures leading up to hospitalization. If possible, patients give consent to treatment medications and methods. When patients are unable to understand and consent, other individuals such as family members, or the court become guardians to give consent (25).

Once in a hospital, the psychiatrist and other team members administer additional assessments to help the psychiatrist make an accurate diagnosis. Assessments such as psychological testing to identify specific cognitive deficits, family evaluation by case managers, as well as, functional and cognitive evaluations by occupational therapists and recreational therapists assist in diagnosis, goal setting and treatment. The psychiatrist orders laboratory tests to rule out physiological causes of symptoms and to serve as a baseline before using medications as treatment: blood cell counts, urinalysis, drug screens, thyroid-stimulating-hormone levels are examples. The psychiatric evaluation may indicate the need for magnetic resonance imaging (MRI) or other imaging diagnostic tools (25).

Pharmacologic Management

Advances in medications in the form of drugs to reduce symptoms revolutionized psychiatric treatment for all mental illnesses but especially for schizophrenia. Before medications, patients were institutionalized for long periods of time with little or no contact with family members and community residents. Lack of familiarity with schizophrenia and other serious mental illnesses created feelings of fear and distrust in community members still seen today. Stigma remains a barrier to good treatment. Residents of a community did not learn about schizophrenia because patients did not live at home for any length of time. Procedures such as physical restraints and seclusion in isolation rooms of hospitals seemed inhumane but patients, family and staff members were trying to reduce agitation, aggression, self-injury, and injury to others. Medications helped individuals with schizophrenia be able to function in the community and in some cases to recover from the brain disorder.

Antipsychotic medications are not a cure but do reduce the positive and negative symptoms. Prescribing, observing, and measuring responses to medications is an art and science. Many guidelines for medication treatment are available for psychiatrists because of the complexities involved. Several studies about the effectiveness of specific drugs on positive and negative symptoms and disordered thinking show long-term, helpful results (28).

Medications for schizophrenia, called antipsychotic medications or drugs, are the first choice of treatment for the symptoms of schizophrenia. Drugs come in several forms depending on the specific medication. About 20% of patients receive more than one antipsychotic medication at a time over a long period of time (29). Because antipsychotic drugs are metabolized by many routes in the brain, drug interactions are of less concern than other types of medications. However, drug interaction studies are few. Once an individual begins medication in treatment, the medication must be taken continuously. Most individuals who have schizophrenia take antipsychotic medication for the rest of their lives. Medications require a period of 4 to 6 weeks to reduce symptoms and stabilize behavior. If the individual does not show the intended response, the psychiatrist will change the medications in about 8 to 12 weeks (18).

All drugs used in the treatment of schizophrenia have side effects. In order to effect change in nerve synapses in the brain to alter brain function in cognition, drugs must be specific, safe, yet powerful. The problems in schizophrenia result from neuronal circuits linking several brain structures which regulate many areas of function. The complex tasks of matching drug action, brain structure and function, and desired treatment results make side effects seem inevitable. A rapidly developing field in pharmacy called pharmacogenomics addresses the science needed to match an individual's genetic code with specific drugs for treatment (30). The brain disorder of schizophrenia shows great variability in individual symptoms, course, and prognosis. Pharmacogenomics will address the problems of side effects and lack of response to medications (29). Until psychiatrists can scientifically make the match between individual symptoms and drugs, consider that the progress to develop antipsychotic drugs is a remarkable scientific discovery.

The first medications developed for treatment of schizophrenia are still used today and are called conventional neuroleptic agents. The term neuroleptic refers to medications that influence neurotransmitters especially dopamine. Pacing, agitation and aggression, and frenetic energy interfere with function for those who have schizophrenia. The excessive production of dopamine stimulates motor symptoms caused by the brain disorder in schizophrenia. Conventional neuroleptic drugs limit the excess production of dopamine and are known as dopamine antagonists because the

Table 5.1 ATYPICAL AND CONVENTIONAL ANTIPSYCHOTIC MEDICATIONS

Medications	Dose in Milligrams/Day	Dose Frequency	Dose Forms	Side Effects
First-Line Atypicals	Start @ 25–30	BID (2x/day)	Tablet	Moderate hypotension, sedation, weight gain.
Quetiapine fumarate	300–800	QD (4x/day)	Tablet	Mild anticholinergic effects and hypotension.
Olanzapine	Start @ 5–10	QD	Disintegrating tablet	Moderate sedation.
Risperidone	15–30	BID	Tablet	Marked weight gain.
Ziprasidone HCL	Start @ 2	QD-BID	Concentrate	Mild sedation.
	2–6	bid-tid (3x/day)	Tablet	Moderate hypotension and weight gain.
	Start @ 40	BID-TID	Tablet	
	80–160	BID		
Other Atypicals	Start @ 25–50	BID	Tablet	Mild hypotension, sedation, and weight gain.
Clozapine	300–600	BID	Concentrate,	
Conventional Low-potency	Start@ 100–200	QID	Injection, suppository	Marked hypotension, sedation and weight gain.
Chlorpromazine	100–600		Tablet,	Moderate EPS and anticholinergic effects.
Thioridazine	Start@ 50–200		Concentrate	
	100–600			
Conventional High-potency	Start @ 2–5		Tablet	Marked hypotension, sedation, and weight gain.
Fluphenazine	2–20		Concentration	Moderate EPS and weight gain.
Haloperidol	Start @ 5–10		Injection	Marked anticholinergic effects, hypotension, and sedation.
Thiothixene	5–20		Depot	Mild sedation, hypotension and weight gain.
Trifluoperazine HCL	Start @5–10		Same as above	Marked EPS
	5–30		Tablet	Same as above.
	Start @ 5–10		Concentration	Same as above.
	5–30		Injection	Same as above.
			Same as above	

References, categories based on effects clinically and functionally.

drugs resist dopamine release. Some conventional medications affect other neurotransmitters (31).

Table 5.1 shows the three groups of antipsychotic medications, first-line atypical antipsychotics, low-potency conventional neuroleptic agents, and high-potency conventional neuroleptic agents (30,31).

Since medications must be taken once or twice a day over long periods of years, the form of the medication such as a tablet or a liquid becomes important to patient treatment.

Some patients prefer to take disintegrating tablets or liquids because they do not like to swallow whole tablets. Other patients require injections because they refuse or are unable to take their medications on schedule. Medication treatment becomes even more complicated because of the cognitive deficits in schizophrenia. Patients can fill a glass of water and then lose track of the intent to take a pill. In community houses for individuals on antipsychotic medications, staff members, often nurses or nurse's aides, administer medications on schedule. Independent community function is limited when individuals must depend on others to give medication. Conventional antipsychotics also come in tablets, concentrated liquids, injections suppositories, and depot forms. Depot forms are dosages injected periodically such as monthly instead of daily dosages with the purpose of improving compliance with medication management (personal communication, MA Kirkpatrick, January 14, 2005).

Medications of any kind, even aspirin, may cause side effects and antipsychotic medications are no exception. Side effects of these medications include sedation, sexual dysfunction, weight gain, cardiovascular, and anticholinergic effects. Sedation makes people look and feel sleepy. Families complain about sedative effects because they cannot rouse their family member off from the couch or bed. The family member seems to sleep life away. Individuals may lose their interest in sexual relationships and may be impotent. Sexual side effects cause serious concern in patients because they want close relationships and families. Weight gain from medication affects body image and health, and the extra pounds are a challenge to lose. A tightly monitored program of healthy eating and exercise may have little effect when body metabolism is altered by medication. Cardiovascular side effects include heart arrhythmias and other problems (30,31).

The term anticholinergic refers to the parasympathetic division of the autonomic nervous system. The parasympathetic nervous system regulates the craniosacral portion of the central nervous system (CNS), which in turn regulates near vision in the eyes, tears, dilation of blood vessels in the brain, narrowing of coronary arteries, narrowing of the bronchi, stomach function, liver function, secretions in the pancreas, bladder function, and blood vessels in sex organs (5). Medications with anticholinergic side effects interfere with the craniosacral functions just mentioned. To reduce some of the anticholinergic side effects, psychiatrists prescribe anti–side-effect medications and help their patients feel more comfortable on the antipsychotic medications.

The three groups of antipsychotic medications differ in their side effects. Atypical first-line antipsychotics have fewer side effects than conventional neuroleptic antipsychotics (31). The latter have more severe extrapyramidal side effects (EPS). The term extrapyramidal refers to the areas of the brain involved in motor activity such as posture and movement. The extrapyramidal system includes the corpus striatum, subthalamic nucleus, substantia nigra, and red nucleus and their connections with the reticular formation, cerebellum and cerebrum (32). Because of the interconnections among the areas of the brain, side effects on the extrapyramidal system cause great discomfort and disability in patients. Patients stop taking their medications, become noncompliant with medications, and the symptoms of schizophrenia return.

Side effects include akathisia, bradykinesia, overall physical stiffness, **cogwheel rigidity** and the most serious of all, tardive dyskinesia. Akathisia is motor restlessness and anxiety. Patients are unable to stand, sit, or lie quietly for any sustained period of time. Therapists may mistake akathisia for a short attention span in patients because they are unable to sit and perform an activity without breaks to stand up and pace. The inattention may be because of a motor side effect of medications as well as the cognitive deficit in attention (2). Bradykinesia, stiffness, and cogwheel rigidity slow down spontaneous movement. Bradykinesia is atypically slow movement and slow thought processes (2). Speech may be slow and labored also. Patients who have bradykinesia look, think, and speak like their bodies are moving through thick syrup. They respond slowly to comments and to directions to move from one space to another. Therapists must speak slowly and patiently wait for patients' responses. Physical stiffness looks different from bradykinesia. Stiffness is when patients have limited movement instead of slow movement. Their bodies appear inflexible and rigid. Some patients have cogwheel rigidity. To visualize cogwheel rigidity, imagine a joint such as an elbow being a hinge with teeth. If a therapist tried to move the relaxed forearm in one direction, the forearm would move stiffly, tooth by tooth.

While the side effect of slowed voluntary movement limits quick spontaneous movement, tardive dyskinesia (TD) causes constant involuntary movements (33). Patients are aware of the uncontrollable movements of the mouth, lips, and tongue, trunk, arms, or legs. The atypical movements seen in TD attract attention because they look strange and unappealing. The movements interfere with the motor performance required to button and zip clothing, eat with utensils, brush teeth, write and sign checks, for example. The effects of the movements on performance in activities of daily living and social participation in the community can disturb patients enough for them to refuse to take medications. Refusal to take medications as prescribed is called noncompliance.

Some patients and families worry about addiction to antipsychotic drugs; however the drugs are neither habit-forming nor mind-altering (21). The purposes and actions of the drugs are symptom and deficit reduction. Patients must take the medications on a regular and prescribed management schedule. Some patients in response to unusual demands in their schedule will skip a dose or two. For example, the sedative effects of some drugs will cause sleepiness during long nighttime drives and patients will go without medications just before and during the drives. It is better to avoid the situations that lead to skipped doses than create circumstances in the CNS leading to return of symptoms, change in mood, and relapse. Both the family and the individual may be unaware of or unable to accept the limitations of schizophrenia. They may expect a full return of function with medications but the expectation is unrealistic.

Family Role in Treatment

When families become involved in treatment, relapse, noncompliance, and rehospitalization rates significantly go down (34). Yet, only 9.6% of families receive education, problem-solving training, crisis intervention training, and support (34). Access to family education and training is uneven across the United States because of differences in state funding for mental health services. Despite the positive support families provide, some families refuse to participate with their family member in treatment. Family refusals can be a result of fear, confusion, and the stigma associated with schizophrenia. In the past, families were blamed for the mental illnesses of their children (35). Recommendations from a large national study, included family intervention for a minimum of 9 months (35). Schizophrenia is not caused by dysfunctional families but can be helped by family support and education. Psychiatrists, psychologists, social workers and other team members, as well as national family and consumer organizations such as the National Alliance for Mental Illness (NAMI), can offer information about diagnosis and treatment, and provide family members with the tools they need to help their child over the course of schizophrenia. Family members become educators of other families and advocates for supportive legislation through organizations like NAMI.

Psychotherapy

Once medications manage patient symptoms, psychotherapy offers support through approaches such as empathy, feedback about thoughts, perceptions, and behavior with the goal of self-understanding. Availability of a psychiatrist, psychologist, or other psychotherapist through office appointments and telephone contact can help individuals cope with real-world challenges most people experience and challenges unique to schizophrenia.

Assertive Community Treatment and Rehabilitation

Assertive community treatment is a program to help individuals who have serious and persistent mental illness remain in the community by providing support and problem-solving 24 hours a day, 7 days a week. The assertive community treatment teams, which may include occupational therapists, focus on changing the environment to help participation and/or on helping individuals compensate for their deficits in performance (36).

Therapy, training, and education occur in rehabilitation programs in in-patient, outpatient, and community mental health programs for patients who have mental illness. Therapy programs conducted by psychologists, art, occupational, and recreational therapists aim to remediate client factors such as cognition and social deficits as well as motor, process, communication, and social interaction skills. One of the real challenges in rehabilitation is to help patients discover their volition in terms of personal causation, goal-directed behavior, meaningful values, and interests for occupational engagement in daily life (37).

Given the cognitive deficits in schizophrenia, life-skills training, such as money management, meal preparation, and transportation, can produce positive results when done in the natural environment where activities occur. In the hospital clinic kitchen, for example, the patient may be trained to make and serve a meal to a small group of five individuals and when discharged the patient may be on a once-a-month rotation to prepare a meal for 8 to 10 other residents.

Impact of Schizophrenia on Client Factors

Schizophrenia can affect both body functions and structures. The following information is a guide to effects of the brain disorder on the body but because the clinical picture of schizophrenia varies widely, the information is a guide only.

Body Function Categories

Mental Functions. Because of the cognitive deficits, positive and negative symptoms, and disordered thinking, schizophrenia affects both global and specific mental functions. Medication side effects also affect mental functions. Examples of affected client factors in mental functions are:

- Consciousness (low or hyperarousal)
- Orientation (confusion because of psychosis)
- Sleep (excessive or diminished sleep, sleep disturbances because of hallucinations.)
- Temperament and personality (emotional instability)
- Energy and drive (anhedonia, impulsivity)
- Attention (interrupted by sensory gating, cognitive deficits, and psychosis)
- Memory (cognitive deficits, psychosis)
- Perception (hallucinations, cognitive and sensory-gating deficits, eye-hand incoordination because of perceptual deficits)
- Thought (delusions, tangential thinking, flight of ideas, and other disordered thought processes)

- Higher level cognitive functions such as judgment, sense of time, and abstract thinking.
- Language (effectiveness of language reduced by idiosyncratic speech patterns and use of words)
- Calculation (arithmetic skills may be intact)
- Sequencing movement (goal-directed or contextual movement affected because the goal itself is lost)
- Psychomotor (agitation and EPS)
- Emotional (blunt or flat affect)
- Experience of self and time (reduced self understand and identity)

Other body functions can be affected by schizophrenia but the problems lie in the brain disorders.

- Sensory—irregular eye movements and reduced awareness of body position in space in sensory functions
- Speech—reduced rate and amount of speech
- Cardiac, circulatory, immune and respiratory functions—medication effects
- Digestive, metabolic, endocrine, genitourinary and reproductive functions—diabetes
- Neuromusculosketal and movement-related functions—vary with the type of schizophrenia and medications. Catatonic schizophrenia has the most obvious muscle and movement dysfunction mostly seen in the atypical postures and lack of movement. They show strong muscular resistance and increased muscle tone; atypical psychomotor activity such as pacing and agitation; extrapyramidal side effects from medications such as involuntary movements in mouth and lips
- Skin and Related Structures—medications can cause burns and irritation with exposure to sunlight

Body Structure Categories

Structure of the Nervous System (reduced size and volume of some areas in the brain in some individuals).

CASE STUDY

Case Illustrations

■ CASE 1

B. is a man with a psychiatric diagnosis of paranoid schizophrenia. His diagnosis which occurred over 32 years ago while he was in military service, led to many psychiatric hospitalizations; some of the hospitalizations lasted for months. From age 21 to 42, he was in and out of hospitals. Then, for a period of 9 years, he remained at home with his parents with no hospitalizations, until the events of September 11, 2001. He reported, "I watched the news day and night for three days and became very upset. I realized America was no longer safe" (personal communication, March 2004, J. Fraker).

Many Americans watched the news of 9/11 on television and came to the same conclusions about the country's safety, but for B., the events began a 3-month period of insomnia, agitation, aggression, and auditory hallucinations, which led to hospitalization.

B. has chronic and persistent schizophrenia and also signs of a mood disorder (Chapter 6). When B. loses close relationships, he withdraws and isolates himself. One such period occurred after a broken engagement when he remained in his room for 8 months, only coming out to eat and use the bathroom. B. was hospitalized after the death of his father and the illness of his mother. At other times, he becomes energized, hyperactive, and manic. During manic periods in the past, he went on spending sprees and showed other excessive behaviors.

At first, B. took his medications for mental illness but over time he blamed visual and other health problems on his antipsychotic medications. As his medication began to control symptoms of psychosis, he stopped taking his medications. Medication noncompliance led to some of his rehospitalizations.

B. requires hospitalization when he becomes agitated, aggressive, suicidal, and homicidal. His intrusive auditory hallucinations cause him to think about committing suicide or killing someone. For example, he heard voices coming from the walls and television set telling him he was in danger from someone coming after him. B. said that the voices cause "tension in his head" (case report). In the hospital, the voices told him that the hospital staff members were going to kill him and in response he carried a Bible around to have his last rites read to him. The voices often occur at night and lead to insomnia which can last for several weeks. Insomnia increases his restlessness and agitation. To calm himself down and escape the voices, he takes long night-time drives, causing his family great concern. B. also tries to remove the voices by inducing pain from banging his body against the wall and other self-injurious actions. The cycle of disturbing voices, agitation, insomnia, and injury affect his ability to function.

Neither parent had a family history of mental illness. However, a younger brother had a psychiatric hospitalization following a divorce. When B was 30 years old, he was married for a period of 3 years. After his divorce, he moved back home where he lives with his mother and spends most of his time in his room. He has remained unemployed throughout his long period of illness, but does receive $2000 in a monthly disability check from the government.

Psychiatrists have changed medications for B. many times since his first psychiatric hospitalization. From his first admission to the present, medications include perphenazine, thiothixene, lithium to manage the mood disorder symptoms, clonazepam (Klonopin), olanzapine (Zyprexa), ziprasidone, and clozapine in addition to medications for high cholesterol, aspirin, and sedatives to aid sleep. Typically, he takes several medications, some twice a day and others less frequently.

Currently, B. attends weekly occupational therapy in a day treatment program at the Veterans Administration Hospital (VA) 1 hour from his home. His occupational therapist and psychiatrist are concerned about his safe driving, given possible visual and cognitive deficits, and medications. In occupational therapy, B. enjoys the educational and current events sessions in the program and especially enjoys the history of United States presidents. He participates with others in structured games like poker and reminiscing about the past. B. talks about learning to play the guitar and playing with his nephews in a grandfather role. The occupational therapist and psychiatrist want B. to remain stable without the symptoms of psychosis returning.

The occupational life for B. has been reduced by mental illness. While he independently performs activities of daily living, he shows limited experiences in the more cognitively complex instrumental activities of daily living. Driving is his primary activity and now that bit of independence may end. He has not successfully fulfilled the typical roles and occupations of adults: career education, uninterrupted employment, sustained relationships beyond his immediate family, and creating his own family. When first diagnosed at age 21 years, the atypical medications for schizophrenia were not available. Newer medications might have prevented hospitalizations and long absences from community life.

Today, individuals who have schizophrenia have brighter futures than they had in the past. Mark, mentioned earlier in this chapter, after 20 years of repeated hospitalizations, returned to community life, bought a car, and just graduated with a bachelor of psychology degree.

Acknowledgment

The author thanks Joyce Fraker, MS, OTR, for providing this case with her remarks on treatment.

References

1. Harvey PD, Walker EF, eds. Positive and Negative Symptoms of Psychosis: Description, Research, and Future Directions. Hillsdale, NJ: Erlbaum, 1987.
2. Sadock BJ, Sadock VA, eds. Kaplan and Sadock's Comprehensive Textbook of Psychiatry. Baltimore, MD: Williams & Wilkins, 2000.
3. Kennedy JL, Farrer LF, Andreason NC, et al. The genetics of adult-onset neuropsychiatric disease: complexities and conundra? Science 2003;302: 822–826.
4. National Institute of Mental Health. Mental illness genetics among Science's top "breakthroughs" for 2003. December 22, 2003. Available at: http://www.nimh.nih.gov/events/runnersup.cfm. Accessed on March 18, 2004.
5. Purves, WK, Sadava D, Orians GH, et al. Life: The Science of Biology. 6th Ed. Sunderland, MA: Sinauer Associates, 2001.
6. Green MF. Schizophrenia Revealed. New York: W.W. Norton & Company, 2001.
7. Walker E, Kestler L, Bollini A, et al. Schizophrenia: etiology and course. Ann Rev Psych 2004;55:401–30.
8. Holden C. Deconstructing schizophrenia. Science 2003;299:333–335.
9. Bowie CR, Harvey PD, Moriatry PJ, et al. A comprehensive analysis of verbal fluency deficit in geriatric schizophrenia. Arch Clin Neuropsychol 2004;19:289–303.
10. Pantelis C, Velakoulis D, McGorry PD, et al. Neuroanatomical abnormalities before and after onset of psychosis a cross-sectional and longitudinal MRI comparison. Lancet 2003;361:281–288.
11. Schmajuk NA. Hippocampal dysfunction in schizophrenia. Hippocampus 2001;11:599–613.
12. Pralong E, Magistretti P, Stoop R. Cellular perspectives on the glutamate-monamine interaction in limbic lobe structures and their relevance for some psychiatric disorders. Prog Neurobiol 2002;67: 173–202.
13. Jentsch JD, Roth RH, Taylor JR. Role for dopamine in the behavioral functions of the prefrontal corticostriatal system: implications for mental disorders and psychotropic drug action. Prog Brain Res 2000;126:433–453.
14. Cannon TD, Rosso IM, Hollister JM, et al. A prospective cohort study of genetic and perinatal influences in schizophrenia. Schizophr Bull 2000;23:351–366.
15. Torrey EF, Miller J, Rawlings R, et al. Seasonality of births in schizophrenia and bipolar disorder: a review of the literature. Schizophr Res 1997;28:1–38.
16. Narrow WE. One-year prevalence of mental disorders, excluding substance use disorders, in the U.S.: NIMH ECA prospective data. Population estimates based on U.S. census estimated residential population age 18 and over on July 1 1998. Unpublished.
17. Evans DL, Cooper KB, Kincannon CL. Statistical abstract of the United States, 123rd ed. Washington, DC: Department of Commerce, 2003.
18. Satcher D, Shalala D. Schizophrenia. Mental health: a report of the Surgeon General, Chapter 4: adults and mental health. December 3, 1999, 1–14. Available at: http://www.surgeongeneral.gov/library/mentalhealth/chapter4/sec4.html. Accessed on January 3, 2005.
19. National Institute of Mental Health. When someone has schizophrenia. 2001:1–4. Available at: http://www.nimh.gov/publicat/schizsoms.cfm. Accessed December 29, 2004.
20. Schwartz RC, Cohen BN. Risk factors for suicidality among clients with schizophrenia. J Counsel Dev 2001;79:314–319.
21. Weiden PJ, Scheifler PL, NcEvoy JP, et al. Expert consensus treatment guidelines for schizophrenia: a guide for patients and families. J Clin Psychiatr 1999:60(supplement 11) 95–100.
22. American Psychiatric Association. Quick Reference to the Diagnostic Criteria from DSM IV-TR. Arlington, VA: American Psychiatric Association, 2000.

23. World Health Organization. The World health report 2001—mental health: new understanding, new hope. Geneva: World Health Organization, 2001.
24. Mishori R. Common problem: skipping doses. Washington Post, Tuesday, February 8, 2005:F5.
25. Brannon GE. History and mental status examination. April 2, 2002: 1–20. Available at: http://www.emedicine.com/med/topic3358.htm. Accessed January 8, 2005.
26. Kelly TA. Policymaker's guide to mental illness. March 7, 2002:1–23. Available at: http://www.heritage.org/Research/HealthCare/BG1522.cfm. Accessed January 2, 2005.
27. Peck MC, Scheffler RM. An analysis of the definitions of mental illness used in state parity laws. Psychiatric Services September 2002; 53:1089–1095. Arlington VA: American Psychiatric Association. Available at: http://ps.pschiatryonline.org/cgi/content/full/53/9/1089. Accessed January 2, 2005.
28. Dossenbach M, Erol A, Kessaci MM, et al. Effectiveness of antipsychotic treatments for schizophrenia: interim 6-month analysis from a prospective observation study (IC-SOHO) comparing olanzapine, quetiapine, risperidone, and haloperidol. J Clin Psychiatr 2004;65:312–321.
29. Tandon R, Jibson M. Pharmacotherapy of schizophrenia. In: Tandon R, Glick I, Goldman, M et al. Managing Schizophrenia: A Comprehensive Primer. New York: McMahon Publishing Group, 2002.
30. Collins FS. The genome era and mental illness. NAMI Advocate 2003;1:29–31.
31. Jibson MD, Tandon R. An overview of antipsychotic medications. In: Managing Schizophrenia: a Comprehensive Primer. New York: McMahon Publishing Group, 2002.
32. Cohen H. Neuroscience for Rehabilitation. 2nd Ed. Philadelphia: Lippincott, Williams & Wilkins.
33. Casey DE. Pathophsiology of anti-psychotic drug-induced movement disorders. J Clin Psychiatr 2004;65(suppl 9):25–28.
34. Olfson M, Mechanic D, Hansell S, et al. Predicting medication noncompliance after hospital discharge among patients with schizophrenia. Psychiatr Serv 2000;51:216–222.
35. Lehman AF, Steinwachs DM. Translating research into practice: the schizophrenia Patient Outcomes Research Team (PORT) client survey. Schizophr Bull 1998;24:1–10.
36. Bond GR, Drakie RE, Meuser KT, et al. Assertive Community Treatment and people with severe mental illness: critical ingredients and impact on patients. Disability Management of Health Outcomes 2001;9:141–159.
37. Kielhofner G. Model of Human Occupation. Philadelphia: Lippincott, Williams & Wilkins, 2002.

Recommended Learning Resources

National Alliance for Mental Illness
Colonial Place Three, 2107 Wilson Blvd, Suite 300
Arlington, VA 22201–3042
Tel: (703) 524–76000
www.nami.org

The organization aims to help families and consumers of mental health services through support, education, and advocacy. To meet the aim, NAMI provides extensive resources by telephone, web site, and through state and local chapters.
The web site provides contact information for state chapters.

National Alliance for Research on Depression and Mental Illness (NARSAD)
60 Cutler Mill Road, Great Neck, New York 11021
Tel: (516) 829–0091; toll free: (800) 829–8289
www.narsad.org

National Institute for Mental Health (NIMH). Available at: http://www.nih.org/nimh.
National Institutes of Health (NIH) Medline database for published articles on schizophrenia research.

Torrey EF. Surviving schizophrenia: a manual for families, consumers, and providers. New York: Harper Collins Publishing, 2001.

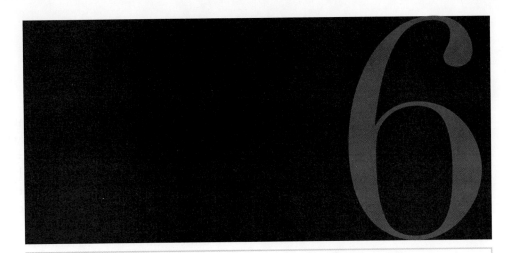

Mood Disorders

Thomas Zelnik and Valerie Howells

Key Terms

Algorithms
Anhedonia
Catatonia
Cyclothymic disorder
Dysthymic disorder
Euthymia
Flight of ideas
Mental disorder
Psychomotor agitation
Psychomotor retardation
Psychosis
Rapid-cycling
Unipolar

"My relationship with depression began long before I noticed it. The first conscious thought that all was not well with me came in 1989, when I was 22. I had been living in Los Angeles for 2 years, working various temporary jobs while trying to establish myself as a writer and performance artist. Out of nowhere and for no apparent reason—or so it seemed—I started feeling strong sensations of grief. I don't remember the step-by-step progression of the illness. What I can recall is that my life disintegrated; first, into a strange cobweb of fatigue. I gradually lost my ability to function. It would take me hours to get out of bed, get bathed, put clothes on. By the time I was fully dressed, it was well into the afternoon. When I went out into the city, I would become disoriented, often spacing out behind the wheel of my car or in the middle of a sentence. My thoughts would just disappear. I'd forget where I was driving to, the point I was about to make in conversation. It was as if my synapses were misfiring, my brain off kilter. . . . After a while I stopped showing up at my temp job, stopped going out altogether, and locked myself in my home. It was three weeks before I felt well enough to leave. During that time, I cut myself off from everything and everyone. Days would go by before I bathed. I did not have enough energy to clean up myself or my home. . . . All I could do was take to my pallet of blankets and coats positioned on the living room floor and wait for whatever I was going through to pass" (1).

Definition

Mood disorders are common, often severe, and sometimes disabling. By definition, this group of **mental disorders is characterized** by a disturbance of mood that is not because of any other physical or mental disorder. The disturbance, generally involving either depression or elation, is prolonged and affects nearly every aspect of daily living. Mood disorders can be effectively treated and managed if appropriately detected and diagnosed. However, many individuals with major depressive disorder (MDD) or bipolar disorder (BPD) may go undiagnosed and untreated or inadequately treated for years. The course of these disorders is often characterized by recurrent episodes of severe mood disturbance separated by periods of normal mood and functioning. It is this recurrent course that paradoxically poses both unique challenges as well as opportunities for persons with mood disorders and for clinicians who work with them. That is, wellness between episodes can reinforce denial and inaction, or it can afford opportunities to better understand those factors that influence future course and prognosis. A comprehensive understanding of biological, psychological, social, and occupational dimensions of recurrent mood disturbances will reward occupational therapists who seek to bring their unique clinical perspectives and therapeutic assistance to patients experiencing MDD and BPD.

Etiology

Feelings of sadness or disappointment, or their opposite, are universal parts of human experience—nearly everyone has experienced feeling down or feeling as if they could accomplish anything no matter the challenges. These feelings are most often associated with identifiable psychological or situational "causes." So basic is this relationship in common human experience that efforts to precisely differentiate between normal and abnormal mood states and their causes have been frustrated by debate and controversy throughout recorded history. Even the term depression itself, by virtue of its wide range of meanings, has contributed to problems of conceptual clarity regarding what causes it and when it is or is not a mental disorder.

A truly comprehensive review of historical and current etiologic models of mood disorders is well beyond the scope of this chapter. Diverse theories of personality and psychopathology (2) and models of mind and brain (3) have clearly influenced conceptual frameworks for understanding causes for mood and other mental disorders. Inherent in debates going back thousands of years has been a seemingly irreconcilable mind/body dichotomy. Greek physicians believed that under the influence of the planet Saturn the spleen of predisposed individuals secreted black bile that influenced the brain and darkened mood. Greek descriptions of what was called melancholy (black bile) are reflected even today in modern diagnostic criteria for MDD. Even so, this early idea of biological causes for depression gave way to other causative theories and reflected prevailing concepts of mind and body of the time (4). Most investigators now agree that a more integrative, nonreductionistic approach should replace the false mind/body dichotomy. Mood disorders are now believed to be caused by a complex set of interactions between genetic/constitutional factors and psychosocial stress factors that combined with individual predispositions lead to a final common pathway of manifest mood disturbances. There is no discrete, single explanation for why some people develop mood disorders and others do not.

An integrative approach is needed to understand the cause, course, and severity of mood disorders. Greden (5) has emphasized the importance of taking a long-term rather than episodic focus when conceptualizing MDD, because a very large proportion of individuals affected with these disorders have a recurrent course. Inherent in this paradigm shift is awareness by clinicians, depressed individuals, and their families that an array of biological, psychological, occupational, and social risk factors must be recognized and managed for optimal long-term outcomes. Risk factors include stressful life events that increase the likelihood of depression and recurrences in individuals who are genetically predisposed (6,7). The death of a loved one or loss of an important relationship is also frequently associated with the onset of a depressive episode (8). The high rate of depression in women in particular, perhaps in part reflecting greater likelihood of help seeking among females, involves a complex interplay of genetic, neuroendocrine, and psychosocial stress factors (9,10). Interpersonal role transitions and losses have also been associated with the onset and persistence of depression in women (11). Thus, while the potential for certain medical conditions and drugs to cause depression via biological mechanisms has been well established (12), it is equally clear that a realistic understanding of the causes of depression will ultimately require a more comprehensive and integrated approach that encompasses numerous psychological and social dimensions as well.

As with major depression, an understanding of the etiology of BPD also requires a longitudinal and multifactorial perspective if there is to be a successful outcome. It has been known for centuries that BPD has a cyclical and recurrent course over a lifetime. Individual episodes may appear spontaneously but there also may be identifiable precipitating factors. Epidemiologic and twin studies clearly suggest that BPD is a heritable disease (13,14), and yet there is not 100% concordance even in identical twins. Therefore, the etiology and manifestations of BPD cannot be exclusively determined by genetics; other contributory factors are clearly operative. The relationship between genetic predisposition and identifiable risk factors in BPD has received a great deal of attention. Disturbances in sleep/wake cycles, exposure to certain drugs, seasonal light changes, hormonal, and other medical conditions are among known biological risk factors in BPD. However, researchers and clinicians have also emphasized the importance of recognition and management of nonbiological, psychosocial stressors over the lifetime course of the illness. It is generally believed that the first and earliest episodes of mania are more likely to be associated with precipitating stress, and that occupation-related events may be particularly important precipitating factors (15). "Kindling" theory suggests that relatively mild, infrequent, and perhaps stress-related mood disturbances early in the course of BPD sensitize affected brain areas such that a firestorm of more severe and more frequent cycles of depression and mania is generated later in life (16). Therefore, the more cycles the individual with a mood disorder experiences, the greater the risk for more frequent and debilitating cycles in the future. As in the case of MDD, a comprehensive understanding of etiology of BPD requires a long-term perspective and awareness of potential precipitating risk factors (15,17).

Incidence and Prevalence

More than 340 million people worldwide and 18 million people in the United States alone have depression at a given point in time (18).

Twelve-month prevalence of MDD for adults in the United States was found to be 6.6% (13.1 to 14.2 million people), and lifetime prevalence was 16.2% (32.6 to 35.1 million people) (19). Methodologic difficulties in precisely quantifying rates of BPD are confounded by the need to differentiate bipolar (having both depressed as well as elevated mood disturbances) from **unipolar** (having recurrences on only one type of disturbance) illness and by the growing recognition that a broad "spectrum" of symptom severity in BPD exists.

Bipolar disorder 1, the most severe form, affects approximately 0.8% of the adult population. With estimates in community samples ranging from 0.4% to 1.6%, these rates are consistent across diverse population groups (20). Some clinical investigators have suggested that there is a complete spectrum of much milder conditions that share with BPD a course characterized by recurrent cycles of mood downturns and elevations. Prevalence rates for more broadly defined "bipolar spectrum disorders" not meeting diagnostic criteria for BPD itself have been reported to be as high as 5% to 7% (21). If the trend to expand the concept of a bipolar diagnostic spectrum continues, to the extent that "even a trace of BPD is BPD" (22), then even these previous prevalence rate estimates will have been considerably too conservative.

For purposes of understanding the etiology and course of mood disorders, incidence rates may be more informative. Severe mood disorders are often recurrent in nature, spanning an entire lifetime for affected individuals. As a result, estimates of incidence rates per se are better considered in specific rather than global clinical contexts. For example, postpartum MDD may emerge after 10% to 15% of all deliveries, making it one of the most important complications of pregnancy. However, MDD following childbirth in women with previous depressive episodes may be as high as 25% to 50% (23). Postpartum relapse in women with BPD is estimated to be 30% to 50% (24). Longitudinal studies of "postpartum **psychosis**" suggest that this condition is not a separate diagnostic entity, but rather a postpartum presentation of an underlying BPD in most instances (25). Incidence rates of severe mood disturbance in women must therefore take into account pregnancy status and personal psychiatric history.

For both MDD and BPD a variety of biopsychosocial risk factors and course modifiers are also known to exist. Furthermore, early course generally differs greatly from later course in terms of episode frequency and severity. As a result, more meaningful incidence and prevalence rates must ultimately be measured and considered in light of more specific clinical contexts.

Signs and Symptoms

Classification of illness (nosology) is necessary to form a conceptual framework for studying disease, to communicate effectively about it, to organize approaches to treatment, and to predict outcomes (26). The *Diagnostic and Statistical Manual of Mental Disorders (DSM IV-TR)* is the classification system that uses a categorical approach and is descriptive in nature, identifying a symptom or a cluster of symptoms that may be present in the individual with a mental disorder (27). It is used by health care professionals to communicate with one another, and to diagnose and treat individuals with mental disorders. It is important to recognize that in the absence of clinically validated laboratory or other physiological diagnostic tests for mood disorders, diagnoses are made based on observable signs (that which the professional sees) and subjective symptoms (those reported by the individual affected with a mood disorder).

DSM IV-TR, published in the year 2000, currently recognizes two broad categories of depressive disorders and BPDs, each with subtypes that reflect differences along a spectrum of course and severity dimensions.

Major Depressive Disorder

MDD is diagnosed when several specific signs and symptoms appear during an episode of at least 2 weeks in duration (Table 6.1). However, the onset of symptoms may be gradual and insidious, and the presence of the illness often goes unrecognized and untreated. In fact, not all persons with MDD experience a sense of sadness or use words like "blue" or "depressed" when describing how they feel. Instead, they may report feeling a "heavy weight," irritability, or a sense of dread. Further, some persons with MDD do not complain of "mood" disturbance at all, but may present with a predominant decrease or inability to experience pleasure **(anhedonia)**. In some instances a family member or friend

Table 6.1 CRITERIA FOR MAJOR DEPRESSIVE EPISODE

A. Five or more of the following symptoms have been present during the same 2-week period and represent a change from previous functioning: at least one of the symptoms is either (a) depressed mood or (b) loss of interest or pleasure.
   (1) Depressed mood most of the day, nearly every day, as indicated by either subjective report (e.g., feels sad or empty) or observation made by others (e.g., appears tearful). Note: In children and adolescents, can be irritable mood.
   (2) Markedly diminished interest or pleasure in all, or almost all, activities most of the day, nearly every day (as indicated by either subjective account or observation made by others).
   (3) Significant weight loss when not dieting, or weight gain (e.g., a change of more than 9% of body weight in a month), or decrease or increase in appetite nearly every day. Note: in children, consider failure to make expected weight gains.
   (4) Insomnia or hypersomnia nearly every day.
   (5) Psychomotor agitation or retardation nearly every day (observable by others, not merely subjective feelings of restlessness or being slowed down).
   (6) Fatigue or loss of energy nearly every day.
   (7) Feelings of worthlessness or excessive or inappropriate guilt (which may be delusional) nearly every day (not merely self-reproach or guilt about being sick).
   (8) Diminished ability to think or concentrate, or indecisiveness, nearly every day (either by subjective account or as observed by others).
   (9) Recurrent thoughts of death (not just fear of dying), recurrent suicidal ideation without a specific plan, or a suicide attempt or a specific plan for committing suicide.

B. The symptoms do not meet criteria for a mixed episode
C. The symptoms cause clinically significant distress or impairment in social, occupational, or other important areas of functioning.
D. The symptoms are not a result of the direct physiologic effects of a substance (e.g., a drug of abuse, a medication) or a general medical condition (e.g., hypothyroidism).
E. The symptoms are not better accounted for by bereavement after the loss of a loved one; the symptoms persist for longer than 2 months or are characterized by marked functional impairment, morbid preoccupation with worthlessness, suicidal ideation, psychotic symptoms, or psychomotor retardation.

Do not include symptoms that are clearly caused by a general medical condition or mood-incongruent delusions or hallucinations.

may be the first to notice the problem. For example, persons with MDD may first appear to be less social and in time may become withdrawn or even isolated. Disinterest in usual occupations and previously pleasurable hobbies and pursuits is not uncommon. To friends and family, an affected individual may simply appear to be "tired," "flat," or "not himself" anymore. Unfortunately, depressed persons may simply feel "blah," deny having any feelings at all, and have little insight into their spiral downward.

In addition to the presence of either depressed mood or loss of interest/pleasure, a diagnosis of MDD according to *DSM IV-TR* requires five or more associated symptoms (Table 6.1). A number of these are commonly referred to as "vegetative symptoms," implying that significant physiological dysfunction is present. Interestingly, the ancient Greek term "melancholic" depression is formally retained in DSM a) when loss of pleasure in all or almost all activities, or "lack of reactivity" (inability to feel better, even temporarily, when something good happens), is present; and b) when three or more of the following is present: distinct quality of mood (not the same as that experienced after the death of a loved one), depression is regularly worse in the morning (diurnal mood variation), early morning awakening, marked **psychomotor retardation** or **psychomotor agitation**, significant loss of appetite or weight loss, and excessive or inappropriate guilt. Although the presence of vegetative symptoms such as these may reflect severe physiological disturbance in MDD and lead to the unmistakable conclusion that something is seriously wrong, depression in the end is also an intensely personal and subjective affliction. Personal accounts of individuals with MDD share many similarities, but at the same time the subjective experience for each person is unique.

MDD may be diagnosed after a single episode, but in many instances subsequent episodes occur and a diagnosis of MDD, Recurrent, is given. Subtypes of episodes of MDD, single or recurrent, are defined in *DSM IV-TR* and may be assigned if specifying features are present. These include psychosis (delusions, hallucinations), **catatonia** (bizarre motor behavior or immobility), melancholia (inability to experience pleasure along with a number of other disturbances that indicate physiological dysfunction), or atypical findings that contrast with those found in melancholia. Course specifiers also exist and are used to describe episodes of MDD that occur within four weeks of childbirth (postpartum onset), or when onset regularly occurs in association with specific months of the year (seasonal pattern). Episodes of MDD may remit completely and be followed by full interepisode recovery, but in some individuals chronic residual symptoms and incomplete recovery are the rule.

Bipolar Disorder

BPD is diagnosed when the clinical course is characterized by the occurrence of one or more episodes of mania, hypomania , or mixed mood states. In contrast to depression, mania is characterized by a persistently elevated, expansive, or irritable mood lasting at least 1 week (Table 6.2, criterion A). In further contrast to depression, persons experiencing clinically elevated mood in BPD often enjoy it and may insist, "There's nothing wrong with me. I never felt better!" Although the elevated, expansive mood may be contagious to others in the short run, for those who are close and know the person well, the ceaseless enthusiasm and confidence become exhausting and overwhelming.

In addition to the hallmark disturbance of persistently elevated mood, three or more associated symptoms must also be present for a diagnosis of BPD (Table 6.2, criterion B). These include inflated self-esteem or grandiosity, excessive involvement

Table 6.2 CRITERIA FOR MANIC EPISODE

A. A distinct period of abnormally and persistently elevated, expansive, or irritable mood, lasting at least 1 week (or any duration if hospitalization is necessary).
B. During the period of mood disturbance, three (or more) of the following symptoms have persisted (four if the mood is only irritable) and have been present to a significant degree:
  (1) Inflated self-esteem or grandiosity.
  (2) Decreased need for sleep (e.g., feels rested after only 3 hours of sleep).
  (3) More talkative than usual or pressure to keep talking.
  (4) Flight of ideas or subjective experience that thoughts are racing.
  (5) Distractibility (e.g., attention too easily drawn to unimportant or irrelevance external stimuli).
  (6) Increase in goal-directed activity (either socially, at work or school, or sexually) or psychomotor agitation.
  (7) Excessive involvement in pleasurable activities that have a high potential for painful consequences (e.g., engaging in unrestrained buying sprees, sexual indiscretions, or foolish business investments).
C. The symptoms do not meet criteria for a mixed episodes
D. The mood disturbance is sufficiently severe to cause marked impairment in occupational functioning or in usual social activities or relationships with others, or to necessitate hospitalization to prevent harm to self or others, or there are psychotic features.
E. The symptoms are not because of the direct psychological effects of a substance (e.g., a drug of abuse, a medication, or other treatment) or a general medical condition (e.g., hyperthyroidism).

Manic-like episodes that are clearly caused by somatic antidepressant treatment (e.g., medication, electroconvulsive therapy, light therapy) should not count toward a diagnosis of bipolar disorder 1.

in pleasurable activities, and an increase in goal-directed activities. In the earlier stages of an episode of mania, affected persons may actually seem quite productive and creative at work or school, or in social situations. If an episode of mania persists, however, the cumulative effects of pressured expansiveness, sleep deprivation, and the negative reactions of others take their toll, and the affected individual him/herself is no longer enchanted with the experience.

Overconfidence often leads to overextension, and impaired judgment may result in painful consequences such as unrestrained spending sprees, sexual indiscretions, and foolish business investments. Some symptoms more directly reflect disturbance of neurophysiologic brain functioning and may include decreased need for sleep, pressure speech, distractibility, racing thoughts, or even frank *flight of ideas* which is seen by others as unmistakable evidence of madness.

An episode of true mania must meet severity criteria and/or include psychotic features (Table 6.2, criterion D). In contrast to mania, hypomania is not severe enough to cause marked impairment in social or occupational functioning or to require hospitalization, and there are no psychotic features. In mixed episodes, criteria for both mania and major depression are met concurrently over a period of at least one week. As with MDD, various course specifiers for BPD, as previously outlined for MDD, may be applied. In addition, the term **rapid-cycling** may be applied in both bipolar disorder 1 (mania) and bipolar disorder 2 (hypomania) when there are at least four episodes of mood disturbance during a 12-month period. The presence of rapid cycling is usually an indication of severe and possibly treatment refractory illness, and the affected individual may feel as though they are unable to depart from an endless ride on a destructive roller coaster.

Dysthymic disorder and **cyclothymic disorder**, not the subject of this review, represent milder but chronic disorders of depressive and bipolar mood disturbance, respectively. These conditions fail to meet diagnostic criteria for MDD or BPD per se, but appear to fall along a larger spectrum of related, albeit milder, mood disorders. Mood disturbances that are secondary to general medical conditions and/or substance abuse are also described in *DSM IV-TR*.

Signs and symptoms, though important in diagnosing disorders, do not address all dimensions of a particular condition. It is also well established that additional aspects of illness (psychological, social, and occupational) are critically important in understanding and treating mood disorders. The *DSM* uses a multiaxial system to address different domains that can affect the individual. These domains of information include medical conditions, psychosocial and environmental problems, and level of functioning. Occupational therapists need to familiarize themselves with the various axes so as to assist in the assessment and treatment planning process.

Course and Prognosis

It is generally accepted that mood disturbance may begin at any age, but formal mood disorders are most commonly first diagnosed in early adulthood. A majority of persons diagnosed with MDD, Single Episode, will go on to have a second episode. With each subsequent episode of depression, the likelihood of having additional future recurrences rises dramatically (28). After three episodes of depression, individuals have a 90% chance of having a fourth, and life-long aggressive treatment is needed. Following a single episode of major depression, as many as 10% of affected individuals go on to develop BPD, long-recognized to be a life-long and recurrent illness as well.

The course of recurrent MDD may be highly variable. Signs and symptoms may develop very insidiously over a period of weeks or even months, but occasionally severe depression may develop suddenly, for instance following a traumatic or psychosocial stressor. Episodes of MDD can resolve spontaneously, but untreated depression may last for many months or never fully remit. Episodes may be separated by a period of several years, or they may cluster and become increasingly frequent over time (29). Current *DSM* classification recognizes a number of course specifiers, including onset of episode within 4 weeks postpartum and onset during a particular season of the year (sometimes referred to as seasonal affective disorder [SAD]). In addition, there are patterns of recurrent MDD that vary according to whether there is or is not full interepisode recovery, and with or without underlying dysthymic disorder (Fig. 6.1).

Greden (30) has emphasized the importance of maintaining a long-term, longitudinal perspective on the treatment of MDD (Fig. 6.2). From this perspective, one can recognize that undetected and untreated depressive disturbances that do not meet the criteria for a formal diagnosis of MDD may evolve into a course of recurrent episodes that are more severe, more frequent, and more treatment resistant. This pattern, coupled with the fact that the disorder is highly prevalent and often early in onset, contributes to the growing awareness that MDD represents a cumulative and overwhelming personal and public health burden.

Similarly, BPD by definition follows a recurrent, often life-long pattern. As with MDD, BPD is also highly variable in onset and course. After a single episode of mania, more than 90% of affected individuals will go on to have future episodes. Most commonly,

A. Recurrent, with full interepisode recovery, with no dysthymic disorder

B. Recurrent, without full interepisode recovery, with no dysthymic disorder

A. Recurrent, with full interepisode recovery, superimposed on dysthymic disorder (also code 300.4)

A. Recurrent, without full interepisode recovery, superimposed on dysthymic disorder (also code 300.4)

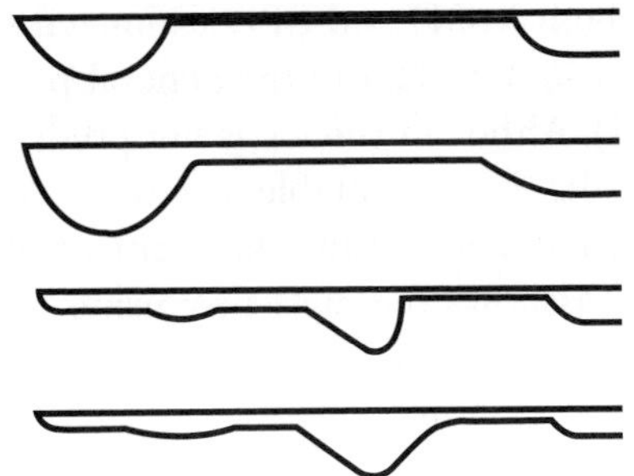

Figure 6.1 Longitudinal course specifiers. (From American Psychiatric Association. Diagnostic and statistical manual of mental disorders text revision (4th ed.). (DSM IV-TR) Washington, DC: American Psychiatric Association. 2000:425)

episodes of mania immediately precede or follow depressive episodes. The onset of symptoms may be gradual or precipitous, and the risk of sudden hypomania or mania may be especially high following significant sleep deprivation in some individuals. The exact sequence of specific symptom onset and constellation in BPD varies considerably from person to person, but the pattern may hold true from episode to episode for a given individual. If this pattern is understood by the individual with BPD, the clinician can help the client to anticipate possible problems that may arise in the future. A commonly held view among most investigators is that cycle length becomes shorter with each recurrence, such that episodes become more frequent over time and eventually level off at some maximal frequency for a given individual (15). Post and others have advanced a "behavioral sensitization" model to explain the observation that course tends to worsen over time (16). A small percentage of individuals with BPD have frequent (four or more per year) cycles of hypomania, mania, depression, or mixed states, and this "rapid-cycling" pattern is generally associated with treatment resistance and a poorer prognosis.

When considering prognosis in mood disorders, it is important to evaluate both acute (pertaining to given episode) and long-term (course over time) perspectives. Major advances have occurred in the diagnosis and treatment of mood disorders in terms of response to both acute phase treatment as well as prevention of future recurrences. Nonetheless, the morbidity associated with recurrent MDD and with BPD over a lifetime remains staggering.

Of course the most costly and tragic outcome associated with mood disorders is suicide. Study after study has confirmed that the presence of a major mood disorder is a significant risk factor for suicide, with lifetime

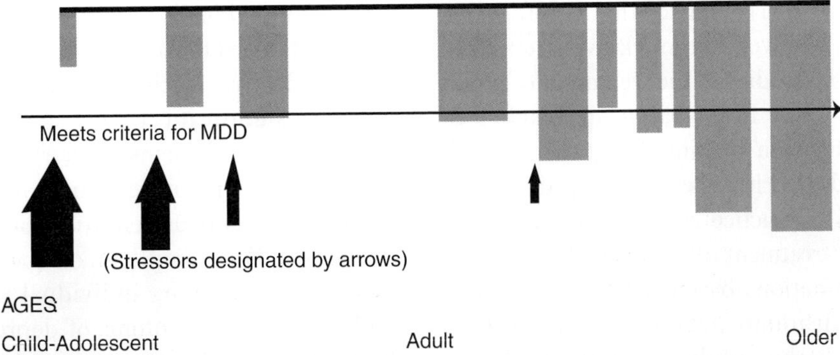

Figure 6.2 Longitudinal course of major depressive disorder. (From Greden, J. F. Treatment of recurrent depression. Washington, DC: American Psychiatric Association. 2001)

risk in both MDD and BPD estimated to be 20 times higher than in the general population (31). Although suicide is not predictable or completely preventable, accurate assessment of risk and careful management of the assessed risk has the most promising potential for reducing suicide rates.

Medical(Psychiatric)/ Surgical Management

Effective treatment for both acute and long-term aspects of mood disorders is essential if prognosis and outcomes are to improve. In the case of MDD, "prevention of recurrences requires a paradigm shift, a call to arms" (5). As discussed below, this will entail a shift in treatment focus from acute intervention to a long-term management perspective. For BPD, contemporary data on course and outcome represent "the baseline, the bare minimum" (15). As with MDD, treatment orientation for BPD must be essentially life-long. Closing the gap between what is known about effective treatment for mood disorders versus how it is actually delivered in the community has become a national health priority.

Optimal management approaches of disorders such as MDD and BPD are based upon current scientific treatment evidence, experience of the treating clinician(s), and informed patient preferences. Informed evaluation of the "evidence" in evidence-based medicine (EBM) requires that careful consideration be given to the relative strength of the available studies in the treatment of mood disorders (32). EBM-based approaches to clinical decision-making for patients with MDD and BPD have been developed and disseminated as practice guidelines (8,17), pharmacologic treatment **algorithms** (33–36) and recommendations based upon expert consensus. Although detailed description of these and other tools to assist in clinical decision-making is beyond the scope of this review, treatment guidelines for MDD and BPD are organized around short-term tactical (Acute and Continuation Phase) as well as long-term strategic (Maintenance Phase) considerations (Fig. 6.3).

The goal in the Acute Phase of treatment (usually the first several weeks) is to achieve complete remission of symptoms and full return of psychosocial functioning. During Continuation Phase treatment (several months), the goal is to maintain **euthymia** (normal mood state) and prevent relapse of the recent mood disturbance. For all patients with BPD and for patients that have recurrent episodes of MDD, the long-term strategic focus during Maintenance Phase treatment (years to decades) is reduction or prevention of future recurrences of illness (8,17,33, 34,35,36).

Treatment recommendations follow from psychiatric assessment which includes biological (severity, pattern, and scope of depressive signs and symptoms, medical status, comorbid psychiatric conditions, laboratory and other diagnostic data, family/genetic history), psychological (developmental history, specific psychological and personality factors, precipitating psychological stresses), and social (past and present levels of functioning in marital, parental, occupational, educational roles) dimensions. The choice of specific treatment modalities will depend in large part upon these patient-specific factors and where the intervention appears in the course of the affected individual's condition. Factors that suggest the need for combination of medication and an effective psychotherapy include presence of significant psychosocial stresses, interpersonal problems, comorbid personality disorder, poor response to previous single-modality treatment trials, or poor compliance (8). For example, an otherwise healthy and well-functioning individual presenting with first onset symptoms of depression following the loss of a loved one may benefit from

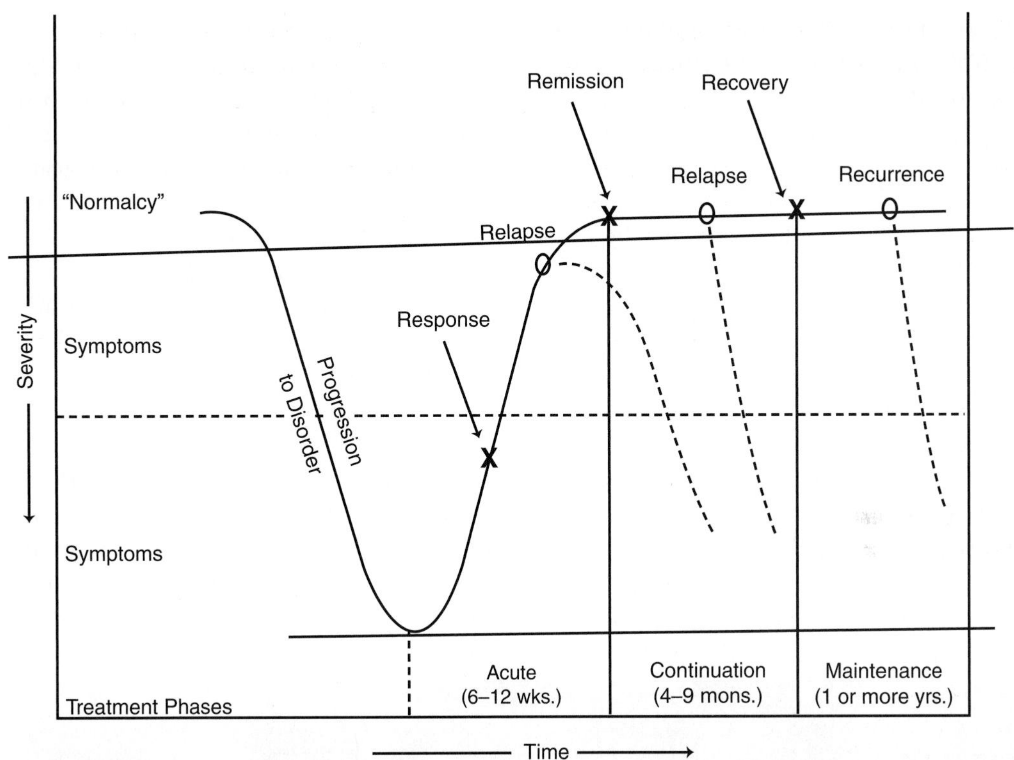

Figure 6.3 Long-term treatment of depression. This requires an illness focus rather than an episode focus. (From Kupfer DJ. Long-term treatment of depression. J Clin Psychiatry 1991:52(suppl 5);28–34. Adapted and reprinted with permission.)

psychotherapeutic assistance alone. On the other hand, a combination of medication and various psychotherapeutic, behavioral, and educational interventions may be required for an individual with a fourth reoccurrence of major depression or for first-time diagnosis of BPD.

The best studied and documented psychotherapeutic methods in the literature shown to be effective in MDD are cognitive behavioral therapy (CBT) and interpersonal therapy (IPT). How to best match specific type of therapy to an individual patient has not yet been determined (8,28). Much of what is known about effective treatment of depression is based upon studies of the Acute Phase of treatment. However, most evidence suggests that combination treatment for recurrent MDD using both medication and psychotherapy is more effective than either medication or psychotherapy alone (5,28).

In BPD, a long-term perspective on treatment must take into account known risk factors such as sleep deprivation, drugs and medical disorders, seasonal light changes, and psychosocial stresses. Relatively little formal study has been published on specific psychotherapies for BPD (32). Given the association between cycling in BPD and occupational stress (15), there is a need for assistance from occupational therapists in addressing associated functional impairment (17). Disturbances of circadian rhythm and sleep/wake cycles in BPD can predispose the individual to mood cycling. "Social rhythm therapy" which combines principles of IPT and CBT has been developed to influence chronobiological and psychosocial factors that disrupt healthy routines (37). Additionally, a novel approach has been proposed that involves phase-specific and sequenced psychotherapies that are delivered in variable patterns and linked to fluctuating mood states in BPD (38).

Pharmacotherapy

Although various medications may be Food and Drug Administration (FDA)-approved, marketed, and even classified according to specific uses (e.g., antidepressants, mood stabilizers, antipsychotics, anxiolytics), it is important to note that medications from any of these as well as other classes are commonly used in the treatment of MDD and BPD. In part, this is a result of the fact that depressed mood, cyclical recurrences, psychotic symptoms, and anxiety may be present in various phases of either condition. It is also increasingly clear that atypical antipsychotics can improve and stabilize mood, and that mood "stabilizers" can be used to treat acute mania or even depression.

Tables 6.3 through 6.5. list medications most commonly used in the treatment of MDD and BPD. It is not currently possible to determine in advance whether a specific medication chosen from a number of available alternatives will be the most effective. Known differences in "side effect" profiles for specific medications influence the initial choice of medication and the order of alternatives if more than one trial is needed. Daily doses of medications fall into usual ranges, but actual dosage requirements may vary widely from one individual to another. For some medications blood levels can be obtained, and these

Table 6.3 COMMONLY USED ANTIDEPRESSANT MEDICATIONS

Generic Name	Usual Dose (mg/day)	Most Common Side Effects
Tricyclics		
■ Amitriptyline	100–300	As a class, tricyclic antidepressants (TCAs) commonly cause dry mouth, constipation, and problems with visual accommodation (focusing). Weight gain is not infrequent. Light-headedness after first standing may also occur. Can be fatal in overdose.
■ Imipramine	100–300	
■ Desipramine	100–300	
■ Nortriptyline	50–200	
SSRIs		
■ Citalopram	20–60	Selective serotonin inhibitors (SSRIs) have largely replaced TCAs as drugs of first choice in depression because of relative safety in overdose. Concerns about possible increase in suicidal ideation have recently been raised Sexual side effects are generally manageable but are not uncommon. Gastrointestinal upset, headache, insomnia, and increased agitation may occur.
■ Duloxetine	60–120	
■ Escitalopram	10–20	
■ Fluoxetine	20–60	
■ Paroxetine	20–60	
■ Sertraline	50–200	
Others		
■ Bupropion SR	150–400	Insomnia, agitation, weight loss, seizures
■ Mirtazapine	15–45	Weight gain, sedation, dry mouth
■ Venlafaxine	75–225	Nausea, sexual dysfunction, dizziness
MAOIs		
■ Phenelzine	15–90	Rarely used as first-line choices because of potential serious drug-drug interactions and strict dietary restrictions that are required.
■ Tranylcypromine	30–60	

Table 6.4 COMMONLY USED MOOD STABILIZERS

Generic Name	Usual Dose (mg/day)	Most Common Side Effects
Lithium	600–2100	Nausea, diarrhea, weight gain, tremor, headache, excessive thirst and increased urination. After long-term use, may cause hypothyroidism and decreased kidney functioning. Requires close blood level monitoring; toxic in overdose.
Divalproex	750–2000	Nausea, sedation, balance problems, hair loss. In some patients, may cause pancreatitis or liver toxicity.
Carbamazepine	400–1600	Drowsiness, headache, nausea, blurred or double vision May suppress bone marrow and in rare instances cause severe reduction in blood cell elements.
Lamotrigine	150–400	Dizziness, nausea, headache, visual disturbances. May cause skin rash and in some instances can lead to potentially fatal dermatologic reactions.

Table 6.5 COMMONLY USED ANTIPSYCHOTIC MEDICATIONS

Generic Name	Usual Dose (mg/day)	Most Common Side Effects
First-Generation		
Antipsychotics	300–1000	The original neuroleptics as a class commonly caused extrapyramidal symptoms (EPS) such as tremor, shuffling gait, and masked facies, as well as motor restlessness (akathisia). Long-term use is associated with permanent movement disorders such as tardive dyskinesia (TD).Sedation often occurs. Weight gain is not uncommon with long-term use.
Chlorpromazine	2–20	
Haloperidol	15–50	
Thiothixene	5–40	
Trifluoperazine	(mg/2–4 weeks)	
Fluphenazine D	6.25–50	
Haloperidol D	50–200	
Second-Generation		
Antipsychotics	15–30	In general, the newer antipsychotics as a class are far less likely to cause EPS and TD. Within the class, clozapine and quetiapine are most likely to cause drop in blood pressure, and along with olanzapine may cause significant sedation. Weight gain (and possible risk of glucose intolerance) is common with clozapine and olanzapine but may occur with the others as well. Clozapine, and to a lesser extent olanzapine, is associated with dry mouth and constipation.
Aripiprazole (Abilify)	12.5–900	
Clozapine (Clozaril)	2–6	
Risperidone (Risperdal)	5–20	
Olanzapine (Zyprexa)	50–750	
Quetiapine (Seroquel)	40–160	
Ziprasidone (Geodon)		

may assist in verifying that doses are being adequately absorbed and distributed.

Availability of effective treatments, however, does not guarantee their use. Noncompliance with treatment recommendations in general medical practice is common, and it may be particularly problematic in persons with mood disorders as a result of the impairment of judgment that may be present, denial that an illness even exists, and shame caused by the stigma of having a mental disorder. It is important to recognize and address treatment noncompliance and to establish a strong therapeutic alliance with the individual with a mood disorder and their family.

It is also important to note that while treatment guidelines and medication algorithms can be helpful in summarizing the findings of clinical studies and the opinions of prominent experts, they cannot define rigid standards of care. Standards of psychiatric care are instead determined on the basis of all clinical data available for an individual case, and ultimate judgments regarding treatment must be made in light of diagnostic and treatment options applicable to that specific situation. Further, given that much about best treatment approaches for these conditions has not yet been delineated, fully informed participation in decision-making by patients and families is essential.

Impact of Mood Disorders on Client Factors

Quotes from personal narratives and the objective data reviewed in this chapter demonstrate the wide variation in presentations of mood disorders from one individual to another (Table 6.6). There is no exact pattern, no uniform mosaic of signs and symptoms that the therapist will observe when evaluating and treating the person with a mood disorder. Virtually any area of occupation, or combination, can be affected in a given individual: Activities of daily living, instrumental activities of daily living, work, education, leisure, and social participation. Therapists may observe problems in the individual's performance skills (motor skill deficits, problems with processing, and difficulty with communicating and interacting) that affect their ability to perform occupations.

Mood disorders have a major impact on an affected individual's quality of life and social functioning (39,40), including the ability to parent (41). Well-studied and quantified is the impact of mood disorders on occupational functioning (42–46). More recent application of an epidemiologic technique called experience sampling suggests that studies based on days missed from work significantly underestimate the lost productivity of depressed individuals who remain on the job, known as "presenteeism" (47). In this study, MDD was more consistently related to poor work performance than any of the seven other chronic physical conditions studied. Even in dysthymic disorder, less severe than MDD, unrecognized work impairment unrelated to work absences has major negative, long-term consequences for affected individuals and their employers (48). Employer concerns about steadily rising health care costs initially led to counterproductive constraints on access to and utilization of mental health benefits over the past decade. Recent studies are now demonstrating, however, that the cost of effective treatments for mood disorders more than offset the direct and indirect costs because of absenteeism and lost productivity (43–47,49).

Although deficits in skills or performance of occupations may occur, the context within which the affected individual exists often plays a crucial role in how they experience and manage their condition and how they function on a daily basis. The availability of support systems, the individual's

Table 6.6 IMPACT OF CONDITIONS ON CLIENT FACTORS

Global Mental Functions	
Orientation functions	In general orientation is spared. However, severe depression or mania accompanied by psychosis can superficially resemble the disorientation seen in organic conditions.
Sleep	Sleep disturbance is a hallmark sign in mood disorders. MDD may be associated with too little or too much sleep. Mania can be associated with decreased need for sleep. Over time sleep deprivation can have profound effects on occupational performance.
Temperament/personality functions	Many functions usually attributed to personality are greatly affected by presence and severity of mood disturbance. These may change according to state of mood.
Energy and drive functions	MDD may be associated with low energy and lack of motivation to engage in previously meaningful activities. BPD may be associated with excess energy, often not goal-directed, and poor impulse control.
Specific Mental Functions	
Attention and Memory functions	Although not always born out by formal testing, people with MDD often complain about inability to concentrate and remember. Individuals with mild mood elevation may subjectively experience improved attention and memory. Severe mania causes objective impairment in these functions.
Perceptual functions	Auditory, and less commonly visual, hallucinations may appear in individuals with mood disorders who are experiencing psychosis. Perceptions in any sensory modality may be muted in persons with MDD and enhanced in individuals with BPD.
Higher level cognitive functions	In mania, impaired judgment can take the form of excessive involvement in pleasurable activities with little regard for the consequences. Individuals with MDD may have unrealistically negative or hopeless outlook.
Mental functions of language	Impairment in mental functions of language may appear as frank disturbance of thought form in severe mood disorders. Individuals with depression may exhibit profoundly slowed speech, muteness, or catatonia. Conversely, people with mania may exhibit rapid or pressured speech, tangentiality, or gross flight of ideas.
Psychomotor functions	Psychomotor agitation or retardation can be present in individuals with MDD. Individuals with psychomotor retardation may exhibit inactivity or slowed movement in MDD. Persons with mania show increased motor activity and often appear driven or extremely agitated.

(Continued)

Table 6.6 IMPACT OF CONDITIONS ON CLIENT FACTORS (*CONT.*)

Emotional functions	Disturbances of emotion are the hallmark of mood disorders. See Signs and Symptoms in the chapter text.
Experience of self and time functions	People who are depressed often feel worthless, guilty, and incompetent. This may reach delusional proportions in some individuals ("My insides are rotting"). Mania is associated with exaggerated self-confidence, and grandiosity can reach psychotic proportions ("I am here to save the world").
Sensory Functions and Pain	
Seeing	Visual acuity may be affected by numerous medications.
Additional sensory functions	Individuals with MDD may complain that food is tasteless and unappealing. Medications may also cause unpleasant or metallic taste and impact eating behavior.
Pain	Perceptions of pain may be enhanced in individuals with MDD, whereas persons with BPD may be less affected by pain sensations.
Functions of Cardiovascular and Hematological Systems	
Functions of the cardiovascular system	Some medications may cause orthostatic hypotension, putting the patient at risk of falling from lightheadedness, especially after stooping or rising to stand.
Functions of the hematological systems	Bone marrow suppression infrequently occurs as a result of some medications.
Functions of the Digestive, Metabolic, and Endocrine Systems	
Functions related to the digestive system	Constipation can become a preoccupation in older persons with depression. Some medications can aggravate dry mouth and constipation. Conversely, other medications may cause nausea and diarrhea.
Functions related to the metabolism and endocrine system	Most medications used to treat mood disorders can cause weight gain, and in some instances increase risk of diabetes. Lithium can cause hypothyroidism.
Genitourinary and Reproductive Functions	
	Some medications may cause urinary retention. Lithium may cause polyuria (production of large amounts of urine per day). Sexual side effects (decreased libido, impotence, anorgasmia) are not uncommon side effects in men or women. Some medications are best avoided during pregnancy, but in some situations, continued treatment is essential to avoid significant clinical relapse.

(*Continued*)

Table 6.6 IMPACT OF CONDITIONS ON CLIENT FACTORS (*CONT.*)

Neuromusculoskeletal and movement-related functions	Lithium, many antidepressants, and mood stabilizers cause tremors; nocturnal myoclonus (leg twitching during sleep) is less common. In toxic amounts, lithium and other mood stabilizers may cause balance problems and incoordination. Antipsychotic medications, sometimes used in mood disorders, may cause Parkinsonian signs and/or akathisia (motor restlessness).
Functions of the skin	Any medication can be associated with allergic skin reactions. Some medications may cause photosensitivity (sunburn).

age and gender, socioeconomic status, resources available to them, social stigma, and their own values and beliefs can profoundly affect how the individual with a mood disorder negotiates the world around them. It is important for the occupational therapist to remember that it is the intersection of multiple factors, not solely the condition, that affects occupational performance.

Having acknowledged that the condition is but one determinant of occupational performance, a review of client factors will assist the therapist in further understanding how specific body functions are influenced by the condition or by treatment interventions and, in turn, how they influence performance. This understanding is of great importance and value to other members of the treatment team and should be actively communicated.

CASE STUDY

Case Illustrations

■ CASE 1

Carolyn is a 42-year-old woman who has a long history of depressive episodes beginning when she was 19 years old. She grew up in a chaotic home with a mother who was an alcoholic and a father who was abusive. Carolyn left home at age 15 and was homeless for a short period of time before being placed in foster care during her high school years. Carolyn has had no contact with her nuclear family or her foster care family since completing high school. After high school she went to work at a local hospital as a clerk and while there she met the head of the radiation therapy department who encouraged her to pursue a degree in the field. Carolyn put herself through college and completed her degree while working full time. She was offered a job at the hospital and quickly became well regarded by the radiologists at this site for her precise work.

Carolyn's depressive episodes recurred throughout her young and middle adulthood. Because of them Carolyn withdrew from others, had limited interactions with other staff when depressed, and had difficulty sleeping and concentrating. In spite of these symptoms, she continued to work and, in fact, excelled at her job. Much of Carolyn's sense of efficacy was related to her view of herself as a competent worker. Over the years, she was given increasingly complex tasks requiring precision and focus and was generally successful in carrying them out.

Carolyn intermittently saw psychiatrists from age 19 to 30 in an attempt to manage her "black moods" and at age 32 she began seeing her present psychiatrist. Rather than focus on only her current episode of depression, they set out to establish a long-term treatment strategy and alliance to help achieve complete remission from her current episode of depression and reduce likelihood of future occurrences. In addition to prescribing an antidepressant medication she had previously found to be helpful, they engaged in interpersonal psychotherapy consisting of cognitive behavioral and psychoeducational approaches. A strong therapeutic alliance was formed and this relationship remains one of the only stable, long-term relationships in Carolyn's life. However, she is inconsistent in keeping her appointments and periodically "disappears" from treatment for months at a time. The other relationship she maintains is with her supervisor at work who originally encouraged her to go to school.

Although she complied with medication recommendations, she was hospitalized for severe depression at age 33 after the breakup of a 5-year relationship with a man who was verbally abusive. She stopped going to work and completely isolated herself, unable to structure her time or perform any household or self-care tasks. She reported she was unable to move or get up from bed except to go to the bathroom. After partial improvement she insisted on leaving the hospital out of concern she would lose her job if she continued to be absent from work. Although her depressive symptoms never completely remitted she managed to return to work and performed adequately until 6 months ago.

Six months ago she began to have difficulty attending to tasks and eventually made a serious error that could have been potentially harmful to a patient. Reluctantly, Carolyn agreed to take a leave of absence. She recontacted her psychiatrist and said that she was fearful she would be fired from her job and did not know what she would do if she couldn't work. Her antidepressant medication was augmented by the addition of lithium. She reported she had not been able to concentrate on any activities since the incident at work. She was encouraged to add meaningful tasks to her daily schedule and began gardening and writing poetry. Her progress was slow and she became convinced she would never be able to resume her role as a radiation therapist. Two weeks ago, she became so despondent that she decided to commit suicide by overdosing on her medication. She left her home determined to follow through with her plan, and she deposited all of her worldly possessions on the curb to be picked up with the trash the next day. She left no notes, but before acting on her plan she called her psychiatrist and after a lengthy discussion agreed to meet him at the hospital and be admitted.

Upon admission, Carolyn presented as very depressed and acknowledged suicidal ideation with a clear plan for harming herself. She reported she had not been able to sleep for more than a few hours each evening for the past month and that she lacked the energy or interest required to initiate everyday activities. She stopped cooking food for herself, cleaning her home, paying bills, and taking care of her beloved cat. Although clean, her appearance was disheveled. She indicated she was never hungry and had lost 10 pounds over the last 2 months.

While in the hospital Carolyn initially remained in bed and refused to take part in ward activities. She was ashamed that she had no clothes and was hesitant to accept those that the nursing staff brought in for her. Instead of socializing she spent most of her time in her bedroom. Having failed to respond to adequate trials of antidepressant medication, and because of ongoing risk of self-harm even while hospitalized, Carolyn's psychiatrist recommended a series of electroconvulsive therapy (ECT) treatments. After 10 treatments over a 3-week period, Carolyn showed dramatic improvement, was discharged, and continued her treatment on an outpatient basis.

■ CASE 2

John is a 59-year-old man who is married and has three adult sons, ages 35, 33, and 29. He was a corporate executive in the health care industry and spent much of his adult life rescuing ailing hospital systems and transforming them into financially successful businesses. John's job required that he travel a great deal and he was often away from home for long periods of time. John was highly respected by those with whom he worked with and was viewed as a source of inspiration to those he mentored.

John first sought help after experiencing what he termed "an abysmal failure in my performance." He was sent to a failing hospital and tried for months to create a change in the organization but he was unsuccessful in everything he attempted. Believing he had failed, he returned to the home office after 6 months, and it was at this point that he first sought psychiatric treatment. He reported that he was a perfectionist and had never felt like a failure before. He was experiencing difficulty sleeping, reduced sexual drive, a lack of interest in work, cessation of leisure pursuits, and trouble recollecting events of the day. He indicated that his bosses were supportive of him but that he was concerned that he had not "lived up to my potential" and that his job could be in jeopardy. He began taking an antidepressant medication, and over the next few weeks noticed his depression had improved. Although concerned about sexual side effects of the medication, he agreed to continue treatment and after 8 weeks started feeling like himself again.

Shortly thereafter John's condition changed abruptly. He became uncharacteristically aggressive in a meeting with coworkers and exhibited pressured speech and distractibility. Against his protests he was asked to leave the building, and when he refused he had to be escorted from the premises. His boss insisted that he seek help before he could return. His diagnosis was revised to BPD, but in his manic state he had little insight and was resistant to starting a mood stabilizer. He said "I need to be at the top of my game" and was fearful that taking the drugs would affect his performance and his energy at work. With the support and encouragement of family and friends, however, he did accept treatment recommendations and over a period of two weeks returned to his previous baseline. He was able to sleep, think clearly, and expressed interest in returning to work. His boss allowed him to return, but he was initially placed in a position that required little contact with others. John reported he had always thrived on the interactions he had with others and missed this desperately. He felt useless in his new position and began to feel depressed again. He expressed vague suicidal thoughts and reported it was "tough to be here" because work had always been "everything to me."

Over the next few months, John continued to experience mild to moderate depression. Discouraged about his job, ongoing problems with mood, and tremor caused by lithium, John discontinued his medication. Within weeks John experienced another hypomanic episode. He began to spend all of his waking hours at home working on the computer. He slept 3 hours a night and often went to the office at 4 o'clock in the morning. He was impatient with everyone at work and unrealistically demanding of his secretary. John felt that the problems he was experiencing in his relationships at work were caused by others' lack of motivation, not his demanding style. He continued to refuse to take lithium as he was convinced it would blunt his creativity. He was becoming increasingly angry and distractible at home as well. John's wife convinced him to see his psychiatrist and at this point he agreed to start an alternative mood stabilizer. Unfortunately, his behaviors at work lead to his dismissal. John and his wife have had to contemplate whether he should seek a comparable position elsewhere or consider retiring earlier than planned. His mood has stabilized, but John remains very conflicted about how he can meaningfully spend his time if he is not working.

References

1. Danquah MN. Willow Weep for Me: A Black Woman's Journey Through Depression. New York: Norton & Company, 1998:27–28.
2. Theories of personality and psychopathology. In: Sadock BJ, Sadock VA, eds. Kaplan's and Sadock's Comprehensive Textbook of Psychiatry. 7th Ed. Philadelphia: Lippincott, Williams & Wilkins, 1999.
3. Contributions of the psychological sciences. In: Sadock BJ, Sadock VA, eds. Kaplan's and Sadock's Comprehensive Textbook of Psychiatry. 7th Ed. Philadelphia: Lippincott, Williams & Wilkins, 1999.
4. Akiskal HS. Mood disorders: introduction and overview. In: Sadock BJ, Sadock VA, eds. Kaplan's and Sadock's Comprehensive Textbook of Psychiatry. 7th Ed. Philadelphia: Lippincott, Williams & Wilkins, 1999.
5. Greden JF. Clinical prevention of recurrent depression. In: Greden JF, ed. Treatment of Recurrent Depression. Washington, DC: American Psychiatric Publishing, 2001.
6. Kendler KS, Neale MC, Kessler RC, et al. A longitudinal twin study of 1-year prevalence of major depression in women. Arch Gen Psychiatry 1993;50:843–852.
7. Kendler KS, Karkowski LM, Prescott CA. Causal relationship between stressful life events and the onset of major depression. Am J Psychiatry 1999;156:837–841.
8. Practice Guideline for the Treatment of Patients with MDD. 2nd Ed. Arlington, VA: American Psychiatric Publishing, 2000.
9. Bifulco A, Brown GW, Moran P, et al. Predicting depression in women: the role of past and present vulnerability. Psychol Med 1998;28:39–50.
10. Heim C, Nemeroff CB. The Impact of early adverse experiences on brain systems involved in the pathophysiology of anxiety and affective disorders. Biol Psychiatry 1999;46:1509–1522.
11. Weissman MM, Markowitz JC, Klerman GL. Comprehensive Guide to Interpersonal Psychotherapy. New York: Basic Books, 2000.
12. Zelnik TC. Depressive effects of drugs. In: Cameron OG, ed. Presentations of Depression. New York: John Wiley & Sons, Inc., 1987.
13. Gershon ES. Genetics. In: Goodwin FK, Jamison KR, Manic-Depressive Illness. New York: Oxford University Press, 1990.
14. Tohen M, Bromet E, Murphy JM, et al. Psychiatric epidemiology. Harv Rev Psychiatry 2000;8:111–125.
15. Goodwin FK, Jamison KR. Course and Outcome. In: Goodwin FK, Jamison KR, eds. Manic-Depressive Illness. New York: Oxford University Press, 1990.
16. Post RM. Transduction of psychosocial stress into the neurobiology of recurrent affective disorder. Am J Psychiatry 1992;149:999–1010.
17. Practice Guideline for the Treatment of Patients with BPD. 2nd Ed. Arlington, VA: American Psychiatric Publishing, 2000.
18. Murray CJL, Lopez AD. The Global Burden of Disease: A Comprehensive Assessment of Mortality and Disability from Disease, Injuries, and Risk Factors in 1990 and projected to 2020, Vol. 1. Cambridge, MA: Harvard University Press, 1996.
19. Kessler RC, Berglund P, Demler O, et al. The epidemiology of MDD—results from the National Comorbidity Survey Replication (NCS-R). JAMA 2003;289(3):3095–3105.
20. Weissman MM, Bland RC, Canino GJ, et al. Cross-national epidemiology of major depression and BPD. JAMA 1996;276:293–299.
21. Hirschfeld RM. Bipolar spectrum disorder: improving its recognition and diagnosis. J Clin Psychiatry 2001;62(suppl 14):5–9.
22. Jefferson JW. BPDs: A brief guide to diagnosis and treatment. Focus 2003;1:7–14.
23. Wisner KL, Perel JM, Findling RL. Antidepressant treatment during breast feeding. Am J Psychiatry 1996;153:1132–1137.

24. Cohen LS, Sichel DA, Robertson LM, et al. Postpartum prophylaxis for women with BPD. Am J Psychiatry 1995;152;1641–1645.
25. Chaudron LH, and Pies RW. The relationship between postpartum psychosis and BPD: a review. J Clin Psychiatry 2003;64:1284–1292.
26. Bogenschutz MP, Nurnberg HG. Classification of mental disorders. In: Sadock BJ, Sadock VA, eds. Kaplan's and Sadock's Comprehensive Textbook of Psychiatry. 7th Ed. Philadelphia: Lippincott, Williams & Wilkins, 1999.
27. Diagnostic and Statistical Manual of Mental Disorders. 4th Ed, revision. Washington, DC: American Psychiatric Publishing, 2000.
28. Boland R, Keller MB. Chronic and recurrent depression. In: Greden JF, ed. Treatment of Recurrent Depression. Washington, DC: American Psychiatric Publishing, 2001.
29. Practice Guidelines for the Treatment of Patients with MDD. 2nd Ed. Arlington, VA: American Psychiatric Publishing, 2000.
30. Greden JF. Recurrent depression: its overwhelming burden. In: Greden JF, ed. Treatment of Recurrent Depression. Washington, DC: American Psychiatric Publishing, 2001.
31. Practice Guideline for the Assessment and Treatment of Patients With Suicidal Behaviors. Arlington, VA: American Psychiatric Publishing, 2003.
32. Bowden CL, Gonzoles CL. Prevention of recurrences in patients with BPD. In: Greden JF, ed. Treatment of Recurrent Depression. Washington, DC: American Psychiatric Publishing, 2001.
33. Trivedi MH, Shon S, Crismon ML, et al. Texas Implementation of Medical Algorithms (TIMA) Guidelines for Treating MDD. In: TIMA Physician Procedure Manual. Dallas, Texas: Depression Module Texas Medication Algorithm Project, 2000.
34. Michigan Implementation of Medication Algorithms (MIMA) Guidelines for Treating MDD. In: MIMA Physician Procedure Manual, 2004.
35. Suppes T, Dennehy EB. Texas Implementation of Medical Algorithms (TIMA) Guidelines for Treating BPD. In: TIMA Physician Procedure Manual. Dallas, Texas: BPD Module Texas Medication Algorithm Project, 2002.
36. Michigan Implementation of Medication Algorithms (MIMA) Guidelines for Treating BPD. In: MIMA Physician Procedure Manual, 2004.
37. Frank E, Swartz HA, Kupfer DJ. Interpersonal and social rhythm therapy: managing the chaos of BPD. Biol Psychiatry 2000;48:593–604.
38. Swartz HA, Frank E. Psychotherapy for bipolar depression: a phase-specific treatment strategy? BPDs 2001;3:11–22.
39. Simon GE. Social and economic burden of mood disorders. Biol Psychiatry 2003;54(3):208–215.
40. Calabrese JR, Hirschfield RM, Reed M, et al. Impact of BPD on a U.S. community sample. J Clin Psychiatry 2003;64(4):425–432.
41. Keller MD, Beardslee WR, Dorer DJ, et al. Impact of severity and chronicity of parental affective illness on adaptive functioning and psychopathology in children. Arch Gen Psychiatry 1986;43: 930–937.
42. Druss BG, Rosenheck RA, Sledge WH. Health and disability costs of depressive illness in a major US corporation. Am J Psychiatry 2000;157:1274–1278.
43. Marlowe JF. Depression's surprising toll on worker's productivity. Emp Benefits J 2002;27: 16–21.
44. Stewart WF, Ricci JA, Chee E, et al. Cost of lost productive work time among US workers. JAMA 2003;289(23):3135–3144.
45. Dean BB, Gerner D, Gerner RH. A systematic review evaluating health-related quality of life, work impairment, and healthcare costs and utilization in BPD. Curr Med Res Opin 2004;20(2):139–154.
46. Elinson L, Houck P, Marcus SC, et al. Depression and the ability to work. Psychiatr Serv 2004;55: 29–34.
47. Wang PS, Beck AL, Berglund, P, et al. Effects of major depression on moment-in-time work performance. Am J Psychiatry 2004;161:1885–1891.
48. Adler DA, Irish J, McLaughlin TJ, et al. The work impact of dysthymia in a primary care population. Gen Hosp Psychiatry 2004;26(4):269–276.
49. Birnbaum HG, Shi L, Dial E, et al. Economic consequences of not recognizing BPD patients: a cross-sectional descriptive analysis. J Clin Psychiatry 2003;64(10):1201–1209.

Recommended Learning Resources

American Psychiatric Association
www.psych.org

American Psychological Association
www.apa.org

National Alliance on Mental Illness
www.nami.org

Depression and Bipolar Support Alliance, formerly known as the National Depressive and Manic-Depressive Association
www.ndmda.org

National Empowerment Association
www.power2u.org

National Mental Health Association
www.nmha.org

National Institute of Mental Health Depression Awareness, Recognition, and Treatment
D/ART
5600 Fishers Lane
Rockville, MD 20857

Substance Abuse and Mental Health Services Administration
www.samhsa.gov

Consumer survivor mental health information
www.mentalhealth.samhsa.gov/consumersurvivor/link.asp

Texas Medical Algorithm Project site
www.mhmr.state.tx.us/centraloffice/medicaldirector/timasczman.pdf

Anxiety Disorders

Christine K. Urish

Key Terms

γ Aminobutyric acid (GABA)
Anxiety
Agoraphobia
Compulsions
Generalized anxiety disorder
Obsessions
Obsessive-compulsive disorder
Panic
Panic attack
Phobia
Posttraumatic stress disorder
Social phobia

As the occupational therapist arrives on the inpatient psychiatric unit, she finds Vera pacing up and down the hallway. Vera was admitted last evening as a result of her significant functional decline in all areas of occupational performance. She has been diagnosed with **generalized anxiety disorder** by her psychiatrist. "I know my psychiatrist has written a referral for me to attend occupational therapy, I know all about occupational therapy," she states. "I have worked in this hospital on the pediatrics unit for quite some time." "I know the occupational therapists come to the pediatrics unit and play with the children and try to get them to move and interact with their parents." "I don't need to play." "I am so anxious, I worry all the time and it seems as if I worry about everything. I don't really think occupational therapy and play will help me at all."

The occupational therapist suggests Vera come with her to discuss occupational therapy services and to complete an initial interview. The occupational therapist wants to determine how Vera's anxiety is impacting her ability to do everyday things. As the occupational therapist walks down the hall Vera responds by saying, "I'm not able to be a nurse anymore, then what will I do?" "This play therapy is not going to help my anxiety, I cannot do anything right and I am certain this is not going to help me." "What in the world was my psychiatrist thinking when he ordered me to attend occupational therapy groups?" "How in the world is this going to help me at all?"

Vera is obviously thinking that occupational therapy is one-dimensional. In her mind, occupational therapy is about play. The occupational therapist knows she will have to explain to Vera how occupational therapy services on the pediatrics unit differ from an inpatient psychiatric setting. She also knows that she will have to do her best to try and convince Vera that occupational therapy can be beneficial to her. The occupational therapist feels that this information could assist Vera in improving her performance skills and decreasing her anxiety.

The occupational therapist looks forward to the challenge of working with Vera. If Vera will learn relaxation techniques and develop her skill at using them, through participation in occupational therapy services, her level of anxiety may decrease. The occupational therapist also has a feeling that Vera may be so focused on her success and performance at work that Vera's leisure lifestyle may be limited. Although Vera thinks all occupational therapy includes is play, this therapist will work with Vera to assist her in understanding that a balance of work, self-care, and leisure is essential to being productive in daily occupations.

This chapter discusses **anxiety** disorders: how they are classified, diagnosed, and differ from "normal" feelings. Evidence-based research on intervention will be presented throughout the chapter. The impact of anxiety disorders upon performance skills in occupation will be examined through the detailed case studies at the end of the chapter. Learning resources for development of additional knowledge are provided at the end of the chapter as well.

Anxiety

Definition

Anxiety is defined as "apprehension of danger, and dread accompanied by restlessness, tension, tachycardia, and dyspnea unattached to a clearly identifiable stimulus" (1). It is important to distinguish fear from anxiety. Fear is similar in that it is an alerting response to a known, external, definite threat. Anxiety is a response to a threat that is unknown, vague, internal, and can lead to conflicted feelings (2). It is normal to have some degree of anxiety in our lives: "Will I get a raise during my review with my boss?" "Will my dress be appropriate for the social occasion to which I am driving?" "Will I get a good grade on the test I recently completed?" Most often, even if we are nervous or anxious about a number of life events, we are able to perform daily activities and occupations without incident (3). In our day-to-day existence we experience anxiety, whether or not we recognize it as anxiety. Anxiety can motivate us into action. For example: "I'm anxious about my performance review at work at the end of the month, so I will go in early or stay late this week to make sure I am caught up on things," or "I think my clothing is getting tighter, I seem to have put on a few pounds. I need to spend more time exercising to lose some weight and improve my physical appearance." Anxiety, however, can also be pathological, when we worry incessantly about things that we cannot control or change. When this incessant worry begins to negatively impact our ability to work, learn, or socialize, anxiety may be considered pathologic. Anxiety symptoms may vary from individual to individual (2).

Classification of Anxiety Disorders

The *Diagnostic and Statistical Manual of Mental Disorders IV Text Revised (DSM IV-TR)* has established criteria to determine if anxiety or anxiety related conditions are pathologic (4). The criteria present both physical and psychological symptoms that must be met for a diagnosis to be made. Anxiety disorders are considered under Axis I in the *DSM IV-TR* multiaxial system. There are eleven anxiety disorders as classified by the *DSM IV-TR*. They include: **panic** disorder without **agoraphobia**, panic disorder with agoraphobia, agoraphobia without history of panic disorder, specific phobia (formerly known as simple phobia), **social phobia** (also known as social anxiety disorder), **obsessive-compulsive disorder** (OCD), **posttraumatic stress disorder** (PTSD), acute stress disorder, **generalized anxiety disorder**, anxiety disorder due to a general medical condition which is specified, and substance induced anxiety disorder. In this chapter the anxiety disorders of panic disorder, **phobia**, social phobia, OCD, PTSD, and generalized anxiety disorder will be presented in a comprehensive fashion.

Occupational therapists treat clients diagnosed with these disorders in a variety of mental health settings including inpatient, partial hospitalization and outpatient settings. Occupational therapists also treat clients in a variety of nonmental health settings in which they observe anxiety symptoms in the clients they treat across the lifespan. Although occupational therapists do not make psychiatric diagnoses, a thorough understanding of the criteria for making such a diagnosis is important information for the clinician to facilitate clinical observations.

Panic disorder includes short, sudden attacks of fear, fear of losing control or terror (5). The diagnosis of panic disorder without agoraphobia (Panic Disorder) includes at least four panic attacks within the last month, ongoing concern of having additional attacks or worry about the implications of having additional attacks (such as concern over health, having a "heart attack," or "going crazy") and a change in behavior as a result of the panic attacks. The absence of agoraphobia (fear of the marketplace) and the panic attack cannot be a result of the physiologic effects of substance(s), other general medical conditions, or be attributed to another mental disorder such as social phobia or OCD, PTSD, or separation anxiety disorder (4).

Phobias are irrational fears that lead individuals to often avoid certain objects and specific situations all together (6). The diagnosis of phobia includes the individual presenting with marked and persistent fear, which is considered excessive or unreasonable in the face of, or when considering the anticipation of a specific object (animals, seeing blood) or specific situation (preparing to fly on an airplane, having blood drawn, receiving an immunization or shot) (4). Exposure to the feared stimulus produces an anxiety response which may present in the form of a situationally bound or situationally predisposed **panic attack**. According to one of the *DSM IV-TR* diagnostic criteria, individuals with phobia should be able to see the fear that they are experiencing is excessive or unreasonable. Individuals may often avoid environments or situations in which the feared stimulus will be present. If they feel compelled to put themselves in uncomfortable situations, they will endure the environment or situation with a great deal of anxiety and distress (4). The avoidance of the feared stimulus, anticipation, or distress experienced as a result of the feared stimulus interferes with the individual's daily routine including occupational or academic functioning, social activities or interpersonal relationships and there is increased distress surrounding having the phobia.

In persons younger than 18 years of age, the duration of the phobia must be present for at least 6 months. Additionally, the anxiety present in phobias and the accompanying panic attacks (or phobic avoidance with a situation or object) cannot be better accounted for by another mental disorder such as OCD, PTSD, separation anxiety disorder, social phobia, or panic disorder with or without agoraphobia.

There are five different types of specific phobias found in adult clinical populations (7). These phobias, in descending order of frequency seen in clinical settings, include: situational, natural environment, blood injection injury, animal, and other types. Situational phobias include fears of tunnels, bridges, using public transportation, flying in an airplane, and being in closed places. Situational phobias are usually more common in adults than children. Natural environment phobias include fears of natural occurrences such as lightening, thunder, heights, and deep water. These fears often present in childhood. Blood injection injury phobias focus on the fear of receiving an injection or treatment, which requires some invasive bodily procedure. The specific phobia of animals is the fourth most frequently seen phobia in adult clinical populations. This phobia includes insects in addition to animals. The final type of specific phobia is categorized as other type which includes loud sounds, falling, contracting an illness, and choking. A fear of costume characters in children is also considered in this category (7).

The diagnosis of social phobia, also known as social anxiety, is a marked, persistent fear in the presence of strangers. People fear being negatively judged by others. The individual experiences anxiety regarding their social interaction or performance and feels their performance will be scrutinized by these people (4). The person fears that he or she will act in a way that will embarrass or humiliate himself or herself. The person is concerned others will perceive them as weak, crazy or stupid. If public speaking is an activity the individual must perform, he or she may fear others will see their hands and voice tremble and fear that he or she will appear inarticulate (8). When an individual is exposed to the feared social or performance situation, he or she experiences anxiety that may appear as a situationally bound or situationally predisposed panic attack. The individual acknowledges and recognizes that his or her fear is excessive or unreasonable, yet feared performance or social situations are avoided. If the individual must attend a social event or perform he or she endures this experience with a great deal of distress. Consequently, people with this disorder experience a marked impact on the quantity and quality of their daily activities. The individual expresses much distress about having the social phobia condition.

In persons younger than age 18 the duration of this condition must exist for at least 6 months for a diagnosis to be made. For the diagnosis of social phobia to be made, the fear or avoidance of the performance or social situations cannot be attributed to the effects of a substance (medication reaction or drug abuse), a general medical condition or another mental disorder. In considering the diagnosis of social phobia, the consideration of avoidant personality disorder should be critically examined.

To be diagnosed with OCD, an individual must experience either **obsessions** or **compulsions** or both that he/she realizes are unreasonable, unnecessary, are intrusive and which he or she cannot resist (4,5). Obsessions are recurrent persistent thoughts, impulses, or images that are experienced as intrusive, inappropriate, and cause significantly increased anxiety and distress. The thoughts, images, or impulses are not excessive worries about day-to-day problems or events. The individual with OCD may attempt to suppress or ignore these thoughts, images, or impulses or try to counteract these thoughts with other thoughts or actions. The individual is aware that the obsessive thoughts, images or impulses are created through his or her own mind, as opposed to thought insertion.

Compulsions are repetitive acts such as handwashing, straightening, checking, or mental activities such as prayer or silently repeating words (4). The individual feels compelled to perform these acts in response to an obsession or according to specific rules which are typically rigidly applied. The behaviors or mental acts performed by the individual are targeted at preventing or decreasing distress or to prevent a negative (or dreaded) event or situation. Unfortunately, the thoughts and behaviors do not logically relate to the objects of distress they hold in their minds.

In addition to causing marked distress the obsessions or compulsions must consume at least 1 hour or more of time daily and interfere in a significant manner with the individual's routine occupational functioning. The obsessive-compulsive behavior is not a result of a general medical condition or a result of the physiologic effects of a substance (4).

Individuals with OCD have obsessions and compulsive behavior, whereas individuals with PTSD have experienced some form of trauma, which causes extreme psychological stress. PTSD is a psychological stress disorder from exposure to traumatic events such as natural disasters, violent crime (e.g. rape, child abuse, and murder), torture, accidents, or war (5). The diagnosis of PTSD is made when an individual has been exposed to a traumatic event in which he or she experienced, witnessed, or was confronted with situations that threatened or involved death or injury or a threat of death or serious injury to himself or herself or to others (4). The individual's response to the event involved intense fear, helplessness, and horror. This traumatic event is re-experienced in a persistent fashion in one of five ways:

1. Intrusive, recurrent, and distressing recollections of the event which may include images, thoughts, or perceptions.
2. Recurrent dreams that cause distress.
3. Experiencing hallucinations, reliving the experience, illusions, or dissociative experiences.
4. Psychological distress that is intense when experiencing internal or external cues that are symbolic of or are similar to a part of the traumatic event.
5. Physiologic reactions upon exposure to internal or external cues that are symbolic of or are similar to a part of the traumatic event (4).

Individuals with PTSD usually avoid stimuli associated with the traumatic event. They may appear numb, in an overall way, and demonstrate at least three of the following seven characteristics:

1. Attempts to avoid thinking about, feeling emotions related to, or discussing the trauma or anything associated to the trauma.
2. Avoidance of activities, locations or individuals who may facilitate recollection of the traumatic experience.
3. Inability to recall events or aspects of the trauma.
4. Significant decrease in interest or participation in activities that were once identified as meaningful.
5. Feelings of estrangement or detachment from other people.
6. Limitations in the individual's affective range.
7. Limited ability to view future or viewing the future as shortened (4).

Additionally, individuals may present with persistent symptoms of increased arousal as demonstrated by two or more of the following symptoms:

- Difficulty attaining or maintaining sleep
- Irritability or angry outbursts
- Concentration difficulties
- Hypervigilance
- Startle response, which is exaggerated

The duration of symptoms presented must be longer than 1 month and the disturbance must cause significant functional impairment in all areas deemed important to the individual (4).

The final anxiety disorder to be presented is generalized anxiety disorder. This disorder is diagnosed when an individual has excessive worry and anxiety, which occurs more often than not for a period of at least 6 months. This excessive worry or anxiety can include a number of events or activities such as school or work performance or family concerns (4). Individuals have difficulty controlling their worry, and they characteristically also have three or more of the following symptoms:

- Feelings of being on edge, restless, or keyed up
- Becoming easily fatigued
- Feeling as if his or her mind is going blank and difficulty with concentration
- Irritability
- Tension in muscles
- Difficulty with sleep, which can include falling asleep, staying asleep, or restless sleep

The concern of the individual with generalized anxiety disorder is not related to another *DSM IV-TR* Axis I disorder such as OCD (anxiety about contamination) or weight gain as in anorexia nervosa (4). The anxiety, worry, and associated physical symptoms cause the individual difficulty in all areas of functioning important to the individual. The generalized anxiety disorder cannot be a result of the physiologic effects of substances or a general medical condition. This diagnosis cannot occur only during a mood disorder, pervasive developmental disorder, or a psychotic disorder. The *DSM IV-TR* does have a characterization for anxiety disorder due to a general medical condition, as well as, substance induced anxiety disorder and anxiety disorder not otherwise specified (4).

Anxiety disorders may co-exist with other disorder such as depression, substance abuse, eating disorders, schizophrenia, personality disorders, or other anxiety disorders (9). Comorbidity of another mental illness was high when individuals were diagnosed with social phobia and generalized anxiety disorder (10). Per the data from the Epidemiologic Catchment Area survey, there are high rates of comorbidity among Axis I disorders, including 46.5% phobic disorder, 31.7% major depression, 24.1% substance abuse (most commonly alcohol abuse) (11). Individuals diagnosed with social phobia also had high levels of comorbidity with avoidant personality disorder (12). Data from the National Comorbidity Survey suggested close to 50% of persons diagnosed with PTSD also had three or more additional diagnoses, most commonly mood disorders, another anxiety disorder, and substance misuse (13). When considering anxiety disorders from a comprehensive perspective it is important to note that anxiety disorders may co-exist with cancer and heart disease as well (9). It is important for clinicians to consider comorbidity to provide the best intervention for individuals with anxiety disorders and other co-existing conditions in everyday practice.

Etiology

The understanding of the causes of anxiety has increased in recent years as neurochemical and physical pathways of fear and anxiety have been critically examined (14). Despite this, more research needs to be done as we are far from having a clear understanding of these complex conditions. In examining the causes of anxiety disorders one must consider the powerful interaction between biology, cognitive/emotional influences, and stress. The likelihood of developing an anxiety disorder includes a combination of life experiences, psychological traits, and genetic factors. Anxiety disorders such as panic disorder have a stronger genetic basis than other disorders, although at this time specific genes have not been identified (15). Women are more at risk for being diagnosed with anxiety disorders than men, although it is not clear as to why. Some researchers suggest the role of gonadal steroid. Other researchers suggest women's response to stress and their exposure to a wider range of life events is different from those experienced by men (15).

There are three major etiologic considerations in examining anxiety disorders. These include biological factors, genetic factors, and psychosocial factors. Three major schools of psychosocial theory have contributed to the understanding of the causes of anxiety: psychoanalytic, behavioral, and existential. Each of these frameworks present conceptual and practice applications for the treatment of anxiety disorders.

According to the biological theories of anxiety, an excessive autonomic reaction is present with increased sympathetic tone. Increased catecholamines are released in addition to increased production of norepinephrine metabolites. **Aminobutyric acid** (GABA) levels are decreased and this causes central nervous system (CNS) hyperactivity. Additionally, a decrease in serotonin causes anxiety, and increased dopaminergic activity is related to anxiety. The temporal cortex activity in those with anxiety is decreased. The center of the brain, locus ceruleus, is hyperactive when anxiety is present, especially during a panic attack (16). Magnetic resonance imaging (MRI) evidence indicates that individuals with panic disorder have pathology in the temporal lobes of the brain in particular in the hippocampus (2).

Research into the neurotransmitters of those diagnosed with OCD has indicated that dysregulation of serotonin is associated with formation of obsessions and compulsions. When critically examining data from brain imaging studies of individuals diagnosed with OCD, one can see altered neurocircuitry between the orbitofrontal cortex, caudate, and thalamus. Positron emission tomography (PET) scans have shown increased metabolism and blood flow in the basal ganglia and frontal lobe. Research indicates an altered noradrenergic system in individuals diagnosed with PTSD (16). Research has also suggested the possibility of opioid system hyperregulation in individuals with PTSD. Biological research into the etiology of generalized anxiety disorder has focused on GABA and serotonin receptors. There are also indications that genetics may play a role in the etiology of anxiety disorders.

Despite the fact that well-controlled research studies into panic disorder are limited, available genetic research has indicated nearly half the individuals with panic disorder have at least one relative affected with an anxiety disorder (2). Approximately 5% of individuals with high levels of anxiety have a variant of the gene associated with serotonin metabolism (16). Phobias also seem to be more common among family members. More specifically the blood–injection-type phobia has a significantly high familial tendency. Further, first-degree relatives with social phobia are three times more likely to be diagnosed with social phobia than those who have first degree relatives without a mental disorder (2). When considering a genetic link in the diagnosis of OCD, available research supports the hypothesis that the disorder has a genetic component. However, the data at this time does not pinpoint the heritable factors from the influence of behavior and culture.

From a psychoanalytic perspective, anxiety is viewed as developmentally related to childhood fears of disintegration and is related to the fear of loss of a loved one, an object, or fear of castration. Clinicians critically examine possible triggers when working with individuals with anxiety disorders. In people diagnosed with phobias, from a psychoanalytic perspective, the individual attempts to repress. When this fails, other defense mechanisms such as avoidance are called upon (2).

Despite the significant biological underpinning of the diagnosis of OCD, one must consider the psychodynamic meaning associated with the obsessions and compulsions and the secondary gain which the individual may experience as a result of his or her behavior. Additionally, one must recognize the situations and experiences which precipitate or exacerbate the individual's obsessions and compulsions. In examining PTSD from a psychoanalytic perspective, the traumatic experience reactivates an unresolved psychological conflict (2). This results in the use of defenses including repression, regression, denial, splitting, dissociation, guilt, reaction formation, and undoing. Individuals diagnosed with generalized anxiety disorder, according to the psychoanalytic perspective, have unresolved unconscious conflicts.

Behavioral theories propose that anxiety is a response that is learned from exposure to parental behavior or through the process of classical conditioning. Anxiety disorders include faulty, distorted, or counterproductive thinking patterns (16). The successes of treating individuals with anxiety disorders using a behavioral approach lends to the credence of this approach in intervention (2). Anxiety is acquired through classical conditioning and observational learning and maintained through operant conditioning. Learning theory is of significance in the treatment of phobias and provides clear explanation for many symptoms experienced by the phobic individual.

When examining OCD through the template of learning theory, obsessions are viewed as conditioned stimuli and are paired through fear and anxiety with an event that is noxious or anxiety producing. Compulsions are viewed as mechanisms that reduce anxiety attached to an obsessive thought. Over time, the compulsions become less effective in reducing the anxiety (2).

From a cognitive behavioral perspective an individual with PTSD cannot process or rationalize the traumatic experience that caused the diagnosis. The individual continues to experience and re-experience the extreme stress and ineffectively use avoidance as a mechanism for dealing with the stressful experience. Some individuals with PTSD may obtained secondary gain related to their diagnosis such as monetary compensation, increased attention, and others fulfilling their dependency needs. These gains need to be critically examined by the health care practitioner.

According to the cognitive behavioral school of thought, an individual with generalized anxiety disorder has an incorrect and inaccurate perception of danger. This inaccuracy is facilitated by selective attention to negative information within the environment, distortion in information processing, and an inability to cope.

From an existential perspective, there is no one specifically identifiable stimulus that facilitates the feeling of chronic anxiety in an individual. Anxiety, according to an existential approach, occurs when the individual becomes aware of profound feelings of a lack of meaning in their lives. This lack of meaning for some individuals is more fear provoking than thoughts of death. With increased concerns of bioterrorism and nuclear attacks, existential concerns in society have been noted to be increasing (2). Occupational therapy professionals are well suited to address anxiety from an existential perspective as we critically examine meaning and occupation in an individual's day-to-day existence.

Stress is the prime cause of PTSD. However, not every individual will experience PTSD after exposure to a traumatic event. The stress experience in and of itself is not sufficient to cause the disorder. Preexisting biological and psychological factors before, during, and after the trauma must be taken into consideration (2). The cumulative and long-term effects of stress contribute to the development of anxiety and anxiety disorders. Chronic stress places an individual at serious risk for physical illness, emotional, social, and spiritual dysfunction. Clearly, unmanaged chronic stress needs to be identified and addressed (14).

Incidence and Prevalence

In the United States more than 15.7 million individuals suffer from anxiety disorders. Another 11.7 million individuals experience both anxiety and at least one other psychiatric disorder (17). The most prevalent psychiatric disorders are anxiety disorders (18). Less than 30% of individuals who suffer from anxiety disorders, however, seek treatment (18). The incidence for anxiety disorders on an annual basis is 16% in the United States (19). Based upon the best estimate of data from the National Comorbidity Survey and the Epidemiologic Catchment Area (NCS/ECA) study for individuals ages 18 to 54 years, the prevalence of anxiety disorders was 16.4% (15).

The annual cost of anxiety disorders is estimated to be $42.3 billion or approximately $1,542.00 per individual diagnosed (20). Of the total cost, $23.0 billion (54% of cost) are spent in nonpsychiatric medical costs (physician office visits, emergency room costs). Approximately $4.1 billion (10%) is spent in indirect workplace costs, $1.2 billion (3%) in mortality costs, and $0.8 billion (2%) in pharmaceutical (prescription) costs. Costs to the workplace are attributed more to lost productivity rather than absenteeism. Other than phobia, all anxiety disorders were found to be associated with impairment in work performance (20).

Panic Disorder

The prevalence of panic disorder was 1.6% (14). Women are two to three times more likely to be diagnosed with panic disorder than men. An underdiagnosis of panic disorder in men however may skew this distribution (2). The male-to-female ratio for panic disorder without agoraphobia is 1:1 and agoraphobia is 1:2 (16). The ethnic differences present in panic disorder are small. One social factor contributing to the development of a panic disorder is relational, for example, experiencing separation or divorce. The mean age for diagnosis of a panic disorder is 25 years of age. This disorder, however, can occur at any age (2).

Phobia

Specific phobia is considered to be more common than social phobia. In women, specific phobia is the most common mental disorder. In men the most common mental disorder is substance-related disorders with specific phobia being the second most common mental disorder (2). Overall, phobias are the most common mental disorder in the United States with 5% to 10% of the population estimated to be affected (2). Despite the fact that phobias are the most common mental disorder, a significant number of persons do not seek help for their phobia(s) or are misdiagnosed upon seeking medical attention (2). The NCS/ECA best estimate of the prevalence of social phobia, also known as social anxiety disorder, ranged from 2.0% to 7.0%. However the lower percentage represents the percentage of people who are significantly impaired as a result of phobia (15).

Obsessive-Compulsive Disorder

The prevalence of OCD is 2.4% based on NCS/ECA data (15). In adulthood both men and women are likely to be diagnosed with OCD. In adolescence, however, boys appear to be more frequently affected than girls. OCD has a male-to-female ratio of 1:1.

The mean age of diagnosis for OCD is 20 years of age. However, this diagnosis can occur as young as 2 years of age. Individuals who are single are more frequently affected with OCD than individuals who are married. Limitations in the access to health care may be a factor as to why OCD occurs less often in blacks than whites (2).

Generalized Anxiety Disorder

When considering NCS/ECA best estimate data for generalized anxiety disorder prevalence is noted to be 3.4% (15). The male-to-female ratio for this diagnosis is 1:2 (2). The lifetime prevalence for this diagnosis is 5%. In anxiety disorder clinics approximately 25% of the clients treated are diagnosed with generalized anxiety disorder (2).

Posttraumatic Stress Disorder

NCS/ECA best estimate data indicated the prevalence of PTSD to be 3.6% (15). Approximately 30% of individuals who served in the Vietnam War experienced PTSD (2). This is of significant concern given recent events, such as the Gulf War and the extended United States conflicts in Afghanistan and Iraq. Men's and women's experiences differ in relation to the trauma to which they are exposed. The lifetime prevalence of PTSD is higher for women than men. Individuals who are diagnosed with PTSD are more likely to be single, divorced or widowed, withdrawn socially, and have low socioeconomic status. The most significant risk factor for this disorder is the duration, severity, and proximity of the trauma to the individual (2).

Age and Sex

When considering individuals older than age 55 the best estimate prevalence rates based on ECA data for anxiety disorders was 11.4% (15). Prevalence of simple phobia in those older than 55 years of age was 7.3%, OCD was 1.5%, and panic disorder was 0.5% (15). The prevalence rates reported indicate that anxiety disorders are common in the general population (21). Prevalence rates for anxiety disorders according to gender are between one third to two thirds higher in women.

Signs and Symptoms

It is important to consider the messages presented by society as we examine the signs and symptoms of anxiety disorders. Messages such as "Don't Worry, Be Happy" abound. Not to say that this mantra is a bad thing, but it is something that individuals may subscribe to in trying to keep their symptoms "under control" so no one will recognize they are experiencing a great deal of internal turmoil and distress (22). In making a diagnosis of an anxiety disorder, presenting symptoms are the primary consideration. Many anxiety disorders may present with similar physical symptoms. In some disorders, however, the symptoms are more severe, whereas in others the symptoms are not as severe. Although all individuals may experience some degree of fear, worry, and anxiety, health care providers need to critically examine the diagnostic criteria relative to the degree of symptoms present and the duration of symptoms.

Panic Disorder

The diagnosis of panic disorder includes experiencing a panic attack. Symptoms of a panic attack include: heart pounding, increased sweating, feelings of trembling or shakiness, feeling short of breath, feeling as if choking will occur, chest tightness, pain, discomfort, abdominal discomfort, distress or nausea, feeling faint, lightheaded or dizzy, feelings of unreality or depersonalization, fear of going crazy or losing control, fear of death, sensation of tingling or numbness, hot flashes, or chills. Individuals who experience at least four of these symptoms, which appear quickly and peak within 10 minutes, are said to have experienced a panic attack. To obtain the diagnosis of panic disorder an individual must have experienced four attacks within 4 weeks or one attack within the last month with ongoing worry or concern of when another attack will strike (6). Panic attacks typically are short lived but can last up to 10 minutes in duration. Rarely, attacks will last up to 1 hour and can occur while sleeping.

Panic attacks are considered according to three categories: unexpected, situationally bound, and situationally predisposed (23). Unexpected panic attacks typically come "out of the blue" without warning and for no specific reason. Situationally bound panic attacks are just that—situational. Individuals may experience a panic attack each time they are exposed to a particular situation such as driving over a bridge, seeing a snake, or visiting the dentist's office (8,23). Situationally, predisposed panic attacks are situations in which an individual may have a panic attack but the attacks are not consistent. An example of this would be when an individual experiences panic attacks when driving (23). Individuals with panic disorder who reported childhood physical abuse were more likely to have additional comorbid Axis I diagnoses including depression and had a higher likelihood of attempting suicide (24).

Phobia

Symptoms of a phobia include many of the physical symptoms previously presented when discussing panic disorder including sweating, increased heart rate, and trembling (6). Phobias are traditionally classified by the specific fear through the use of Greek or Latin prefixes. For example, acrophobia is the fear of heights, ailurophobia is the fear of cats, pyrophobia is the fear of fire, and xenophobia is the fear of strangers (2). Diagnosis of a phobia should indicate which type of phobia (animal, natural environment, blood injection, situational, other) (4). If the person experiences extreme anxiety when faced with the feared situation or object, the individual's daily routine, social activities, and interpersonal relationships are impacted and, because of these fears, a diagnosis may be made by a qualified and trained professional. Phobias may impact many different areas of occupation depending on the specific feared stimulus of the individual.

In social phobia, the symptoms present are similar to those for specific phobia. In addition the extreme anticipatory anxiety regarding performance or social situations negatively impacts cognition and leads to actual or perceived poor performance in the situations evoking fear, which only further perpetuates the cycle of anxiety (8).

Obsessive-Compulsive Disorder

OCD is characterized by an individual's repetitive thoughts (obsessions) or behaviors (compulsions), or both (5). Individuals may verbalize obsessions as recurrent thoughts, ideas, or images (which can be aggressive or violent in nature) that occupy the individual's consciousness (e.g., arm being attacked by flesh-eating bacteria, obsessing about germs). As much as the individual may try to counteract these thoughts, ideas or images, they remain ever present. Compulsions are repetitive behaviors that are ritualistic and performed according to rules or stereotypical patterns. Excessive behavior (e.g., hand washing to counteract previously presented obsession) may temporarily relieve the tension brought about by the obsessions (5). Common obsessions include fears of germs and contamination; fear of harm to self or others; excessive concern for orderliness; fear of making a mistake or losing a valuable item; constant thoughts of a number, sound, word, or image; or fears of social embarrassment (5).

Symptoms presented by an individual with OCD can range from mild to severe. Some individuals may only experience obsessions and may be able to control their obsessions and associated compulsions for a short period of time, thus hiding the condition from friends, family, and coworkers. This diagnosis is characterized by symptoms that the client perceives as excessive or unreasonable. However, there is a wide range of insight that individuals have in relation to their obsessive-compulsive symptoms. Therefore a subtype of OCD, "poor insight," has been introduced to the *DSM IV-TR* criteria for the diagnosis (25). Clients who demonstrate poor insight tend to overestimate the likelihood of harm and are less likely to benefit from behavioral interventions but can benefit from pharmacologic interventions (26).

Although a common societal misperception exists that OCD focuses exclusively on hand washing, this is only one of many potential compulsive behaviors. Common compulsive behaviors include hand washing and excessive cleanliness of the skin, checking and rechecking of appliances to assure they are turned off and of doors to assure they are locked, counting to a specified number repeatedly, repeating words or specific actions several times in a row throughout the day, arranging of items in a rigid and specific order, and hoarding and collecting items that are no longer needed such as mail or newspapers (5).

Posttraumatic Stress Disorder

People with PTSD may relive the traumatic event over and over to the point of becoming emotionally numb. They can experience chronic anxiety, exaggerated startle response, trouble with concentration on tasks, nightmares, and insomnia. Individuals with this diagnosis may vehemently avoid situations that would remind them of the traumatic event as this will cause increased distress and could cause a panic attack (6). Symptoms that last less than 3 months are considered acute PTSD. Symptoms that last longer than 3 months are considered chronic in nature (4). Individuals with PTSD may use alcohol or drugs to self-medicate and try to "forget" about the traumatic experience. This compounds the problems experienced in the areas of occupation for the person as not only are they dealing with the symptoms of PTSD, but they are also dealing with the negative effects of drug and alcohol use. Depression is comorbid with PTSD and suicide risk associated with this diagnosis is one to which practitioners need to be attentive (2).

Generalized Anxiety Disorder

Symptoms of generalized anxiety disorder include chronic tension, exaggerated worry, and irritability. These symptoms that do not appear to have a cause, present as more intense than a situation would warrant. Physical symptoms can include restlessness, difficulty with sleep (both falling asleep and staying asleep), increased headaches, trembling, muscle twitches, tension, and sweating. A diagnosis can be made when an individual has been worried excessively about everyday problems for greater than 6 months (6).

The *DSM IV-TR* diagnostic criteria are most commonly used in examining the signs and symptoms of anxiety disorders to make a diagnosis. Other psychological tests that may be used include: Rorschach test, thematic apperception test, Bender-Gestalt, draw a person, the Minnesota multiphasic personality inventory II, state-trait anxiety inventory, hamilton anxiety rating scale, and the zung self rated anxiety scale (16,19). At present there are no specific laboratory tests that can be used to diagnose anxiety.

Course and Prognosis

Despite a specific course and prognosis identified for each anxiety disorder, health providers should carefully consider the unique characteristics of each client when establishing intervention plans.

Panic Disorder

The age of onset for panic disorder is typically early to middle adulthood (27). However, onset can occur at childhood, early adolescence, or midlife (2). Panic disorder is associated with increased risk of agoraphobia and depression. Panic disorder is more common in young or middle-aged individuals and those who live alone (28). One relationship factor identified as contributing to panic disorder is the history of a recent divorce or separation (2). Comorbidity of depression, substance abuse, and other anxiety disorders are associated with poor prognosis.

Considered a chronic condition, the course of panic disorder is variable across clients as well as within a single individual. Studies that have examined intervention for panic disorder are not easily interpreted because of the inability of researchers to control for the effects of treatment (2). However, 30% to 40% of individuals have presented as symptom free after long-term follow-up. One half of individuals with this diagnosis continue to have symptoms but these symptoms are mild enough to not significantly impact their lives. Approximately 10% to 20% of individuals continue to have symptoms despite treatment (2).

It is important that clinicians use a psychometrically sound instrument such as the Panic Disorder Severity Scale to monitor clients and determine if symptoms are reoccurring to facilitate treatment modification. By responding to recurrence of symptoms, a complete relapse may be avoided (29). Full remission of all symptoms is the goal for individuals diagnosed with panic disorder, and individuals are considered to have met this standard when they no longer meet the diagnostic criteria in the *DSM IV-TR* for 6 months or longer (29).

Phobia

The most common phobia among women is a fear of animals and among men is a fear of heights (30). Phobias are the most common anxiety disorder. Individuals may commonly avoid the feared stimulus and may go to extreme lengths to avoid the feared stimulus (2). Depression is a comorbid condition in approximately one third of people with phobia. Animal phobia, natural environment phobia, and blood-injection phobia appear to peak at childhood. Other phobias have a peak onset at early adulthood. Phobias have been found to run in families, especially blood-injection phobia (16).

Limited data exist regarding the course of specific phobia despite being the most common anxiety disorder. Individuals frequently do not seek treatment for this condition and may live with anxiety for many years. The condition appears to remain constant and does not appear to have the waxing and waning progression that is seen in other anxiety disorders. For individuals who do seek treatment, a positive response to intervention was associated with better long-term outcomes (31). One study that examined outcomes of individuals diagnosed with phobia 10 to 16 years after treatment challenged the notion that recovery from this diagnosis is characterized by complete and lasting remission from symptoms (31).

Social Phobia. The most misunderstood and least studied of the anxiety disorders is social phobia (32). The age of onset for individuals with social phobia is childhood or adolescence and the individual may experience symptoms of the disorder for many years. Parental psychopathology, including social phobia, depression, and parenting style (overprotection or rejection), have been associated with development of social phobia in youth (33). This disorder is commonly associated with substance dependence, depression, avoidant personality disorder, panic disorder, and generalized anxiety disorder (34).

Social phobia is more common in women than in men. Social phobia has onset before other psychiatric conditions (35). Additionally, psychiatric conditions complicate approximately one third of those diagnosed with social phobia. Early intervention of social phobia may prevent the onset of other psychiatric conditions (35). Without intervention the course of social phobia is chronic and unremitting. A significant concern relative to this disorder is the strong tendency of society, including mental health professionals, to trivialize this disorder (32).

Obsessive-Compulsive Disorder

OCD is typically diagnosed in adolescence or early adulthood. Over half of the individuals with OCD experience sudden onset of symptoms. Between 50% to 70% of the symptoms occur after a stressful event such as death of a loved one, pregnancy, or sexual problems (2). If untreated, however, as the condition progresses individuals may become so consumed by obsessions and compulsions that they are unable to function in work or complete daily living activities because so much time is spent engaged in rituals (36). Because of the desire of the individual to "hide" their condition, diagnosis and treatment are challenging. Individuals with OCD often do not receive intervention until as many as 5 to 10 years after the initial onset of symptoms (2). Between 20% to 30% of individuals can experience significant improvement in their symptoms, 40% to 50% may experience moderate improvement and the remaining 20% to 40% may have continuation or worsening of symptoms (2). One third of individuals diagnosed with OCD also are diagnosed with depression. Suicide is a significant risk for this comorbidity (2).

OCD can be accompanied by depression, eating disorders, substance abuse, attention deficit hyperactivity disorder, and other anxiety disorders. Effective intervention for these conditions is essential for the successful treatment of OCD (9). Poor prognosis is associated with the following characteristics: yielding to compulsions, childhood onset, bizarre compulsions, delusional beliefs, and comorbid personality disorder. The content of an individual's obsessions does not appear to be related to prognosis (2).

Posttraumatic Stress Disorder

The course of PTSD can be from as short as 1 week after exposure to a trauma to as much as 30 years after exposure. Therefore, PTSD can be diagnosed at any age at which an individual experiences an extreme trauma. The male-to-female ratio for this diagnosis is 1:2 (16). Symptoms may vary with time and may be most extreme in cases of increased stress. Without treatment, 30% of individuals who would have been diagnosed with PTSD will recover, whereas 40% will continue to experience mild symptoms, 20% moderate symptoms, and 10% will remain the same or experience a worsening of symptoms (2). Of individuals diagnosed with PTSD, 50% will recover within 1 year.

Individuals who are very young and individuals who are very old have more difficulty with traumatic events than do those individuals at midlife (2). This is associated with the fact that the young person may not have yet developed effective coping strategies to deal with the trauma and the older individual may have more rigid coping strategies that may be ineffective when presented with a traumatic experience. Individuals who experience rapid onset of symptoms of short duration, who had good premorbid functioning and experience positive social supports are more apt to experience a good prognosis. Furthermore, individuals who do not have a co-existing physical disability, substance-related disorder, or other medical condition are also more likely to have a good prognosis (2).

Generalized Anxiety Disorder

The age of onset for generalized anxiety disorder is variable and difficult to pinpoint. It can occur as early as childhood (2). Individuals, when questioned about their symptoms, often recall feeling anxious as long as they can remember. This condition tends to worsen without treatment and especially during times of increased stress (7). One third of individuals with generalized anxiety disorder symptoms seek psychiatric intervention. More often these individuals present to family practitioners, cardiologists, internists, or gastroenterologists from whom they are seeking relief for the somatic concerns that they are experiencing as a result of this condition (2). Because of a high incidence of comorbidity of generalized anxiety disorder with other psychiatric conditions, a specific course and prognosis are difficult to identify. Generalized anxiety disorder can be viewed as a chronic condition in which the individual may experience symptoms which can be lifelong (2).

Medical/Surgical Management

Society has become more aware and accepting of identification and treatment of mental illness over the last several years. This is apparent through public health initiatives targeted at addressing mental health concerns such as national mental illness awareness week, anxiety screening day, and depression screening day as well as through the increasing amount of information regarding mental illness, diagnosis, and treatment available via the Internet (37,38).

Current guidelines for treatment of severe mental illness can be found in four different categories (39). These categories vary depending on the score and stringency for which the guidelines rely on research evidence. The categories include:

- Recommendations
- Comprehensive treatment options
- Algorithms
- Expert consensus guidelines

In 1998, comprehensive treatment options were developed for panic disorder by the American Psychiatric Association (APA) (40). However, the strength of evidence presented in support of these treatment options is less stringent than Patient Outcomes Research Team (PORT) recommendations. PORT treatment recommendations for schizophrenia were developed by the United States Agency for Health Care Policy and Research. The PORT project critically examined literature, which was then followed by expert review. The PORT recommendations contain very specific evidence of efficacy of treatment interventions that supported the utilization of these interventions. The APA guidelines developed for panic disorder were by a professional organization and did not require the evidence considered for inclusion to be as stringent as the guidelines used for the development of PORT. As a result, the APA treatment guidelines are less prescriptive than the PORT treatment recommendations. Treatment guidelines have also been developed for PTSD by the International Society for Traumatic Stress Studies. These guidelines strongly endorse the use of specific serotonin re-uptake inhibitors as a first-line medication for the treatment of PTSD (41).

Algorithms, a single rule or set of rules, are used when solving a problem. Medication algorithms are considered within practice guidelines. Algorithms provide practitioners with a step-by-step approach to clinical decisions considering medications. At present the Texas Medication Algorithm Project has the most extensive collection of medication algorithms for persons with mental illness. Unfortunately, there are no algorithms for anxiety disorder treatment. Algorithms do exist, however, for schizophrenia, bipolar disorder, and major depressive disorder (39).

The last category is expert consensus guidelines. These are recommendations based upon surveys completed by a comprehensive array of experts in the treatment of identified conditions. These guidelines do not rely on critical analysis of research literature. The rationale provided for the development of these expert guidelines is related to the fact that research literature at times does not address specific points in treatment decision making. At present, expert treatment guidelines exist for OCD and PTSD. In addition to expert treatment guidelines for practitioners, guidelines have been developed for patients and families regarding these diagnoses (39).

People with anxiety disorders are three to five times more likely to seek the care of a physician and six times more likely to be hospitalized for a psychiatric disorder (23). From an occupational therapy perspective their functional abilities would be assessed and it would be determined how their anxiety was impacting activities of daily living, Instrumental activities of daily living (IADLs), education, work, play, leisure and social participation. The occupational therapist may consider administering an activity configuration, role checklist, interest checklist, or self-assessment of occupational functioning to determine functional deficits (42).

Most common treatments for anxiety disorders include a combination of pharmacologic and psychological interventions with the exception of specific phobia for which there is no good pharmacologic treatment (7). Remission is the ultimate goal for the treatment of anxiety disorders (43). Occupational therapy intervention would be targeted at changing performance deficits in areas of occupation as a result of the symptoms experienced by the person (42). Although some individuals may continue to experience symptoms of anxiety throughout their lives, occupational therapy intervention can be focused toward the development or reestablishment of meaningful daily routines. Engagement in meaningful occupation can serve to facilitate adaptation, which can lead to improved health and wellness, quality of life, and positive life satisfaction. It is important to remain client centered as interventions that may reduce anxiety in one individual may prove ineffective for another.

Medications utilized to treat anxiety disorders include anxiolytics and antidepressants, specifically serotonin re-uptake inhibitors (2). One should be cautious when working with clients who are on benzodiazepines who have addiction concerns as these medications are highly addictive. Further, older adults are at risk of falls when on benzodiazepines because of side effects impacting balance as a result of the half-life of the medication. Side effects of benzodiazepines include sedation and fatigue, cognitive and memory impairments, delayed reaction time, impaired balance and coordination, hangover effects, withdrawal, and abuse potential.

For individuals diagnosed with panic disorder, antidepressant medication such as paroxetine hydrochloride (Paxil), which is a selective serotonin re-uptake inhibitor, or benzodiazepines such as alprazolam (Xanax) are approved by the Food and Drug Administration (FDA) and are often prescribed (2,7). Paxil has been shown to be effective with individuals diagnosed with social phobia. Benzodiazepines may be used for social phobia on a very short-term basis. For the pharmacologic treatment of OCD, antidepressant medications such as fluvoxamine maleate (Luvox) and clomipramine hydrochloride (Anafranil) have been shown to be effective interventions (7). Caution should be exercised when pharmacologic interventions are considered with individuals diagnosed with PTSD as substance abuse disorder can complicate the pharmacologic choices (44). Antidepressants such as sertraline hydrochloride (Zoloft), anticonvulsants such as carbamazepine (Tegretol), and antipsychotic medications such as olanzapine (Zyprexa) are considered for individuals with PTSD (7). With the use of consistent and ongoing antidepressant therapy, the remission rate of anxiety disorders is improved. However, response to medications is very individualized and many clients may need extended time in treatment before a benefit is obtained (43).

Some research has indicated cognitive behavioral interventions are superior to pharmacologic approaches whereas other research indicates the contrary (2). In considering cognitive behavioral interventions for anxiety disorders, a variety of interventions exist. Findings from one study indicated when treating individuals with panic disorder, progress can be obtained through the use of a self-help workbook and brief therapist contact (45). An emphasis on family and client psychoeducation focusing on symptomatology, nature and course of panic disorder, and lifestyle modifications have been suggested as evidence based intervention which cost less (in Australia) than the cost of drug therapy over a 1-year period of time (46).

The APA's comprehensive treatment guidelines for panic disorder indicate most individuals can be treated on an outpatient basis and may rarely require hospitalization (40). Cognitive behavioral interventions suggested by the APA include the use of psychoeducation, panic monitoring, breathing monitoring, anxiety management skill development, cognitive restructuring, and in vivo exposure. Establishing and maintaining a therapeutic alliance with the individual diagnosed with panic disorder was viewed as a key element in successful intervention. Educating the individual on the early signs of relapse was considered a significant consideration for successful outcome of remission of panic symptoms.

Panic Disorder

From an occupational therapy perspective, individuals with panic disorder may need assistance in the area of IADLs. People may be fearful of leaving the house and therefore community mobility may be impaired. Systematic desensitization can be useful, but very stressful for individuals in addressing this fear (47). Relaxation training including deep breathing, progressive muscle relaxation, visualization and autogenic training are effective interventions utilized by occupational therapy practitioners for individuals with panic disorder and phobias (48).

Phobia

When considering other available interventions for phobia, 70% to 85% of individuals responded with clinically significant improvement when exposure was used as a behavioral intervention. The addition of cognitive components appeared to add little efficacy (21). Therapist-directed exposure was suggested rather than self-directed exposure to the feared stimulus. Although some studies have used virtual reality techniques as intervention for the treatment of phobias, this may be cost prohibitive and technically challenging but could provide a clinic with the ability to expose the client to a wide range of feared stimuli (21).

Social Phobia. When considering evidence-based intervention for social phobia, five cognitive behavioral treatments including exposure therapy, cognitive restructuring, exposure coupled with cognitive restructuring, social skills training, and relaxation were compared and found to be moderately effective with no differences obtained at the end of the study or at the follow-up (49). Further, both individual and group interventions were found to be equally beneficial to individuals with this diagnosis. Some obstacles to effective treatment for social phobias are:

- The individual's avoidance of treatment because of fear, shame, or stigma.
- Limited screening to assess social phobia are available at present.
- Assessment and intervention may be directed toward somatic complaints expressed by the individual rather than the social phobia syndrome.
- Physicians lack knowledge of effective treatment options or they trivialize the client's concerns or view them as unchangeable (50).

Despite these facts, cognitive behavior therapy is useful when treating social phobia (9). Both cognitive therapy and exposure therapy present good efficacy and the combination present the largest effect sizes in meta-analytic reviews (21). There is limited research on the efficacy of social skills training with social phobia.

Obsessive-Compulsive Disorder

Expert treatment guidelines exist for the treatment of OCD (50,51). These guidelines address specific cognitive behavioral strategies, medications, maintenance of treatment, treatment of comorbidities, and minimizing medication side effects. Guidelines for families and patients have also been developed. Treatment for OCD commonly combines medication and behavioral intervention to achieve effectiveness.

Exposure and response prevention has been identified as the most useful intervention in treating this condition. In this approach the individual is deliberately and voluntarily exposed to what triggers their obsessive thoughts. The individual is then taught techniques to avoid performing the compulsive behaviors and how to cope with the associated anxiety (9). Although exposure and response prevention has been shown to be effective, it is important to note it may facilitate a reduction in symptoms, rather than a removal of symptoms. Some individuals continue to display ongoing distress even after intervention (21).

Posttraumatic Stress Disorder

Medications are used with caution in individuals with PTSD because of the concern of self-medication and the potential for substance abuse. Specific serotonin re-uptake inhibitors (SRIs) are suggested for individuals with this diagnosis (7,41). Expert consensus guidelines exist for the treatment of PTSD. These guidelines provide insight into recommended treatment interventions based on the most prominent symptoms present. For example, if an individual experiences intrusive thoughts, exposure therapy is suggested. If irritability and/or angry outbursts are present, cognitive therapy and anxiety management are suggested. Anxiety management training as specified in the guidelines includes relaxation training, breathing retraining, positive thinking and self-talk, assertiveness training, and thought stopping (41).

Cognitive therapy focusing on assisting people in modifying their unrealistic assumptions, beliefs, and automatic thoughts can be implemented by trained professionals. Exposure therapy, play therapy, and psychoeducation are examples of effective intervention for individuals with PTSD. Group therapy in which the individual can talk with others who have had similar experiences has been found to be effective intervention. Opportunities to express emotion are valuable. Activities including drawing emotions and experiences can be viewed by the individual as both relaxing and cathartic (47). Individuals may need assistance in re-establishing social relationships, work, and leisure participation.

Limited research has been completed examining the link between sensory defensiveness in adults and increased anxiety (52). It is hypothesized that many symptoms of sensory defensiveness may be interchangeable with psychiatric disorders including generalized anxiety disorder. Research has explored the use of sensory integration interventions for decreasing anxiety levels by using deep pressure, tactile, and proprioceptive activities (53).

Generalized Anxiety Disorder

Generalized anxiety disorder can be addressed using cognitive therapy focusing on education and lifestyle alterations focusing on how the external environmental influences internal feelings. Addressing diet (caffeine intake), medication use (over-the-counter [OTC] medications may increase anxiety), and the need for regular exercise can also be helpful in addressing generalized anxiety disorder (42). Further, rational/ cognitive approaches which focus on assisting the person in replacing negative self statements with more positive ones can be effective with individuals diagnosed with generalized anxiety disorder. Time management activities that assist the individual in prioritizing activities may assist in decreasing anxiety as well. Expressive activities such as journal writing, drawing, or other craft activities can provide a mechanism for the individual to communicate their feelings and may assist in the development of coping skills (42).

Clinicians should be mindful regarding the length of intervention provided to individuals with anxiety disorders. Outpatient sessions between 6 and 7 weeks were deemed too short by clients in two different studies (54,55). Structured course content should include opportunities for skill development, communication, and practice with ongoing monitoring by the clinician. Cognitive aspects of intervention such as relaxation training and assertiveness were found to be most beneficial per client report. An 8-week course was felt to allow more time for learning and practice of the cognitive aspects of the course deemed most important by those diagnosed with anxiety disorders.

Impact of Conditions on Occupational Performance

The impact of anxiety disorders on client factors is dependent on the specific disorder with which the client is diagnosed. In the area of mental functions, specifically global mental functions, sleep, temperament, and energy can be impacted by the diagnosis of an anxiety disorder. In the area of specific mental functions, the following areas are impacted:

- Attention
- Reduced recall (memory)
- Impaired ability to make associations
- Time management
- Problem solving
- Decision making
- Emotional functions in the area of self control (2)

From a sensory perspective, individuals with an anxiety disorder may demonstrate increased startle response. Physical signs present in anxiety disorder from a neuromuscular and movement-related perspective include: feeling shaky, muscle tension, backache, headache, and fatigue. From a cardiovascular and respiratory perspective, symptoms include tachycardia and hyperventilation, which can lead to syncope (passing out). From a gastrointestinal (GI) perspective clients may experience signs of diarrhea and have the feeling of an upset stomach or "butterflies" in the stomach. When considering the genitourinary system and reproductive functions, clients may experience urinary frequency and decreased libido, which could relate to reproduction or lack of desire for sexual relationships (2,4,7).

Panic Disorder

The symptoms an individual may experience during a panic attack can have a negative impact upon the many different areas of occupation, including care of others, care of pets, child rearing, community mobility, safety and emergency response, educational participation, job performance, and leisure and social participation. A common concern of individuals who experience panic disorder is *when* the next attack will occur. This fear can significantly alter daily routines and habits. This can have a negative impact upon his or her ability to initiate performance in daily activities. The individual who experiences a panic disorder and has children may worry about the wellbeing of his or her children. He or she may feel as if he or she is dying while having an attack. Those experiencing symptoms of panic disorder may begin restricting themselves to their residence for fear of having a panic attack while in public and this behavior can facilitate another diagnosis, agoraphobia.

Phobia

Social phobia impacts the areas of educational participation, such as having to get up in front of class and give a presentation. Their job performance, as well as other social roles and responsibilities, may be impaired. Communication skills may be negatively affected because of the individual's significant level of anxiety. Individuals with social phobia may experience low self esteem due to their inability to perform up to self-imposed standards yet they frequently do not seek assistance for their concerns. Individuals with this disorder may be characterized by others as "nervous" or "ineffective" in social situations.

Obsessive-Compulsive Disorder

Areas of occupation impacted by OCD can include activities of daily living, instrumental activities of daily living, education, work, play, leisure, and social participation. OCD has a negative impact upon the individual's process skills. Typically motor and communication skills are not impacted (47). The obsessive and compulsive rituals engaged in by the individual can occur indirectly in any of these areas or can indirectly negatively affect another area. For example a client who obsesses about turning off all the lights in the house prior to leaving for work may be frequently late to work, which will most likely have a negative impact on his or her work performance. The obsession and compulsion are related to home management but may negatively impact job performance because of the poor work habit of arriving late. Occupational therapy interventions can assist the individual with OCD to develop improved coping skill, and to explore issues related to the obsessive thoughts and compulsive actions. Performance patterns are seriously impacted in individuals diagnosed with OCD. Occupational therapy interventions can work to facilitate change in this area (47). Client motivation is a significant factor in the success of behavioral interventions for OCD (56).

Posttraumatic Stress Disorder

PTSD can impact activities of daily living to the point where the person does not care about their personal hygiene and grooming. Sleep is of significant concern as the person may experience nightmares and flashbacks. IADLs can be negatively impacted in the areas of care of others, care of pets, child rearing, financial management (especially if alcohol and drug use/abuse are present), health management/maintenance, home management, educational participation, job performance, leisure performance, and all aspects of social participation. Roles, routines, and habits can be negatively impacted through flashbacks and re-experiencing the trauma. Process skills are negatively impacted because of intrusive thoughts experienced by the individual. No concerns are typically present in motor and communication skills (47). Family and friends may notice these problems and try to provide assistance. Denial, however, is common and the person may refuse assistance or treatment.

Generalized Anxiety Disorder

Any area of occupation can be impacted by generalized anxiety disorder. The individual may express excessive worry about himself or herself and his or her own health and well-being (IADLs) or his or her educational participation, job performance, as well as social participation. This anxiety disorder is one that many people express as similar to the gray cloud of worry that follows them everywhere and as such impacts every area of occupation.

CASE STUDY

Case Illustrations

■ CASE 1—GENERALIZED ANXIETY DISORDER

Vera is a 34-year-old registered nurse. She has worked in nursing for 13 years on a hospital pediatrics unit. For the last 7 months, for more days than not, Vera finds it difficult to control her level of anxiety and worry. She is worried about getting along with coworkers, pleasing the physicians with whom she works, and interacting appropriately with the parents of the children for whom she is providing care. Additionally, Vera has been worrying about her children's school performance and the fact that many companies in her community are downsizing. Although her husband has frequently reassured her that his position is stable, she cannot help but worry that he will lose his job or be demoted.

Vera also worries about her difficulty attending to her tasks as a nurse. She finds her mind going blank and she has difficulty concentrating on what a physician is saying to her while she is doing rounds. Three times during the last month she has recorded physician's orders incorrectly. The unit secretary has *caught* these errors and brought them to Vera's attention. Vera is demonstrating difficulty responding in an appropriate fashion to safety concerns, which are typically presented in her workplace such as "Code Blue." She feels others know of her problems. She is concerned about her relationships with her coworkers since she is so preoccupied by her anxiety, she finds herself irritable at work and has "snapped" at a several different coworkers over the last few months.

Vera has been having difficulty falling and staying asleep. She has been awakening 2 to 3 hours early and is not able to fall back to sleep. As a result she feels fatigued and has been experiencing increased muscle tension, backaches, and frequent headaches. Vera describes her *keyed-up* feelings of restlessness like "walking on eggshells." Vera expresses frustration in her lack of ability to relax and inability to decrease her anxiety. Vera expresses decreased appetite and has experienced noticeable weight loss over the last 7 months.

At home, Vera has not been preparing meals for her family as she had in the past, rather has been relying solely on frozen dinners and take out food for family dining. Vera *picks up* the house but does not clean per se. She verbalizes feelings of fatigue and lack of desire to keep things clean in her home. Although she expresses numerous interests including sewing, cooking, reading, and walking she has not been able to participate in these leisure activities because of her anxiety level and accompanying fatigue. Vera had previously been active as a volunteer at her church and involved in activities at her children's school, but at this time she feels so overwhelmed she is unable to complete these tasks. She has been caring for her children marginally. She has experienced difficulty helping them with their school work and has been distant or short with them in her communication.

Vera's husband and friends have noticed a change in Vera's behavior, as well. Although they have been supportive and encouraging of Vera, they do not know what to do or how to assist her in diminishing her level of worry. Vera agrees to go on family outings in the community with her husband and children, but at the last minute, she backs out. Infrequently she will speak to friends on the phone but has not gone to social activities with her friends in months.

Financially, Vera and her family have money in their savings, live comfortably, and have been saving for their children's college education and their retirement. Despite these facts, Vera spends between 4 to 6 hours each weekend reviewing the financial status of the family and constantly worrying about expenses that are considered by many others to be *routine* expenditures.

Vera has seen a psychiatrist who has prescribed medication and supportive psychotherapy 1 week ago. Despite Vera's complaints of fatigue the psychiatrist encouraged her to try to walk one to two times per week as physical exercise is beneficial to those with generalized anxiety disorder. Additionally, deep breathing exercises were reviewed in attempts to decrease her level of anxiety. Vera plans to continue to pursue therapy on an outpatient basis with a psychologist and occupational therapist for relaxation training and to critically examine life stressors and coping mechanisms to deal with her current level of anxiety.

■ CASE 2—OBSESSIVE-COMPULSIVE DISORDER

Lisa is a 28-year-old female who ruminates about the potential for her car and other valuable items in her possession to catch fire. In preparing to leave to go anywhere she repeatedly walks around the car and opens and closes the hood several times before getting in the car. Once she starts the car, she allows the car to idle for a few minutes but then turns off the car, walks around the car and then again opens the hood. She repeats this routine at least three times before she is able to drive anywhere. It is not uncommon for Lisa to pull off the road and repeatedly turn her car off and on and open the hood to make sure the car is not on fire. Lisa is constantly late to work and social engagements because of her obsessive and compulsive routine regarding transportation. Lisa vehemently refuses to ride with others because they will not stop when she wants to stop to allow her to get out and check their car for signs of fire. Recently the police followed Lisa and pulled her over for her erratic behavior in driving and her frequent stops on the side of the road to check her car for signs of fire.

In her home, Lisa is constantly plugging and unplugging in electrical appliances because she is fearful that if she leaves them plugged in her home will catch fire. Lisa lives alone in a single-family home. Her family is unaware of her behavior as she is estranged from her parents and is an only child. Lisa frequently stares at light bulbs to make sure that the light is off despite the fact that she had turned off the light switch. This delays Lisa's ability to leave her home in a timely fashion.

As a result of being home a great deal of time, Lisa has become a compulsive shopper using television shopping channels for leisure and entertainment. She has numerous items that she has ordered and not taken out of the boxes that are piled in the corner of her living room. Lisa is also experiencing difficulties in the area of financial management because of her compulsive shopping behaviors and her inconsistent employment status. She has recently begun a new job as a customer service representative for a telemarketing company. She has been recently reprimanded several times for spending excessive time speaking with older adult customers who call in to the center.

Lisa does not eat healthy meals and does not like to leave her house to purchase food. As a result she is gaining weight and her blood pressure is elevated. In the area of self care, Lisa is meticulous about her personal appearance spending great lengths of time to make sure her hair, makeup, nails, and clothing are coordinated and appropriate for the event.

After 7 years of college, Lisa graduated with a bachelor of arts degree in English from a private college. She has never been able to secure the type of employment she desires, which would be creative writing. It took Lisa longer to graduate as she would frequently drop classes mid-semester if she did not attain the grade that she felt she should have been receiving from the course instructor. Lisa has held seven jobs since she graduated from college 2 years ago. She is often fired for absenteeism, tardiness, or decreased productivity on the job because of her obsessive-compulsive behavior at work.

Socially, Lisa does not participate in community activities, is estranged from her family and relies on her coworkers as friends. As a result of her frequent job changes she has a limited number of friends. Lisa has alienated herself from college friends and roommates who have tried to provide caring feedback about her behavior.

■ CASE 3—POSTTRAUMATIC STRESS DISORDER

Eric is a 23-year-old male who served in the war in Iraq. He is a member of the United States Marine Corps Reserve and was responsible for delivering equipment and supplies along various routes in Iraq. During his 18 months in Iraq, he was in several convoys that were shot at by insurgents. On one occasion, despite orders to not leave his vehicle, Eric ran to a vehicle in need of emergency assistance. Upon arrival at the vehicle which was engulfed in flames, Eric removed two of the four passengers who were already deceased as a result of an insurgent attack. After this event, Eric began having flashbacks, seeing the faces of his dead comrades in his dreams. Each time Eric would leave his base for a delivery of supplies after the event, he would be hypervigilant because of his fears of his convoy being attacked. While in Iraq, he reported auditory flashbacks of the attack on his convoy in which he tried to rescue his fellow soldiers. As a result of this experience, Eric reported decreased ability to sleep while in Iraq and now that he is home he continues to demonstrate an inability to obtain a restful night's sleep. After this incident, Eric was noticed to be isolative from the other members of his unit. His superior noticed this behavior and attempted to get assistance for Eric, but he vehemently refused. Upon arrival in the United States, Eric's family and friends hosted numerous celebrations for him. Prior to his tour of duty in Iraq, Eric was a friendly and outgoing individual. Since his return, he does not like to have attention drawn to himself and his family is concerned about his "loner" behavior as he has been isolative since his return from Iraq. Eric has not been participating in community activities at this time. Prior to going to Iraq, Eric was active in his church and was a member of the Jaycees. However, at present, he rarely goes out with "the gang from work," an activity in which he participated regularly prior to going to Iraq. When friends call and ask him to participate in social activities, he states he will, but then fails to follow though and attend these events.

In the area of work, upon his return to civilian life, Eric has returned to his position as a journeyman and he is working toward becoming an electrician. Eric has been home nearly 2 months. The attack he continues to re-experience occurred 4 months ago. He has experienced difficulty on the job in the areas of concentration, exaggerated startle response and irritability with his coworkers. Eric has been calling in sick as a result of his excessive drinking behavior, has been showing up for work late, and has gotten into arguments with supervisors and coworkers who have expressed concerns about his behavior. Eric has not been completing tasks as assigned, rather he is verbalizing "he knows a better way" to do things. Eric has experienced difficulties in the area of safety procedures/emergency response during the fulfillment of his duties as an electrician.

Eric is single, and lives on his own. His parents and siblings reside in the same community. Eric has expressed his difficulty with sleep to his mother who is a nurse. He states he has difficulty falling asleep and often wakes up with vivid dreams of the attack on his convoy in which his comrades were killed. Eric has been lifting weights by himself at home. He has not been participating in any social or community leisure activities aside from an occasional beer and game of darts at a local tavern. After the attack, Eric was noted to be using alcohol on an increased basis to cope with the stressful event he experienced.

References

1. Dirckx JH. Steadman's Concise Medical Dictionary for the Health Professional. Philadelphia: Lippincott, Williams & Wilkins, 2001.
2. Sadock BJ, Sadock VA. Kaplan & Sadock's synopsis of psychiatry. 9th Ed. Philadelphia: Lippincott, Williams & Wilkins, 2003.
3. Grey House Publishing. The Complete Mental Health Directory. New York: Sedgwick Press, 2004.
4. American Psychiatric Association. Diagnostic and statistical manual of mental disorders IV. 4th Ed., text revision. Washington: American Psychiatric Association, 2000.
5. John Hopkins. Anxiety Disorders. Available at: http://www.hopkinsafter50.com. Accessed September 20, 2004.
6. Substance Abuse and Mental Health Services Administration. Anxiety Disorders. Available at: http://www.mentalhealth.org/publications/allpubs/ken98–0045/default.asp. Accessed August 26, 2004.
7. Fadem B. Behavioral Science in Medicine. Philadelphia: Lippincott, Williams & Wilkins, 2004.
8. American Psychiatric Association. Diagnostic and statistical manual of mental disorders. 4th Ed. Washington: American Psychiatric Association, 1994.
9. National Institute of Mental Health. Facts about Anxiety Disorder. Available at: http://www.nimh.nih.gov/publicat/adfacts.cfm. Accessed March 28, 2005.
10. Brown TA, Campbell LA, Lehman CL, et al. Current and lifetime comorbidity of the DSM-IV anxiety and mood disorders in large clinical sample. J Abnorm Psychol 2001;110:585–599.
11. Karno M, Golding JM, Sorenson SB, et al. The epidemiology of obsessive-compulsive disorder in five US communities. Arch Gen Psychiatry 1988;45: 1094–1099.
12. Rettew DC. Avoidant personality disorder, generalized social phobia, and shyness: Putting the personality back into personality disorders. Harv Rev Psychiatry 2000;8:283–297.
13. Kessler RC, Sonnega A, Bromet E, et al. Posttraumatic stress disorder in the national comorbidity survey. Arch Gen Psychiatry 1995;52: 1048–1060.
14. Brantley J. Calming Your Anxious Mind. Oakland: New Harbinger Publications, 2003.
15. United States Surgeon General. Epidemiology of Mental Illness. Available: http://www.surgeon-general.gov/library/mentalhealth/chapter2/sec2_1.html. Accessed February 21, 2005.
16. Sadock BJ, Sadock VA. Kaplan & Sadock's Pocket Handbook of Clinical Psychiatry. 3rd Ed. Philadelphia: Lippincott, Williams & Wilkins, 2001.
17. Miller, CR. Patients with anxiety disorders: a challenge for primary care. American Acad Ambul Care Nurs 2001:2:1–16.
18. Lepine JP. The epidemiology of anxiety disorders: Prevalence and societal costs. J Clin Psychiatry 2002;63(Suppl 14):4–8.
19. Family Practice Notebook.com. Anxiety Disorders. Available: http://www.fpnotebook.com/PSY1.htm. Accessed January 20, 2006.

21. Greenberg PE, Sisitsky T, Kessler RC, et al. The economic burden of anxiety disorders in the 1990s. J Clin Psychiatry 1999;60:427–435.
22. Roth A, Fonagy P. What Works for Whom: A Critical Review of Psychotherapy Research. 2nd Ed. New York: 2004: Guilford Press.
23. Copeland ME. The Worry Control Workbook. Vermont: Peach Press, 2003.
24. Anxiety Disorders Association of America. Panic Attack. Available: http://www.adaa.org/AnxietyDisorderInfor/PanicDisAgor.cfm. Accessed March 29, 2005.
25. Friedman S, Smith L, Fogel D, et al. The incidence and influence of early traumatic life events in patients with panic disorder: a comparison of other psychiatric outpatients. J Anxiety Disord 2002;16: 259–272.
26. Matsunaga H, Kiriike N, Matsui T, et al. Obsessive-compulsive disorder with poor insight. Compr Psychiatry 2002;43:150–157.
27. Stekette G, Pigott T. Obsessive-Compulsive Disorder: The Latest Assessment and Treatment Strategies. Missouri, Kansas city: Compact Clinicals, 2003.
28. Weissman MM, Bland RC, Canino GJ, et al. The cross national epidemiology of panic disorder. Arch Gen Psychiatry 1997;54:305–309.
29. Rouillon F. Epidemiology of panic disorder. Encephale 1996:5:25–34.
30. Shear MK, Clark D. The road to recovery in panic disorder: response, remission and relapse. J Clin Psychiatry 1998;59(Suppl 8):4–8.
31. Curtis GC, Magee WJ, Eaton HU, et al. Specific fears and phobias. Epidemiology and classification. Br J Psychiatry 1998;173:212–217.
32. Lipsitz JD, Mannuzza S, Klein DF, et al. Specific phobia 10–16 years after treatment. Depress Anxiety 1999;10:105–111.
33. Judd LL. Social phobia: a clinical overview. J Clin Psychiatry 1994;55(Suppl):5–9.
34. Lieb R, Wittchen HU, Hofler M, et al. Parental psychopathology, parenting styles, and the risk of social phobia in offspring: a prospective-longitudinal community study. Arch Gen Psychiatry 2000;57:859–866.
35. Long PW. Internet mental health: Anxiety Disorders. Available at: http://www.mental-health.com/whtdhtml.htm. Accessed August 18, 2004.
36. Weissman MM, Bland RC, Canino GJ, et al. The cross national epidemiology of social phobia: a preliminary report. Int J Clin Psychopharmacol 1996;11(Suppl 3):9–14.
37. Hwang MY. I can't stop myself: the devastation of obsessive-compulsive disorder. JAMA 1998;280: 1806.
38. Wang PS, Berglund P, Kessler RC. Recent care of common mental disorders in the United States prevalence and conformance with evidence based recommendations. J Gen Intern Med 2000;15: 284–292.
39. Richards J, Klein B, Carlbring P. Internet based treatment for panic disorder. Cog Behav Ther 2003;32:125–135.
40. Mellman TA, Miller AL, Weissman EM, et al. Evidence-based pharmacologic treatment for people with severe mental illness: a focus on guidelines and algorithms. Psychiatric Services 2001;52:619–625.
41. American Psychiatric Association. Panic Disorder Comprehensive Treatment Guidelines—1998. Available at: http://www.psych.org/psych_pract/treatg/pg/pg_ panic_ 1.cfm?pf=y. Accessed March 29, 2005.
42. Foa EB, Davidson JRT, Frances A. The expert consensus guideline series: Treatment of posttraumatic stress disorder. J Clin Psychiatry 1999;60(Suppl 16): 1–69.
43. Reed KL. Quick Reference to Occupational Therapy. 2nd Ed. Frederick, Maryland: Aspen Publishers, 2001.
44. Kjernisted KD, Bleau P. Long term goals in the management of acute and chronic anxiety disorders. Can J Psychiatry 2004;49(Suppl 1):51S–63S.
45. Read JP, Brown PJ, Kahler CW. Substance use and posttraumatic stress disorders: Symptom interplay and effects on outcome. Addict Behav 2004;29: 1665–1672.
46. Hecker JE, Losee MC, Roberson-Nay R, et al. Mastery of your anxiety and panic and brief therapist contact in the treatment of panic disorder. J Anxiety Disord 2004;18:111–126.
47. Andrews G, Oakley-Browne M, Castle D, et al. Summary of guidelines for the treatment of panic disorder and agoraphobia. Australas Psychiatry 2003;11:29–33.
48. Bonder BR. Psychopathology and function. 3rd Ed. New Jersey: Slack, 2004.
49. Levitt VB. Anxiety disorders. In: Cara E, MacRae A, eds. Psychosocial Occupational Therapy: A Clinical Practice. 2nd Ed. New York: Thomson Delmar Learning, 2005.
50. Federoff IC, Taylor S. Psychological and pharmacological treatments of social phobia: A meta analysis. J Clin Psychopharmacol 2001;21:311–324.
51. Thomsen PH. Obsessive-compulsive disorder: pharmacological treatment. Eur Child Adolesc Psychiatry 2000;9:76–84.
52. Bruce T, Saeed A. Social anxiety disorder: A common underrecognized mental disorder. Am Fam Physician 1999;60:2311–2320.
53. Kinnealey M, Fuiek M. The relationship between sensory defensiveness, anxiety, depression and pain in adults. Occup Ther Int 1999;6:195–206.
54. Kinnealey M, Oliver B, Wilbarger P. A phenomenological study of sensory defensiveness in adults. Am J Occup Ther 1995;49:444–451.
55. Rosier C, Williams H, Ryrie I. Anxiety management groups in a community mental health team. Br J Occup Ther 1998;61:203–206.
56. Prior S. Determining the effectiveness of short term anxiety management course. Br J Occup Ther 1998;61:207–212.

Recommended Learning Resources

Hyman BM, Pedrick C. The OCD Workbook: Your Guide to Breaking Free From Obsessive-Compulsive Disorder. Oakland: New Harbinger Publications, 1999.

Bourne EJ. The Anxiety and Phobia Workbook. Oakland: New Harbinger Publications, 1995.

International Society for Traumatic Stress Studies.
www.sanctuaryweb.com/main/istss.htm.

Anxiety Disorders Association of America
www.adaa.org

Expert Consensus Guidelines Treatment of Obsessive-Compulsive Disorder
www.psychguides.com/ecgs8.php

Expert Consensus Guidelines Treatment of Obsessive-Compulsive Disorder for Patients and Families
www.psychguides.com/pfg10.php

Expert Consensus Guidelines Treatment of Posttraumatic Stress Disorder
www.psychguides.com/ecgs10.php

Expert Consensus Guidelines Treatment of Posttraumatic Stress Disorder for Patients and Families
www.psychguides.com/pfg12.php

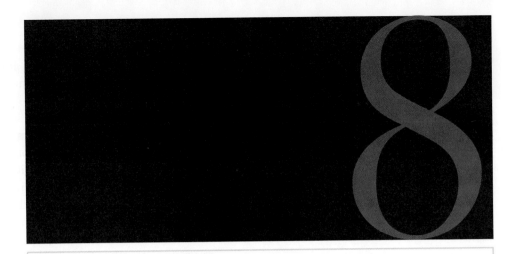

8 Dementia

Joyce Fraker

Key Terms

Agnosia
Analgesic
Anomia
Aphasia
Apraxia
Asterixis
Beta-amyloid plaques
Bradykinesia
Circumlocution
Disinhibition
Dysnomic aphasia
Dysphagia
Executive function
Extrapyramidal symptoms
Hyperflexia
Hyperorality
Hypersexuality
Lability
Long term memory
Neurofibrillary tangles
Neuroleptic
Paraphasia
Paratonia
Personal episodic memory
Procedural memory
Prodromal
Recent memory
Remote memory
Semantic memory
Short term memory
Sundowning
Tau
Topographical orientation

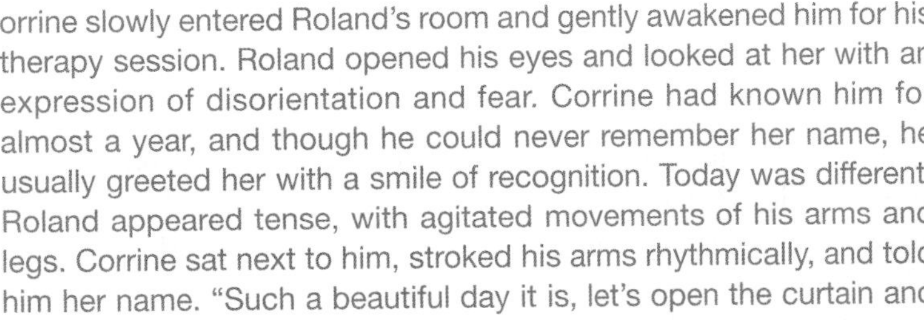

Corrine slowly entered Roland's room and gently awakened him for his therapy session. Roland opened his eyes and looked at her with an expression of disorientation and fear. Corrine had known him for almost a year, and though he could never remember her name, he usually greeted her with a smile of recognition. Today was different. Roland appeared tense, with agitated movements of his arms and legs. Corrine sat next to him, stroked his arms rhythmically, and told him her name. "Such a beautiful day it is, let's open the curtain and look at the view," she told him. She opened the curtains and handed him his glasses. Roland put them on without difficulty and turned his vacant gaze toward the window. Within moments, Roland relaxed, and his limbs calmed.

Corrine said, "Let's get dressed. I will help you put on your clean pants." She lightly touched a leg to cue him to lift it so she could place his foot in the pant leg. Roland looked at her, anxious and bewildered. "What do you want me to do?" he cried.

Corrine lightly touched his foot, directing him to lift it. Roland tightly gripped his upper thighs and he began to shake. He pleaded, louder this time, "I can't move them, what do you want me to do?" Corrine gently took his hand and began stroking his arm. "Let's just rest for a moment," she said. After he had visibly calmed, Corrine gently lifted each foot and placed them into the pant legs. She positioned his walker and said, "You can help us stand." She lightly guided him by the elbow, and he came to a stand. "Thank you for doing such a good job," Corrine told him, and helped him pull on the pants. "Now all we need are shoes, and then we can get some breakfast." Roland looked at her, again without recognition, the fear now replaced with calm.

Cognitive Disorders

Dementia, as defined by the *Diagnostic and Statistical Manual of Mental Disorders, 4th Edition (DSM IV-TR)*, is a condition characterized by multiple cognitive deficits, with the main deficit being impairment of memory. Alzheimer's disease is the most prevalent form of dementia. Dementia, an often misunderstood disorder, has been variously identified in the past as organic brain syndrome, organic mental disorder, or senile dementia. The American Psychiatric Association no longer classifies dementia as an organic disorder, because "organic" implies that only dementia, and not other mental disorders, has a biological basis (1). Senile dementia is a term that was used when the medical community believed that memory loss was a normal part of the aging process. "Senile" literally means age 65 or older, but the term conjures up negative images of one who is weak and incompetent. Some memory loss may occur as a normal part of aging; this varies from person to person and should not interfere with occupational performance. In fact, well into late old age, individuals can learn new things (2). Memory loss that impairs function is a serious concern that calls for medical investigation.

Serious and persistent memory loss is the hallmark, or most significant symptom, of dementia. However, because memory loss is a symptom seen in other disorders, it is useful to review cognitive disorders in general. The *DSM IV-TR* includes dementia in the chapter "Delirium, Dementia, and Amnestic and Other Cognitive Disorders." These disorders are grouped together because they share the symptom of a significant deficit in cognition or memory that represents a decline from a previous level of occupational function.

Delirium and dementia are the cognitive disorders most commonly seen by occupational therapists. Although they differ greatly in their course and prognosis, they can easily be mistaken for each other. Therefore, the occupational therapist must be able to differentiate between them.

Delirium

The diagnostic criteria for delirium are as a) disturbed consciousness (reduced level of arousal) with decreased ability to focus, sustain, or shift attention; b) change in cognition (such as memory loss, disorientation, language disturbance) or the development of perceptual disturbance (hallucinations, paranoid thoughts) that cannot be explained by a pre-existing, established, or evolving dementia; c) the disturbance quickly develops, usually within hours or days, and symptoms fluctuate throughout the course of a day; and d) there is medical evidence that the disturbance is either caused by a medical condition or developed during intoxification or withdrawal from a substance, including alcohol, illegal substances such as cocaine or hallucinogens, or prescription medications (1).

It is not unusual for delirium to occur when a person is being treated, or is in need of treatment, for an acute physical condition. A high fever can bring on delirium, causing the person to be confused, to misinterpret shadows, to be disoriented (especially in a hospital environment, which is unfamiliar and possibly frightening), and to be unable to express thoughts and needs clearly. These symptoms might fluctuate, just as the degree of a fever might fluctuate during the course of a day. An asymptomatic urinary tract infection is often suspected when a delirium occurs without clear signs of a medical problem. The delirium ends as the acute medical condition clears.

Etiology. Delirium is caused by one or more underlying medical conditions. Although a fever can bring on a delirium, the rise in body temperature is in itself merely a symptom of an underlying medical condition. Medical conditions associated with delirium are many and varied. They include infection, burns, and recovery from surgery. Delirium can also be the result of an adverse reaction to medication or the use of a toxic substance, including alcohol or illegal substances. Risk factors for delirium include increased severity of physical illness, older age, and the presence of a baseline cognitive impairment, such as dementia (3).

Delirium can manifest in confusion and disorientation following surgery. In fact, delirium is a frequent finding during recovery for cardiac surgery (4). Persons with acquired immune deficiency syndrome (AIDS) are vulnerable to delirium, as are persons with drug dependency experiencing withdrawal.

Incidence and Prevalence. There is no way to estimate the incidence of delirium, as it can occur during an illness such as influenza, in which the person is not hospitalized, or during a period of heavy drinking. In hospitalized populations, 10% to 15% of inpatients are delirious at some point during hospitalization. For acutely ill geriatric patients, that number increases, with 30% to 50% becoming delirious at any given time during their hospital stay (3).

Signs and Symptoms. The **prodromal** symptoms of delirium can include restlessness, anxiety, sleep disturbance, and irritability. Clinical features of delirium include altered arousal and disturbance of the sleep-wake cycle. The person may be easily awakened, quickly fall asleep, or sleep restlessly. Perception may be altered, with misperceptions, illusions, delusions, or hallucinations. The wrinkled pattern of a blanket may appear to be an object; a shadow in the corner seems to move and is perceived as threatening. The person will likely have decreased attention, impaired memory, disorientation to time or place, and disorganized thinking and speech (4). Neurological abnormalities can include: dysgraphia (inability to write a sentence); constructional **apraxia** (evidenced by inability to draw a clock face); **dysnomic aphasia** (difficulty naming objects); motor abnormalities (tremor, **asterixis**, or hand-flapping tremor;) myoclonus or muscle spasms, and reflex and tone changes) (4). Additionally, there can be psychomotor agitation, psychomotor retardation, sadness, irritability, anxiety, anger, or euphoria.

Course and Prognosis. Delirium has a rapid onset. For persons who have delirium, 50% meet diagnostic criteria within the same day that they developed their first symptoms; 86% meet criteria within 48 hours of emergence of symptoms (4). There is a fluctuating course. There can be lucid intervals as well as periods of confusion and anxiety within the course of a day or even hours. It is not unusual for symptoms to worsen in the evening or at night, and this phenomenon is known as **sundowning** (3).

Delirium usually has a brief duration of days to weeks. It is a transient condition that ameliorates as the underlying medical condition resolves. The following is a list of the possible outcomes for delirium (4):

1. Full recovery
2. Progression to stupor and/or coma
3. Development of seizures, more commonly in drug or alcohol withdrawal
4. Progression to chronic brain syndromes
5. Death
6. Associated morbidity, such as fractures or subdural hematomas from falls

It should be noted that a person does not die from delirium. For a person who is declining with a terminal illness, it is not uncommon for delirium to develop as the body's life-sustaining systems begin to fail. It is also important to note that there is a risk for falls that accompanies delirium. The person hospitalized postoperatively or for a serious illness may attempt to get out of bed even though he or she may not have the needed strength, balance, or coordination.

Medical Management. Treatment for delirium involves treating any underlying cause or medical condition. It is important to withdraw any sedatives or medications that act on the central nervous system (CNS). The exception to this rule is when the delirium is related to withdrawal from alcohol or sedatives, in which case the use of anxiolytics is indicated. The person with delirium requires extra supportive physical care, including attention to nutrition and hydration, and maintenance of a safe and quiet environment. If hospitalized, it is also helpful for the person to have positive orienting cues, such as familiar pictures or things nearby, and frequent contact with family or loved ones (3).

For a person who is normally alert with intact memory, the symptoms of delirium are significant cause for concern. If the person is recovering from a medical condition that resulted in delirium, care should be taken that long-term decisions, such as guardianship and nursing home placement, be avoided until the delirium has cleared. Consider the possibility of an individual who has a delirium caused by a prescribed medication, such as a sedative. If the delirium is not accurately diagnosed and the medication routine changed, the person could be assessed as being unable to live independently. Delirium is a temporary condition whose course usually ends as the person becomes medically stable.

Dementia

Memory impairment is the first and most prominent symptom to emerge in most cases of dementia. **Recent memory** is affected first, often manifested as the person uncharacteristically misplaces things. In addition to memory impairment, other cognitive deficits may emerge. These include **aphasia, apraxia, agnosia, or a disturbance in executive functioning.** For an individual to be diagnosed as having dementia, these deficits must be severe enough to impair occupational performance and represent a decline from a previous functional level (1).

A person who has dementia may experience other cognitive and personality disturbances as well. **Topographical orientation** may be affected, which, compounded by memory loss, can result in the person easily becoming lost. A disturbance in spatial relations creates difficulty with spatial tasks. The person with little or no awareness of memory loss, and who has other impairments, often displays poor judgment or poor insight. One who has awareness of cognitive deficits may become anxious or defensive. Dementia may be associated with gait disturbances that lead to falls, disinhibited behavior such as making inappropriate jokes, and psychotic symptoms such as delusional thinking or hallucinations (1).

The *DSM IV-TR* differentiates between the types of dementia based on their etiologies. Table 8.1 lists the causes of dementia. Dementia of the Alzheimer's type is more

Table 8.1 CAUSES OF DEMENTIA

Degenerative Brain Diseases
Alzheimer disease
Parkinson disease
Pick disease
Frontotemporal degeneration
Huntington disease
Progressive supranuclear palsy
Spinocerebellar degeneration
Multiple sclerosis

Multiple Infarct Diseases
Binswanger disease
Subcortical leukoareosis
Thalamic infarct

Cerebral Vasculitides
Lupus erythematosus
Giant cell arteritis

Infectious Diseases
Syphilis (general paresis of the insane)
Tuberculosis
HIV disease (AIDS dementia complex)
Prion disease (Jakob-Creutzfeldt disease)
Fungal encephalitides
Viral encephalitides

Psychiatric Disorders
Major depressive disorder
Schizophrenia

Traumatic Brain Injuries
Closed head injury
Open head injury
Subdural hematoma

Vitamin Deficiencies
Vitamin B12 deficiency (subacute combined sclerosis, pernicious anemia)
Vitamin B6 deficiency (pellagra)
Vitamin B1 (thiamin) deficiency

Endocrine Diseases
Hyperthyroidism
Hypothyroidism
Growth hormone deficiency
Hyperparathyroidism
Cushing disease (hyperadrenalism)
Addison syndrome (hypoadrenalism)

Cerebral Tumors
Intrinsic brain tumor
Metastatic cancer

(Continued)

Table 8.1 CAUSES OF DEMENTIA (*CONT.*)

Toxin Exposure
Alcohol
Heavy metals (lead, arsenic, mercury)
Volatile hydrocarbons
Medications
Others
Normopressure (communicating) hydrocephalus

Reprinted with permission from Goldman LS, Wise TN, Brody DS. Psychiatry for Primary Care Physicians. 2nd Ed. Atlanta: American Medical Association, 2004.

commonly known as Alzheimer's disease (AD). The cause of AD is the subject of much debate and the diagnosis is made after ruling out other types of dementia. Vascular dementia was formerly referred to as multi-infarct dementia. Dementias that result from other general medical conditions may be diagnosed when one of the following medical conditions is present: human immunodeficiency virus (HIV) disease, head trauma, Parkinson's disease, Huntington's disease, Pick disease, Jakob-Creutzfeldt disease, normal pressure hydrocephalus, hyperthyroidism, brain tumor, vitamin B12 deficiency, and intracranial radiation. Substance-induced dementia may be diagnosed when there is evidence that cognitive deficits are related to the effects of substance use, such as a drug of abuse or a medication. The *DSM IV-TR* lists alcohol, inhalants, sedatives, hypnotics, and anxiolytics as substances that may induce dementia.

This chapter will focus on the most commonly seen dementias. AD is by far the most common form of dementia and accounts for 50% to 70% of all cases of dementia. Vascular dementia is the second most common form of dementia and comprises 15% to 25% of dementia cases (3). This chapter also briefly discusses frontotemporal dementia otherwise known as Pick disease, and dementia with Lewy bodies. Recent research has focused attention on these forms of dementia, and the possibility that they may be more commonly occurring than was previously understood (5,6).

Alzheimer's Disease

Etiology. There is no known cause for AD, and at present, there is no widely accepted biological marker that is diagnostic of AD in a living person (1). The clinical diagnosis can be made only after ruling out the etiologies, such as cardiovascular disease or Parkinson's disease, for other dementias. However, much research has focused on associated features and laboratory findings relevant to AD in an attempt to discover its origin(s). This chapter will review some of the major findings now being studied.

Neuropathology. Neuroimaging tools, such as magnetic resonance imaging (MRI), are being used to detect the earliest changes of AD or to differentiate AD from other forms of dementia (7). Some of these physical findings are cortical atrophy, widened sulci, and ventricular enlargement (4). This shrinking of brain structure is a result of neuronal loss, which seems to be caused by **neurofibrillary tangles** and **β-amyloid plaques.**

β-amyloid plaques are caused by a chemical accident, or the defective breakdown of a benign substance known as amyloid precursor protein (APP). APP lives in various parts of the body, including the brain, and its role in cellular function is unknown. As part of its mysterious function, APP regularly gets broken down into much smaller soluble components and is washed away with other decomposed tissues and chemicals. Under some conditions that are not understood, the breaking apart does not proceed correctly. The outcome produces sticky, insoluble shards of β-amyloid. These shards stick to each other, attracting fragments of dead and dying neurons, and slowly decline into dense, misshapen plaques (8). β-amyloid plaques collect outside and around the neurons. It is believed that this accumulation causes physical damage to axons, and that prolonged neuronal response to this injury ultimately leads to the development of neurofibrillary tangles and neuronal death (9).

Neurofibrillary tangles are made up of another contaminated protein called **tau**. Tau normally serves as connectors or "railroad ties" for a track like structure that transports nutrients and other important molecules throughout the cell body of every neuron. The contaminated or tangled tau somehow becomes hyperphosphorylated, a corruption resulting in several extra molecules of phosphorous. Without the stabilizing railroad ties of normal tau, the tracks bend into a twisted mess. Under the weight of the nutrients being transported, the tracks buckle, and the damage increases. Inside the neuron, this twisted debris gets worse as the filaments of track keep twisting around each other. As cell communication and nourishment is lost, the neuron begins to wither. The neuron, axon, and dendrites disintegrate, and as a result, thousands of synapses vanish (8,10). It is well documented that the brains of persons with AD have an abundance of the abnormal structures of β-amyloid plaques and neurofibrillary tangles (11).

The structural changes just described do not cause AD, but are the end-product of a pathological process. The challenge for researchers is to discover what causes this degeneration. The loss of neurons occurs throughout the brain but is significant in the cerebral cortex. The cerebral cortex is responsible for higher brain functions, including thinking, judgment, reasoning, speech, and language. Plaques and tangles are also dense in the hippocampus, which plays a role in attention and memory (12).

It is possible that amyloid has a function as a repair protein. Amyloid levels have been noted to increase when there is some injury to the brain. Some researchers contend that β-amyloid plaques do not lead to AD, but in fact, might be a byproduct of the AD process (8).

Genetic Predisposition. Unlike some diseases, AD is not caused by a single gene. More than one gene mutation is seen in AD, and genes on multiple chromosomes are involved. In most cases, genes alone are not sufficient to cause AD. The two types of AD are early onset and late onset. Early onset refers to AD that manifests before the age of 65, and late onset refers to AD seen at or after age 65. Less than 5% of AD is early onset, and this form of the disease is often inherited (13,14).

Three genes have been identified as responsible for the rare early onset familial form of AD. Mutated chromosome 21 causes an abnormal amyloid precursor protein to be produced. Mutated chromosome 14 causes an abnormal protein called presenilin 1 to be produced. Mutated chromosome 1 causes yet another abnormal protein, presenilin 2, to be produced (11). It appears that these mutations increase the likelihood that β-amyloid will be snipped from the APP, causing more of the sticky β-amyloid to be formed (12). Even if only one of these genes inherited from a parent is mutated, the person will almost certainly develop early onset AD. This means that in these families, children have a 50% chance of developing early onset AD if one parent has this disease.

In the more common late-onset AD, a polymorphism in the apolipoprotein E gene is associated with increased susceptibility (15). The apolipoprotein E gene is found on chromosome 19. This gene codes for a protein that helps carry cholesterol in the bloodstream. The apolipoprotein E gene comes in several forms, called alleles. The three most common alleles are apolipoprotein E 2, apolipoprotein E 3, and apolipoprotein E 4. A person inherits one apolipoprotein E allele from each parent. One or two copies of the 4 allele increases the risk of getting AD. However, having the 4 allele does not mean that AD is certain, as some persons with even two of the 4 allele do not develop the disease. The rarer 2 allele may be associated with having a lower risk for AD (14,16).

Down syndrome is a risk factor for AD. In fact, all individuals with Down syndrome, who carry an extra copy of chromosome 21 and overexpress APP several-fold in the brain, develop AD if they live past the age of 40 (17).

Neurotransmitter Abnormalities. There is some evidence that the neurotransmitter acetylcholine is implicated in the progression of AD. Neurons that contain acetylcholine are known as cholinergic neurons, and many of these are bunched together to form tracts. Cholinergic tracts radiate throughout the entire brain. Autopsy shows that for a person with AD, many cholinergic tracts throughout the entire brain have been destroyed. Several chemical changes occur in the cholinergic nerves before they die. First, the enzyme choline acetyltransferase (CAT) is needed to form acetylcholine, and there is a serious reduction of CAT in the brains of persons with AD. Second, this reduction of CAT is greatest in areas of the brain where there is a dense amount of plaques and tangles (14).

Cardiovascular Risk Factors. Although vascular dementia accounts for 15% to 25% of all dementia cases, there is now a concern that cardiovascular disease is also linked to AD. As people are living longer with AD, and living long enough to be diagnosed with AD at age 80 and 90, these groups are also at risk for developing cardiovascular disease. Some see this group as having a mixed dementia, or a combination of AD and vascular disease (12). Epidemiologic studies suggest that risk factors for cardiovascular disease and stroke are associated with cognitive impairment and AD, and that the presence of these factors intensifies the severity of symptoms in AD (14). In autopsy studies, 60% to 90% of AD cases exhibit variable cerebrovascular pathology (21). Researchers have also found that the use of statins, the most common type of cholesterol-lowering drug, is associated with a lower risk of developing AD (13).

Other Potential Causes. One of the theories of aging suggests that over time, damage from a kind of molecule called a free radical can build up in neurons and cause a loss of function. Free radicals can be helpful in fighting infection but too many can injure cells by changing other nearby molecules, such as those in the neuron's cell membrane or in DNA. This can lead to a chain reaction, releasing more free radicals, and causing more damage. This is called oxidative damage and may contribute to AD by upsetting the proper flow of substances in and out of cells (11). Some researchers are focusing on a possible connection between oxidative stress and amyloid β-peptide, the principle component of plaques found in the brain of the person with AD (20).

Researchers are also studying the possible role of inflammation, because cells and compounds that are known to be involved in inflammation are found in AD plaques. Some scientists think that inflammation is harmful and sets off a cycle of events that lead to the death of neurons. Others believe that some aspects of the inflammatory process may be a helpful part of the brain's natural healing efforts (11).

Research is focused on even more factors that may be related to AD, including trace elements, the role of the immune system, and the possibility of a viral connection (12).

Incidence and Prevalence. In the next 50 years, the prevalence of AD in the United States is expected to nearly quadruple. This means that 1 in every 45 Americans would meet the diagnostic criteria (21). This phenomenon is largely a result of the fact that the baby boom generation will be elderly, and that life expectancies are increasing with medical advances. The *DSM IV-TR* states that, while the prevalence increases with age, women tend to have a higher incidence of AD. By age 65, 6% of males and 8% of females will have AD; by age 85, 11% of males and 14% of females have AD; at age 90 these figures increase to 21% of males and 25% of females (1). The National Institutes of Health (NIH) finds that for every 5-year age group older than age 65, the percentage of persons with AD doubles. By 2050, 14 million older Americans are expected to have AD unless preventative treatment becomes available (11).

In addition to age, there are numerous factors that appear to create a higher risk for AD (4). These factors include the following:

1. Low educational level
2. History of head trauma with loss of consciousness
3. History of depression
4. Late maternal age
5. Environmental and occupational exposure (e.g., to aluminum)
6. History of electroconvulsive therapy
7. Alcohol abuse
8. **Analgesic** abuse
9. Long-standing physical inactivity

Signs and Symptoms. Although the hallmark symptom of dementia is memory impairment, the signs and symptoms of AD impact virtually all performance skills. Since AD is a progressive disease, the first signs can be mistaken for normal aging. Even though there are small changes in process skills with normal aging, a healthy older adult can continue to learn and problem solve at any age. Researchers are generating new information on normal aging versus mild cognitive impairment (MCI). A person with MCI will have more impairment of process skills than is expected with normal aging, but will not yet meet the diagnostic criteria for dementia. Table 8.2 lists the prominent cognitive symptoms and the neuropsychological profile associated with normal aging, MCI, AD, and other dementias.

Defining the progressive stages of AD is an arbitrary process, and various researchers use different ideologies. Reisberg, a prominent researcher in the study of AD, has proposed seven stages (22). These stages range from stage 1, in which there is no impairment, to stage 7, which is very severe decline. Most researchers use a three-stage approach (4,8,23). The Clinical Dementia Rating (CDR) is used to measure dementia (24). This scale defines three levels of dementia as mild, moderate, and severe.

This chapter will use the three stage approach, with the stages being defined as early, middle, and late. We will also briefly review mild cognitive impairment, as it is possibly a precursor to dementia. It is important to remember that each person with AD is a unique individual, with unique concerns, needs, and strengths. Although such individuals do not always fit into a rigid classification system, using the three stages will give the reader general guidelines for better understanding the problems facing the person with AD and his or her caregivers.

Mild Cognitive Impairment. MCI is defined as the clinical state of individuals who are memory impaired but are functioning well and do not meet the criteria for dementia (25).

Table 8.2 CLINICAL COGNITIVE SYNDROMES AND ASSOCIATED NEUROPSYCHOLOGICAL PROFILES

Cognitive Syndrome and Characteristics	Neuropsychological Profile
Normal aging	
Subjective memory complaints Annoying but not disabling problems Frequent problems with name retrieval Minor difficulties in recalling detailed events	Impaired fluid abilities (novel problem solving) Deficiencies in memory retrieval Decreased general speed of processing Lowered performance on executive tasks and visuospatial skills/visual motor speed
Mild Cognitive impairment	
Subjective memory complaints Noticeable change in memory as noted by informants Clinical Dementia Rating score of 0.5 (mild, questionable dementia) (24) Problem is not disabling	Memory performance 1.5 standard deviations below age-matched peers Otherwise intact neurocognitive function Functional disorder limited to mild interference from the memory difficulty
Alzheimer's disease	
Insidious onset Progressive impairment Prominent memory impairment Possible disorders: aphasia, apraxia, agnosis	Impaired memory consolidation with rapid forgetting Diminished executive skills Impaired semantic fluency and naming Impaired visuospatial analysis and praxis
Frontotemporal dementia	
Prominent personality/behavior change Disinhibition or apathy Impaired judgment, insight Normal mental status initially	Cognitive inflexibility Impaired sequencing Perseverative, imitative, utilization behaviors Poor use of feedback Prone to interference Less obvious memory impairments
Lewy body dementia	
Fluctuations in alertness/acute confusional state Visual hallucinations Memory impairment Parkinsonian signs Neuroleptic sensitivity Falls resulting from orthostatic hypotension	Memory impairment of Alzheimer's disease but with some partial saving Pronounced apraxia; visuospatial difficulties Rapidly increasing quantifiable deficits in many cases
Vascular dementia	
Variation of symptoms with subtype Focality on examination Abrupt onset In multi-infarct dementia, stepwise progression	Language/memory retrieval difficulties common Benefit from structural support/cueing Asymmetric motor speed/dexterity Executive inefficiencies

(*Continued*)

Table 8.2 CLINICAL COGNITIVE SYNDROMES AND ASSOCIATED NEUROPSYCHOLOGICAL PROFILES (*CONT.*)

Cognitive Syndrome and Characteristics	Neuropsychological Profile
Parkinson's disease dementia	
Extrapyramidal motor disturbance Gait dysfunction and frequent falls **Bradykinesia** Bradyphrenia	Slowed performance Retrieval memory deficits Executive deficiencies (slowed sequencing, impaired lexical fluency) Impaired fine motor speed (asymmetry common) Constructional deficits
Huntington's disease	
Early age at onset (midlife) Choreiform movements Dementia Bradyphrenia	Slowed performance Memory difficult in retrieval Benefit from retrieval supports (recognition OK) Executive compromises Poor verbal fluency/preserved naming
Progressive supranuclear palsy	
Extrapyramidal syndrome but no impaired tremor Ophthalmic abnormalities (limited downgaze) Axial rigidity Pseudobulbar palsy Frequent falls	Mild dysexecutive symptoms: sequencing, fluency, flexibility Motor slowing Memory weakness characterized as inefficiencies in storage and retrieval
Hydrocephalus	
Memory impairment Gait disturbance Incontinence	Slowed information processing Memory retrieval problems Benefit from retrieval supports
Jakob-Creutzfeldt disease	
Rare Typically, rapid onset and course Dementia with pyramidal and extrapyramidal signs Transient spikes on electroencephalogram	Rapidly evolving dementia Subtypes include a profile akin to Alzheimer's disease, or pronounced complex visuospatial disorder (Balint's syndrome)
Dementia and geriatric depression	
Affective disorder Psychomotor slowing Memory complaints Cognitive complaints linked temporally to the depressive disorder	Impaired performance on tasks involving effortful processing Impaired attention, concentration, sequencing, cognitive flexibility, and executive control Retrieval memory difficulty cueing/recognition Memory improvement with poor motivation Behavioral tendencies to abandon tasks,

Reprinted with permission from Blazer DG, Steffens DC, Busse EW. The American Psychiatric Publishing Textbook of Geriatric Psychiatry. 3rd Ed. Washington, DC: American Psychiatric Publishing, Inc., 2004.

MCI appears to be a prodromal stage of AD. It is a stage of mild but persistent memory loss and is often seen with word naming difficulties. According to Cohen, the diagnosis of MCI includes five criteria:

1. The individual complains of memory problems.
2. Memory loss is abnormal for the person's age.
3. Activities of daily living are not affected.
4. Other cognitive abilities are intact.
5. There is no dementia.

For individuals given a diagnosis of MCI, 40% show progressive impairment and are diagnosed with AD within 3 years. This is significantly higher than the expected 3% of healthy 65-year-olds who will develop AD within 3 years (12).

Early Stage. The early and mild stage usually lasts 2 to 3 years (26.) The cognitive changes in the early stage can be divided into three groups: memory, language, and visuospatial.

Memory. **Short-term memory** is significantly impaired, which makes new learning very difficult. The person forgets tasks, loses the thread of a conversation, and misplaces things. **Long-term memory** begins to be impaired (4). The person might be able to remember a phone number long enough to repeat it, but will forget it if there is any delay in using it. **Procedural memory**, such as knowing how to write, will remain intact. However, other types of memory begin to show deficits including **personal episodic memory**, which is time-related information about one's self, such as where and if one ate breakfast; **semantic memory**, such as remembering the name of a common object; and general knowledge, such as remembering the name of the highest mountain in the world (14).

Language. Aphasia, an abnormal neurological condition in which language is impaired, appears in the early stage. The person can usually maintain sentence structure, though it becomes less complex. Poor semantic memory leads to difficulty with word retrieval (the ability to name an object when shown a picture of it) and word list generation (being able to quickly name words in a common category or beginning with the same letter, for example.) When forgetting a word, the person may substitute inappropriate words, making sentences incomprehensible (14). This would be an example of **paraphasia**, which means saying the wrong word, substituting a word that sounds alike, or using a word in the same category as the intended word. **Anomia** is the phenomenon in which a person searches in vain for a word, and says "thing-a-ma-jig" or just gives up. **Circumlocution** may occur, in which the person tries to express an idea by talking around the intended word with extensive description and elaborations (29).

Visuospatial Skills. Visuospatial abilities decline in early AD. The person starts to get lost in a familiar neighborhood, or does not recognizing a familiar intersection. There may be some disorientation within the home, with the person putting the frying pan in the freezer, or the wallet in the dishwasher (10).

Executive Functions. In addition to these classic symptoms, the person in the early stage of AD begins to have difficulty with instrumental activities of daily living (IADL). Balancing the checkbook is impossible, and bills may be forgotten. The family notices that the person is more rigid and irritable, and less spontaneous or adventurous. Problems with planning, organizing, sequencing, and abstracting become apparent, as the person begins to have difficulty in the workplace or following a recipe. The person may begin to prepare a meal, become distracted, and forget to complete it (4).

The person may recognize that memory has become impaired or may not have the judgment needed for such insight. It is not unusual to see personality changes. Some persons with AD become suspicious, thinking that one's things are being stolen, or that his or her spouse is being unfaithful. Depression is seen in up to 25% of people in the early stage of AD. Confusion or anxiety may lead to withdrawal from routine social activity. In some cases, delusional thinking may emerge (28).

Middle Stage. In the middle stage of AD, which can last from 2 to 10 years, there is continued decline in memory, visuospatial skills, and language. All areas of performance skills begin to show deficits, psychiatric symptoms increase, and behavior disturbances arise.

Memory. Recent and **remote memory** worsens. The person may think he or she is back at an earlier stage of life and become focused on a past worry, such as getting the children to school on time. The person is no longer bothered by the memory loss. There is disorientation to place and time, and at times the person may not recognize his or her own face in the mirror, much less friends or family members. New information is not retained for more than a few moments. There is difficulty organizing thoughts and thinking logically, and inability to cope with new or unexpected situations. Thinking is concrete, with no ability to take into account ideas or objects that are not present (8,11,27).

Language. Aphasia worsens, and the person loses fluent language. Language is limited to the concerns of the moment or reminiscing about the past. There may be diminished verbal responsiveness, or verbalizations may be impulsive and inappropriate. There is difficulty understanding simple questions or instructions. The person has trouble following a conversation and may be unable to keep track of his or her own thoughts or words (6).

Internal speech is part of the complex process used when an individual makes plans or mentally solve problems. A person who can no longer use words effectively loses this ability of rational planning and problem solving. His or her actions will become impulsive and disorganized, requiring step-by-step direction and supervision for any occupation (27).

Visuospatial Skills. Visuospatial abilities continue to decline. Visual inattention which is seen in the early stage begins to seriously limit function in the middle stage (29). The person gets lost in familiar environments, and is unable to become oriented if he or she moves to a new environment. Constructional skills are compromised, and the person is unable to sort out the arms and legs of garments while trying to get dressed. There is a loss of ability to judge depth and distance. The person may step highly over a mark on the ground, or choose to walk around it. He or she may not be able to distinguish furniture from designs on the carpet, or interpret changes in flooring. These visuospatial impairments can lead to falls. Judging direction and distance is problematic, resulting in knocking something over when trying to grasp it, or grasping at thin air (27).

Psychiatric Symptoms. Psychiatric symptoms that emerged in the early stage worsen. Depression and anxiety are frequently seen and the presence of depression is associated with increased mortality. The person may lose control over his or her emotions, having outbursts of fear or anger. Visual hallucinations are not uncommon, and auditory hallucinations can also occur. Sleep is disturbed, with increased daytime napping, and frequent night time wakefulness (28).

Behavior Disturbances. Behavior disturbances increase the likelihood that the individual will need nursing home placement. It is in the middle stage of AD that wandering and agitation becomes a problem (11). The person paces, seemingly without a goal or destination.

Pacing could be a sign of stress or anxiety or perhaps it is the person's need for activity and exercise. Agitation could be the person's only way to respond to fear or frustration (28). Loss of impulse control manifests in sloppy table manners, undressing at inappropriate times or places, and vulgar or rude language (9). There is a loss of social propriety and inhibition, a failure, so to speak, of the filtering system that determines which thoughts to keep to one's self and which thoughts or actions should be acted upon. This inability to inhibit impulses can cause offense to others, or become dangerous if the person with AD acts upon aggressive impulses. (27).

Late Stage. The late stage of AD can last from 8 to 12 years. At this stage, the person with AD is fully dependent on others for basic activities of daily living (ADLs), such as bathing, dressing, and eating. Motor skills are affected, and the person becomes immobile and incontinent.

Memory. There is no ability to create new memories, and little or no recognition of close family members. All process skills are seriously impaired, and purposeful, goal-directed occupation is lost.

Language. Speech is limited to one or two words, or speech and vocabulary may be totally intelligible. Over time, speech will decline to the point where there is none. The person no longer smiles or communicates with facial expression (8). There can be instances of moaning or crying, and since these are universal sounds of distress, it is important for caregivers to explore the possible causes of discomfort. Receptive language is also seriously impaired. The person cannot process the meaning of words but may respond to a calm and soothing tone of voice.

Motor Skills. The person becomes bed bound with eventual loss of postural control. Neurological symptoms develop, including **hyperflexia**, apraxic gait, and frontal release signs (grasp and snout reflexes). **Paratonia** is a primitive reflex in which there is involuntary resistance in an extremity in response to a sudden passive movement. Thus, if a caregiver quickly moves the person's arm, he or she automatically resists the movement (23).

Seizures may occur, and contractures, pressure ulcers, urinary tract infections, and pneumonia may develop from immobility. There is incontinence of bladder and bowel. Appetite decreases, and eventually the person develops **dysphagia**, or the loss of ability to chew and swallow (28).

Psychiatric Symptoms. The sleep cycle is very disturbed as the person spends 60% of time sleeping, including much of the daytime hours. Hallucinations persist for some (28).

Course and Prognosis. The course of AD tends to be slowly progressive, with the loss of 3 to 4 points per year on the Mini Mental State Examination (MMSE), a standard cognitive assessment instrument (1,30). The stages outlined in the previous section of this chapter illustrate the progression of the signs and symptoms of AD. Some researchers have found that the person with AD lives a median of only 3.3 years after first seeing a doctor regarding memory problems. This statistic can be misleading, as there are many difficulties in establishing the date of onset for this disease (23). The majority of people with AD have symptoms for several years before receiving a diagnosis. The time from diagnosis to death can be as little as 3 years if the person is older than 80 years of age when diagnosed, or as long as 10 or more years if the person is younger at the time of diagnosis (11).

This disease progresses until death. Death is usually a result of complications such as infection, or the eventual inability of the individual to maintain nutrition and hydration.

Medical Management.

Diagnosis. There are three primary criteria in the diagnosis of AD. First, there is the development of multiple cognitive deficits manifested by both memory impairment and at least one other cognitive disturbance. These cognitive disturbances include aphasia, which is language disturbance; apraxia, which is impaired ability to plan motor activities despite intact motor function; agnosia, which is failure to recognize or identify objects despite intact sensory function; and disturbance in executive function, such as problems with planning, organizing, sequencing, and abstracting.

The second criterion for AD is the finding that the multiple cognitive deficits cause significant impairment in social or occupational functioning and represent a significant decline from a previous level of functioning. The third criterion is having a course characterized by gradual onset and continuing cognitive decline (1).

The *DSM IV-TR* uses the first two criteria in diagnosing all other dementias. In addition to the aforementioned criteria, the clinician must eliminate other possible causes of dementia for the diagnosis of AD to be made. A definitive diagnosis of AD is possible only after death, when an autopsy can reveal the physical findings of plaques and tangles in the brain.

The diagnosis is a time-consuming process, but an important one, as the thorough medical investigation may reveal a condition that can be treated. The possibility of reversible dementia will be discussed later.

The National Institutes of Health (NIH) has outlined the following steps in diagnosing AD:

1. A detailed patient history should include a description of how and when the symptoms developed, the patient's and family's medical condition and medical history, and an assessment of the patient's emotional state and living environment.
2. Interviewing family members or close friends can provide information on how behavior and personality have changed.
3. Physical and neurological examinations and laboratory tests help determine neurological functioning and identify possible non-AD causes of dementia.
4. A computerized tomography (CT) scan or an MRI test can reveal changes in the brain's structure and function that indicate early AD.
5. Neuropsychological tests that measure memory, language skills, and other cognitive functions help indicate what kind of cognitive changes are occurring.

Treatment. Goldman describes the following four pillars of complete dementia care:

1. Supportive care for the patient
2. Supportive care for the family and/or caregiver
3. Disease treatment
4. Symptom treatment, including cognitive, mental, and behavioral symptoms

Supportive care includes assessing the environment for aspects of safety, as well as looking at how the environment can improve function and well being. Very early in the disease process, the person with AD needs to discuss financial and medical concerns such as wills and advance directives. It is important to determine the level of care that is needed, who will provide the care, and additional supports such as day programs. The family may need to help make decisions regarding ability to drive and work. Maintaining the person's dignity and privacy is always important. The person with AD will also need ongoing medical care and evaluation of vision and hearing.

Support for the caregiver is critical. Caring for someone who is progressively losing memories and skills can be stressful, sad, and frightening. Care giving can become a 24-hour-a-day job. The Alzheimer's

Association can refer caregivers for support, resources, and advocacy.

Disease treatment is meant to target the etiology or cause of the progressive decline in AD. Although the etiology of AD is unknown, medical management of the vascular process is important not just for persons with vascular dementia, but also for AD.

Treatment targets symptoms such as the cognitive decline, psychiatric symptoms such as psychosis or depression, and behavior disturbances. Pharmacotherapy is useful for these symptoms. The use of medications will not stop the disease process, but relieving the associated symptoms can comfort the person with AD and the caregiver, as well as improve the quality of life.

Former President, Ronald Reagan brought national attention to the disorder when, in 1994, he announced that he had been diagnosed with Alzheimer's disease. Since his death, his widow, Nancy Reagan, has publicly campaigned for increasing dementia research funds, and for limiting obstacles to stem cell research.

Pharmacotherapy. Prescription drugs are frequently used in managing symptoms such impaired cognition, depression, delusions and hallucinations, and agitation or aggression. Some of the newest medications are those used in treating cognitive symptoms, and work as cholinesterase inhibitors. These include donepezil (Aricept), rivastigmine (Exelon), and galantamine (Reminyl). Inhibiting acetylcholinesterase leaves more acetylcholine in the synapse, which facilitates activity of the remaining neurons. These medications do not inhibit cell loss. Research does show that there is modest cognitive improvement in about a third of the persons taking these medications; this improvement is seen in increased function in ADLs and in delaying placement in nursing homes (25). Some studies show that treatment with cholinesterase inhibitors can bring cognition back to the level seen about 6 months prior to the start of treatment (29). What this means is that the person may be able to again do the things he or she could do half a year ago, such as dressing with verbal prompts only. However, these treatments cannot halt the progression of AD, and cognitive decline will continue.

Cholinesterase inhibitors are indicated in the early and middle stages of AD. Memantine (Namenda) is also used in the middle stage for moderate to severe symptoms of AD. This medication works by regulating excess glutamate, a chemical involved in memory function (11).

Depression is seen in as many as 25% to 30% of persons with dementia. Depression can occur in the early stage of AD, and if untreated, can lead to earlier institutionalization and death, aside from the mental suffering. Select serotonin re-uptake inhibitors (SSRIs) are the first line of treatment for depression, followed by the use of agents with dual effects on the serotonin and norepinephrine systems (25).

Delusions and hallucinations can begin in the early stage of AD, and are more common in the middle stage. Low-dose **neuroleptics** are used, and the newer, atypical neuroleptics such as risperidone (Risperdal) and olanzapine (Zyprexa) are less likely to cause side effects (25).

Disruptive behavior such as agitation and aggression is often a sign of a medical problem. Urinary tract infections or pneumonia can create delirium with agitation or aggression. Ruling out these and other concerns such as environmental stress or pain is the first step in reducing problem behaviors. If the behavior is truly caused by the underlying dementia, low-dose neuroleptics and mood stabilizers can be beneficial (23).

Impact of Condition on Client Factors.

Early Stage. With the progressive loss of performance skills, AD impacts on increasing areas of occupation and performance patterns. Although this section outlines the expected impact of AD on client factors, it is important to remember that each individual will perform differently. Someone who has always been flexible and adaptive may compensate in ways that support function; another person who is prone to anxiety or has fewer coping skills might have more significant functional losses.

In the early stage, ADLs remain intact. The first signs of memory impairment manifest in IADL. The person experiencing memory loss cannot adequately or safely fulfill the responsibilities of child rearing or caring for others. Memory impairment affects orientation to place, and so community mobility is impaired. The person easily becomes lost in a new environment. The person with early AD will be disoriented while vacationing or traveling away from home, and sometimes this is when family members begin to note the symptoms of AD. Financial management begins to deteriorate. There is decreased ability to do math, and so the checkbook is not balanced correctly. The person may forget to pay a bill or misplace it. Shopping becomes a problem when the person is disoriented, loses track of what he or she is trying to purchase, and has difficulty making the money transactions. Compensations can include shopping only in the neighborhood and using a credit or debit card.

Other IADL may be impacted. Meal preparation can be a problem if the person starts the task, gets distracted, and then forgets to finish preparing and even eating the meal. Health management can be a problem if the person forgets to make or keep appointments, or forgets to take medication. Home management may not be a problem if there are well-established routines and no unexpected problems arise. However, routine car maintenance might be neglected, and response to problems and emergencies might be less organized.

The ability to drive is an IADL that deserves special attention. As a general rule, persons with early stage dementia who wish to continue to drive should have their driving skills evaluated. Many states offer driving assessments through their state departments. The Family Caregiver Alliance advises families to observe for behavioral signs that the person with dementia is no longer able to drive with safety (32). It is possible to determine a person is no longer safe to drive when he or she:

1. Has become less coordinated
2. Has difficulty judging distance and space
3. Gets lost or feels disoriented in familiar places
4. Has difficulty engaging in multiple tasks
5. Has increased memory loss, especially for recent events
6. Is less alert to things happening around him or her
7. Has mood swings, confusion, irritability
8. Needs prompting for personal care
9. Has difficulty processing information
10. Has difficulty with decision making and problem solving

Memory loss impacts performance in education. Learning becomes very difficult, if not impossible. Reading is problematic. The person is likely able to read, but will have difficulty retaining or remembering what is read. Work is also seriously impacted. Tasks that are routine may remain intact, but forgetfulness will impact the ability to get work started, attend to all details, and to follow the task through to completion. As job performance deteriorates, relationships with coworkers and supervisors can become strained. Some employers make efforts to arrange work loads and expectations in order to maintain the worker in employment as long as possible. In other cases, the person in the early stage of AD may have to seek early or medical retirement. The person will likely need assistance in determining benefits and making plans for productive retirement. Volunteer exploration and participation will be difficult. New routines are difficult to establish, and the task demands, as with regular employment, may be too high for the person with memory and other cognitive impairments.

Leisure exploration will be difficult for the same reasons. Learning new tasks or routines, even for leisure, will be very difficult. The person might be able to maintain established leisure patterns that have little demand for problem solving. Other activities may be given up; attending the bridge club becomes stressful instead of relaxing when it is hard to remember your partner's name, or what cards were just played.

The person with early stage AD will find social participation no longer easy nor enjoyable. The family begins to notice that the person avoids social contact, is rigid or irritable, and no longer spontaneous. He or she may drop out of community and family events, or attend without actually participating. The changed behavior could be a result of depression, deteriorating language skills, or fear of embarrassment because of forgetfulness. For the same reasons, intimacy and sexual expression will be diminished.

In the early stage, performance skills will be unaffected. As cognition declines, the process skills of temporal organization are impacted. It is easy to be distracted in the middle of a task and then forget to continue, sequence, and properly terminate it. If the task is new or unfamiliar, adaptation may be too demanding. Communication and interaction skills are impaired as language problems develop, and the person may no longer be able to clearly articulate thoughts and needs.

Performance patterns begin deteriorate. The person might rigidly cling to habits or routines, as he or she becomes aware of and attempts to compensate for memory loss. Another person may begin to neglect habits and routines; the garbage is not taken out, or the person stops going to church. Roles begin to change: a grandmother can no longer babysit, but needs help to go shopping; a father can no longer help his family do the taxes, even though he worked all of his life as an accountant.

Cultural and spiritual contexts remain strong, but participation begins to decline, as a result of memory impairment and communication difficulties. Family and friends need to provide ever increasing support to ensure the person is included in family, cultural, and spiritual events.

Client factors that are impacted in the early stage are the mental functions: memory, orientation, perception, higher level cognition, mental functions of language, and calculation. Self concept will be impacted as the individual fears embarrassment or worries that his or her competence is declining.

Middle Stage. In the middle stage of AD, there is impairment in all areas of occupation, and the person can no longer live alone. ADLs are not always attended to, and when attempted, performance may be poor or inadequate. The person may attempt to shower, but have difficulty setting the water temperature. Showering may consist of just getting wet, with no attention to the need for soap or shampoo. If shampoo is used, regulation is poor, with too much or too little, using it on the top of the head only, or forgetting to rinse. Dressing requires decision making such as choosing attire based on weather and occasion, and the sequence of donning each article. The person with AD might make mistakes in these decisions, as well as in understanding the need to remove dirty clothing and replace with clean. Although the person begins misplacing glasses and dentures in the early stage, by now these articles might be lost as well as unnoticed. Toilet hygiene is no longer productive, as the person may neglect to clean the body or properly refasten clothing. The sleep-wake cycle is often disturbed, and wandering in the night can create a crisis for caregivers.

IADL are neglected or performed without proper sequence and completion. Home management tasks that are repetitive, such as folding towels can be performed after someone else has sorted, laundered and dried them. The person is dependent in areas of community mobility, financial management, and shopping. Some cleaning and cooking tasks may be done with supervision and direction. Safety is a major concern for the person in the middle stage of AD. At first, he or she may be safe if left home alone for an hour. As the symptoms progress, there can be risk for wandering, letting a stranger in the house, or setting a fire while trying to cook.

There is no ability to perform in areas of work or education. Leisure participation is limited to activities that do not require problem solving or decision making, such as singing or going out with a friend or family member to church or a restaurant. In fact, friends or family are needed for any social participation, as the person will have difficulty initiating or organizing social interaction outside of his or her immediate environment.

Performance skills remained intact in the early stage. By the middle stage, some of these skills are affected. The decline in visuospatial skills leads to many problems. Positioning and reaching are not always effective. Poor judgment of distance, direction, and floor or ground surfaces creates fall risk. By the middle stage, all process skills are impacted. Attention is limited, and serious memory impairment compromises all aspects of knowledge, temporal organization, organizing space and objects, and adaptation.

In the early stage, the person begins to have problems with communication and interaction skills. By the middle stage, information exchange is limited because of memory impairment and aphasia. As a result, social interactions are affected, often becoming limited to caregivers. Communication may be driven by anxiety, and it is not unusual for the individual to perseverate, asking the same question or expressing the same worry over and over again.

Performance patterns are severely limited. The individual may attempt to engage in habits, and may be successful in some, such as brushing hair or teeth. Habits that require problem solving or adaptations, such as setting an alarm clock or sewing a button, will be less productive, if attempted at all. While most people have established routines for workdays, weekends, and holidays, the person in the middle stage of AD can no longer differentiate days. This loss of routine can contribute to the person's anxiety and depression. Caregivers can help by maintaining structure in the day as well as creative use of meaningful occupations. Roles continue to be lost, and family and friends need to support the most significant roles by reminiscing and affirming the individual's importance.

Cultural contexts begin to diminish in middle stage AD. Personal and temporal contexts may be confused, and some days the person may believe he or she is in an earlier stage of life. At first, cultural, social, and spiritual contexts may be intact. As the condition progresses, there is less attention given to beliefs and values that defined the individual.

Client factors of mental functions are seriously impaired. Orientation to person, place, and time is affected. Personality changes; instead of spontaneity, there is disinhibition; instead of motivation and goal direction, there is apathy or anxiety; instead of fluent verbal and nonverbal communication, there is disinterest or perseveration. There is progressive impairment in all cognitive functions. The person may have hallucinations or delusional ideas. Emotions are not well regulated, and there can be outbursts of anger, fear of an imagined threat, or crying spells that come and go suddenly.

Late Stage. During the late stage of AD, all areas of occupation diminish and are lost. The person is fully dependent in all ADLs and can no longer ambulate with safety. All performance skills and patterns are impaired, and eventually the person loses all functional capacity. Speech is reduced to a few words, and then entirely lost. The person may moan or cry, and caregivers need to assess this as a possible response to pain, discomfort, or psychosis. There is no awareness or understanding of cultural, social, or spiritual contexts. Mental functions are completely impaired, and now there is serious impact on neuromusculoskeletal and movement-related functions. Nerve cell damage takes a toll on muscle strength and tone, and voluntary movement is limited. Once the ability to swallow is lost, the family must make the decision to provide artificial life support, or allow the natural course of the illness to proceed to death.

It is important to note that individuals with AD will show a wide variance in the signs and symptoms within these stages. This is true for several reasons. An individual with a strong set of beliefs and values may maintain these ideas longer than expected; the woman who always took care and pride in her appearance will maintain grooming habits in the middle stage; someone who has always been organized may adapt for memory loss more productively. A formerly shy person may become very impulsive and disinhibited, or become even more withdrawn. The course of the disease is also dependent upon the extent and the areas of neuronal damage.

Vascular Dementia

Etiology. Vascular dementia is caused by one or more strokes that occur when blood cannot get to the brain. Blood clots or fat deposits can block a vessel from delivering oxygen and nutrients to part of the brain. A stroke can also occur when a blood vessel in the brain bursts. High blood pressure, diabetes, heart disease, and high blood cholesterol levels cause strokes.

Vascular dementia can be caused by large multi-infarcts, which are blockages in the large vessels of the brain. Lacunar strokes, in which the small arteries are affected, also cause vascular dementia. Lacunar strokes affect very small areas of tissue, and people with a history of arrhythmias, or irregular heart beat rhythms, may be especially at risk for this problem (12).

Incidence and Prevalence. Goldman states that vascular dementia accounts for 15% to 30% of all dementia cases. As many as 10% of patients first diagnosed with stroke will show signs of dementia within 6 months, and one third will develop dementia in 4 years (23). While there is a slightly greater risk of AD for women, vascular dementia is more likely to occur in men.

Signs and Symptoms. Signs and symptoms vary depending on the area and extent of damage to the brain. When damage in the deep brain areas leads to degeneration of the subcortical white matter, prominent symptoms are memory disturbance, changes in executive function, apathy, and amotivation. Thrombotic or embolic strokes in the large or small cerebral blood vessels produce a different pattern of symptoms. These symptoms include amnesia, receptive or expressive aphasia, constructional or other types of apraxia, and disturbance of executive function (23).

The first two criteria that the *DSM IV-TR* gives for dementia are the same for all the dementia types. These criteria are:

1. There is development of multiple cognitive deficits manifested by memory impairment and at least one other cognitive disturbance (such as aphasia, apraxia, agnosia, and disturbance of executive function).

2. These cognitive deficits cause significant impairment in social or occupational function.
3. For the dementia to be a vascular dementia there is a third criteria, in which signs and symptoms of cardiovascular disease are judged to be related to the cognitive deficits.

Although there are similarities between AD and vascular dementia, some symptoms are more prominent with vascular dementia. The person with vascular dementia tends to have more apraxia, moving with rapid, shuffling steps, and have more falls. Emotional lability is also more common, causing the person to laugh or cry inappropriately (33).

Course and Prognosis. Because strokes occur quickly, symptoms will appear suddenly. The classic course of vascular dementia is a step-wise pattern of increased symptoms. This means that a small stroke can suddenly cause some memory impairment; there may be no new symptoms arising for weeks or even months until another small stroke suddenly worsens memory or causes a new symptom. A slow, progressive course, much like that of AD, can also occur in vascular dementia (23). Controlling the risk factors and treating cardiovascular disease can reduce the progression of vascular dementia.

Medical Management. It is important for someone who may be having a stroke to get emergency treatment. The signs of a stroke are sudden numbness or weakness on one or both sides of the body, and difficulty speaking, seeing, or walking. Immediate treatment can re-open a blocked blood vessel and reduce the severity of the stroke.

The diagnostic process for vascular dementia is similar to the process used to diagnosis AD. The clinician will assess cardiovascular risk factors including high blood pressure, diabetes, high cholesterol, and heart disease. Assessment should also include diet, medications, sleep patterns and stress factors. A CT scan or MRI test can identify signs of stroke as well as tumors or other sources of brain injury. Differentiating vascular dementia from AD can be difficult, and it is possible for an individual to have both diseases (33).

Treatment for cardiovascular risk factors may prevent further strokes, and therefore halt the progression of the disease. High blood pressure is the primary risk factor, and can be treated. Treatment needs to include strategies for managing diabetes, high cholesterol, and heart disease. The doctor may prescribe aspirin or other drugs to prevent clots from forming in small blood vessels. In some cases, the doctor may even recommend surgical procedures to improve blood flow or remove blockages in blood vessels (33).

Frontotemporal Dementia

Memory impairment is considered the hallmark symptom of dementia. However, memory impairment is not the first symptom of frontotemporal dementia (FTD). This form of dementia was first identified by Pick in 1906, and was known as Pick disease (34). Some researchers refer to this condition as Pick's complex and believe that it includes an overlapping of the following syndromes: primary progressive aphasia, corticobasal degeneration, progressive supranuclear palsy, and motor neuron disease (35).

Etiology. Findings on autopsy include bilateral atrophy of the frontal and anterior temporal lobes and degeneration of the striatum (36). Researchers have discovered a link with chromosome 17 as well as the finding of tau mutations (34). These genetic factors continue to be the subject of research.

Incidence and Prevalence. FTD accounts for 5% of all dementias and up to 20% of early onset dementia. It occurs most commonly between the ages of 45 and 65 years, though it can develop before the age of 30 or after the age of 65. There is an equal incidence in men and women, and there is a family history of dementia in about half of the cases (36).

Signs and Symptoms. The most prominent feature of FTD is a change in character and social conduct. There is a decline in personal grooming and hygiene. Mental rigidity and inflexibility combined with distractibility can cause the person to appear memory impaired, when in fact memory may yet be intact. There may be **hyperorality**, which is overeating, or restrictive dietary patterns. There may be perseverative and stereotyped behavior, such as humming or hand rubbing. Utilization behavior refers to touching or grasping anything within sight, and inappropriate use of objects, such as trying to drink from an empty cup. Speech is affected; there can be aphasia, stereotyped speech, echolalia, perseveration, and eventual mutism (34).

A striking feature of FTD is the combination of disinhibition with apathy, although at various stages of the disease, one or the other symptom may predominate. Disinhibited behaviors manifest as **hypersexuality**, hyperorality, and utilization behavior. For the middle age or older person, hypersexuality may consist of verbalizations or gestures. Hyperorality can be seen in excessive overeating, or in developing a limiting food preference, such as eating only milk and bananas. Some may grab food, eat from other's plates, or eat inedibles. Another group of behaviors can be considered negative, including apathy, amotivation, indifference, and flat affect. There may be striking disinterest in the affairs of the family. The person may neglect to change clothing, or lack the ability to attend to any task to completion. There is often decreased language and communication (5).

Course and Prognosis. This disorder was often mistaken for Alzheimer's disease, as its course is progressive. There is a great variation in the symptom patterns of FTD, so the course will vary between individuals.

Medical Management. Treatments for FTD require further research. Since there seems to be no abnormality in the cholinergic system, the cognitive medications used for AD are not likely to be effective. Some of the disinhibited behaviors may be treated with SSRI (36).

Dementia with Lewy Bodies

Dementia with Lewy bodies (DLB) has often been misdiagnosed as AD, delirium, or viewed as Parkinson's disease plus AD. Lewy bodies are microscopic spherical neuronal inclusion bodies within the cytoplasm of a cell. In DLB, Lewy bodies are found in the brainstem and cerebral cortex (3).

Etiology. Just as with AD, the etiology of DLB is unknown. Examination at autopsy reveals, in addition to Lewy bodies, the presence of senile plaques. Unlike the findings of AD, there are sparse neurofibrillary tangles (5).

Incidence and Prevalence. DLB occurs in 10% to 20% of late onset dementias. The mean age of onset is between 75 and 80 years of age. There is a slightly higher risk for males (6).

Signs and Symptoms. An international consortium established guidelines for the diagnosis of DLB (6). According to this guide, the central feature is progressive decline of cognition resulting in impaired social or occupational function. Secondary features include: fluctuation in cognition, alertness, and attention; recurrent visual hallucinations; and motor parkinsonism. In addition to these symptoms, there may be:

1. Repeated falls
2. Syncope

3. Transient loss of consciousness
4. Neuroleptic sensitivity
5. Systematized delusions
6. Hallucinations in other sensory modalities
7. Rapid eye movement (REM) sleep behavior disorder

Course and Prognosis. The course of DLB can be variable and differ from person to person, depending on the location of neuropathology. Some persons have more **extrapyramidal symptoms** (EPS). These include bradykinesia of the extremities or the face, rigidity of the limbs, resting tremor, and gait disturbance. Other persons may have hallucinations more prominently. Mean duration of the disease is five to six years, with a range of 2 to 20. The rate of progression is typically measured by a loss of 4 to 5 MMSE points per year. This is thought to be a more rapid decline than in AD, but this finding has not been validated as yet by research (5).

Medical Management. Clinical management is similar to that of AD, with a need for family involvement and assessment of safety. Medication management requires extreme care, as neuroleptics can result in serious side effects. Any medications with anticholinergic side effects should be avoided. The use of antiparkinsonian medication for motor symptoms is unproven. Research is beginning to show some effectiveness in the use of cholinesterase inhibitors for the treatment of neuropsychiatric and cognitive symptoms of DLB (5).

Reversible Dementia

The idea that dementia may be reversible is a topic of debate. Most researchers today believe that reversible dementia is very uncommon (38). In many cases, what seemed to be a reversible dementia was simply some other cause for cognitive impairment that was misdiagnosed as dementia. Burke et al. refers to the term of reversible dementia as a misnomer, and states that dementia should only be used to identify cognitive impairment in cases of irreversible degenerative brain disease (39).

It is a fact that cognitive impairment can be misdiagnosed as dementia. Having a potentially treatable impairment misidentified, and left untreated, could have drastic and dire consequences for the person's function and way of life. And so it is important to review what some may refer to as reversible dementia, and others see as reversible cognitive impairment.

Hejl et al. states that the most frequently encountered potentially reversible conditions are depression, normal pressure hydrocephalus, alcohol related conditions, space-occupying lesions, epilepsy, and metabolic conditions (40). Depression is sometimes known as pseudo-dementia when it presents with cognitive impairment in an elderly person. The National Institute of Aging also places depression high on their list of treatable causes of dementia (11). Their list is as follows:

1. Medication side effects
2. Depression
3. Vitamin B12 deficiency
4. Chronic alcoholism
5. Certain tumors or infections of the brain
6. Blood clots pressing on the brain
7. Metabolic imbalances, including thyroid, kidney, or liver disorders

Cohen also discussed reversible causes of dementia (10). Asymptomatic infections can cause a delirium that could be misdiagnosed as dementia. In addition to metabolic disorders, there may be nutritional disorders leading to a false diagnosis of dementia. A disturbance in electrolytes or uncontrolled diabetes can cause impairment in cognition. Cardiovascular and pulmonary changes can reduce oxygen and nutrients needed by the brain for normal cognition. Medication related problems may be the most common cause of cognitive impairment, and yet are the most easily treated. Lastly, impaired vision or hearing can create the impression that the person's functional loss is a result of impaired cognition. It is for these reasons that any change in cognition must be treated as a serious, but possibly treatable symptom of disease.

CASE STUDY

Case Illustrations

■ CASE 1: ALZHEIMER'S DISEASE

Mrs. L. was born in South America. She was bilingual, speaking her native Spanish as well as flawless English. In her early years, she had the luxury of maids and a cook. She was a widow before her two children were grown. At age 60, her adult daughter died, leaving Mrs. L. as the primary caregiver for her two young grandchildren. Soon after her daughter's death, Mrs. L. fled her native land for political reasons, bringing her orphaned grandchildren to live in New York. After raising them, she continued to live with her adult granddaughter, G.

EARLY STAGE

When Mrs. L. was 82, G. married and her new husband moved into their home. Mrs. L. had always told G. that "when you marry and no longer need me, it will be my time to die." She seemed angry at G. and showed her irritation by complaining. Nevertheless, she continued to prepare the family meals, make beds, and do some of the laundry. In spite of failing vision, she was aware of the need to dust. She continued to take impeccable care of her appearance, always setting her hair at night and never going out without wearing hose and high heels. Her social life was full, with friends and neighbors frequently visiting. She took pride in serving tea and dessert to her weekly women's support group who met at her apartment. There were times when Mrs. L. misplaced her dentures (in odd places such as in a plant pot) or forgot to use detergent when washing the dishes. She was often anxious and needy when G. came home from work, and she became defensive and easily upset when questioned about mistakes. Her granddaughter attributed these aberrations to Mrs. L.'s increased stress as a result of the marriage.

MIDDLE STAGE

At age 86, Mrs. L. broke her hip, her granddaughter had a new, colicky baby, and the family moved to a larger apartment in the same complex. As a result of these crises, Mrs. L. seemed to have slowed down and became more dependent on G. She began making more obvious mistakes, such as using the toilet brush to scrub the floor and neglecting to wash the dishes before putting them away. G. took over the housekeeping and cooking duties.

Mrs. L.'s hearing and sight continued to decline, and she complained about "nothing ever being right." G. got her books on tape, but Mrs. L. could not learn to operate the tape player. She continued to entertain her weekly women's group, basking in the compliments from her friends for the tasty desserts that they knew were now being made by G.

Mrs. L. became a picky eater, putting catsup on everything, including salads and fruit. She was still very particular about her appearance, but she began to need help doing her hair and became neglectful of her denture care. She could still fold laundry, make beds, and take her bath independently.

There were times when Mrs. L. became fearful of G.'s husband, accusing him of wanting to hurt her granddaughter.

At age 91, the family moved out of the apartment complex, where they had lived for many years, to a new home. Mrs. L. was no longer able to make impromptu visits to her neighbors, and her circle of friends now rarely visited. Mrs. L. was afraid to use anything in the new kitchen, especially the unfamiliar gas stove. Her appetite continued to be poor, and she was losing weight. Strategies to enable her to make her own tea and toast were unsuccessful, and she would forget to eat food left for her in the refrigerator when G. went to work.

Mrs. L. began to have incontinence of bowel and bladder, yet she would resist her granddaughter's suggestions that she needed to shower or bathe. Ironically, when Mrs. L. fell and broke her wrist, she became amenable to assistance. Insurance covered about 6 weeks of home health care, and Mrs. L. seemed to enjoy the attention.

Late Stage

At age 92, it was clear that Mrs. L. could not be left alone. She continued to be incontinent; she couldn't lift herself from the toilet and seemed afraid to use a bedside commode. When her granddaughter came home from work, she would follow her about, repeating the same question over and over. She was not eating lunch or dinner. Her granddaughter, pregnant with her second child, was having difficulty bathing Mrs. L. On one occasion they both ended up falling on the bathroom floor during a bathing session. In-home care proved unaffordable, and G. made the difficult decision to place Mrs. L. in a nursing home. The nursing home, known for its excellence, proved to be a positive move for Mrs. L. She regained some of her weight and seemed much less anxious. Mrs. L.'s deep-rooted social personality and gift for charming those around her made a reappearance. This served to ensure that a constant stream of staff and residents dropped by her room for brief chats. When G. and her family visited, Mrs. L. remained cool, as if to reprimand G. for sending her away.

Within a year, Mrs. L. was not always able to recognize G. when she came to visit. Sometimes she mistook G. for her daughter. Eventually she completely lost the ability to recognize G. Her granddaughter continued to visit with her own children, who delighted in playing word games with Mrs. L. The youngest child, himself learning to speak, would say a few words or phrases to Mrs. L., which she would mimic. This would set both children to giggling, in turn pleasing Mrs. L. to have had such an amusing effect on the children.

At age 94, Mrs. L. seemed no longer able to speak English. Her verbalizations in Spanish were limited to a few words, which were sometimes unintelligible. She was no longer able to ambulate and needed total care for feeding. Shortly after her 95th birthday, Mrs. L. died peacefully of heart failure.

■ CASE 2: VASCULAR DEMENTIA

Mr. B. is a 71-year-old African American who is cared for at home by his wife. Mrs. B. describes him as having been a quietly dignified person before the onset of his illness. He enjoyed spending time with his family, including his four children and other members of his extended family.

As a young college graduate, Mr. B. was unable to find work in his field of engineering but did get an unskilled job with the phone company. His supervisor recognized his talents and abilities, and over time, he had a series of promotions that eventually took him to the position of personnel manager.

When Mr. B. was 60, his company was bought out and he was given an early retirement. Soon after this, he started taking classes in cabinet making, and began working for an architect who was building a local church.

At age 64, Mr. B. began making errors in measurement in his work. He was aware of, and troubled by this difficulty. He decided to cut back his hours at work. Mrs. B. noted at this time that he sometimes appeared confused. During family gatherings he was not only quieter than his usual self, but he would actually distance himself by sitting in another room. Although he was still driving, he began misplacing things. Mrs. B. had some concerns about these behaviors but attributed them to the stress of life changes.

It was when Mr. B. was no longer able to read a ruler that Mrs. B. began to realize something was seriously wrong. At about this time, Mr. B. had an episode in which he got lost on the way to the dentist. Mrs. B. turned to her family physician for help, and an 18-month period of medical and neurological testing ensued.

At age 66, Mr. B. had a stroke. During hospitalization, the diagnosis of vascular dementia was finally made. When Mr. B. left the hospital, he was able to walk and perform his self-care activities independently.

At first, things went well at home. Both Mr. and Mrs. B. adjusted to a routine in which she would make sure that he was up, dressed, and had breakfast before she left for work. His lunch was prepared and left for him to retrieve from the refrigerator. One day Mrs. B. came home from work and found that the stove had been left on. At this point, she realized that Mr. B. was no longer safe when left alone, and she enrolled him in a day-care program.

About 8 months later, Mrs. B. made the decision to stop working. The day program cost almost as much as her pay. It was becoming more and more difficult to help Mr. B. get dressed and out of the house every morning. In fact, Mr. B. started choosing to undress himself several times a day. He began having problems speaking and understanding what others said to him. Mrs. B. felt he was losing his personality; he wasn't able to focus on conversation or show interest, even when his grandchildren visited. He was still ambulating with help. He began having difficulty swallowing, was losing weight, and was having bladder infections. He was no longer continent of bowel or bladder.

At age 69, Mr. B. had another stroke. Despite the efforts of the rehabilitation service, he could no longer ambulate. He returned home in a wheelchair. His home did not have a ground floor bedroom, so Mrs. B. converted the living room to his bedroom. For about 1 month, his insurance provided a home health aide who would give Mr. B. a weekly bed bath. Eventually Mrs. B. took over this responsibility, along with complete care for dressing and feeding him. Mr. B. often did not recognize Mrs. B. and no longer recognized his children.

During a recent visit to the outpatient clinic, Mrs. B. talked about the difficulty of getting through each day. "I rarely get out unless one of the family members can stay with my husband, and even then I'm just too tired. I think about the reality that someday I may need to put him in a nursing home. I'll do it when it gets to the point where I'm no longer able to take care of him or if my health goes bad. But if that happens, I'll lose our life savings—it's not much, but enough to help pay bills with my social security check." She also related an incident that illustrated the small daily frustrations of caring for her husband: "I was feeding him lunch, and he reached for the glass of milk with his left hand. I helped place the glass in his outstretched hand, but he began raising his right hand to his mouth as if to drink. Obviously that wasn't working, so I took the glass out of his left hand and put it in his right hand. This must have totally confused him, and he just looked at me as if to say 'what did you do that for?' I felt so helpless, and so bad that I couldn't even help him."

Mr. B., who at 71 is still handsome, sits straight and tall in his wheelchair, appearing to emanate dignity and calm, faintly smiling and nodding as his wife tells their story.

References

1. Diagnostic and Statistical Manual of Mental Disorders. 4th Ed., text revision. Washington, DC: American Psychiatric Association, 2000.
2. Van Wynen EA. A key to successful aging: learning-style patterns of older adults. J Gerontol Nurs 2001;27(9):6–15.
3. Sadock BJ, Sadock VA. Kaplan and Sadock's Comprehensive Textbook of Psychiatry. 7th Ed. Philadelphia: Lippincott, Williams & Wilkins, 2000.
4. Hales RE, Yudofsky SC, Talbott JA. The American Psychiatric Press Textbook of Psychiatry. 3rd Ed. Washington DC: American Psychiatric Press, 1999.
5. Mosimann UP, McKeith IG. Dementia with Lewy bodies-diagnosis and treatment. Swiss Med Wkly 2003;133:131–142.
6. Frank C. Dementia with Lewy bodies. Can Fam Physician 2003;49:1304–1311.
7. DeCarli C. The role of neuroimaging in dementia. Clin Geriatr Med 2001;17(2):255–279.
8. Shenk D. The Forgetting. New York: Anchor Books, 2003.
9. Vickers JC, Dickson TC, Adlard PA, et al. The cause of neuronal degeneration in Alzheimer's disease. Prog Neurobiol 2000;60(2): 139–165.
10. Bear MF, Connors BW, Paradiso MA. Neuroscience: Exploring the Brain. 2nd Ed. Baltimore: Lippincott, Williams & Wilkins, 2001.
11. National Institute on Aging. Alzheimer's Disease: Unraveling the Mystery. Washington, DC: National Institutes of Health, 2003.
12. Cohen D, Eisdorfer C. The Loss of Self. New York: W.W. Norton & Co., 2001.
13. Rocchi A, Pellegrini S, Siciliano G, Murri L. Causative and susceptibility genes for Alzheimer's disease: a review. Brain Res Bull 2003;61(1): 1–24.
14. Alzheimer's Disease Education & Referral Center. Alzheimer's Disease Genetics: Fact Sheet. Washington DC: U.S. Department of Health and Human Services, 2004.
15. Tanzi RE, Bertram L. New frontiers in Alzheimer's disease genetics. Neuron 2001;32(2):181–184.
16. Blazer DG, Steffens DC, Busse EW. The American Psychiatric Publishing Textbook of Geriatric Psychiatry. 3rd Ed. Washington, DC: American Psychiatric Publishing, Inc., 2004.
17. Neve RL, McPhie DL, Chen Y. Alzheimer's disease: a dysfunction of the amyloid precursor protein (1). Brain Res 2000;886(1–2):54–66.
18. Breteler MM. Vascular risk factors for Alzheimer's disease: an epidemiologic perspective. Neurobiol Aging 2000;21(2):153–160.
19. Kalaria RN. The role of cerebral ischemia in Alzheimer's disease. Neurobiol Aging 2000;21(2): 321–330.
20. Varadarajan S, Yatin S, Aksenova M. Review: Alzheimer's amyloid beta-peptide-associated free radical oxidative stress and neurotoxicity. J Struct Biol 2000;130(2–3):184–208.
21. Kawas CH, Brookmeyer R. Aging and the public health effects of dementia. N Engl J Med 2001;344(15):1160–1161.
22. Reisberg B, Sclan SG. Functional assessment staging (FAST) in Alzheimer's disease; reliability, validity and ordinality. Int Psychogeriatr 1992; 4(Suppl 1):55–69.
23. Goldman LS, Wise TN, Brody DS. Psychiatry for Primary Care Physicians. 2nd Ed. Atlanta: AMA Press, 2004.
24. Hughes CP, Berg L, Danziger WL, et al. A new clinical scale for the staging of dementia. Br J Psychiatry 1993;140:566–572.
25. Peterson RC, Stevens JC, Ganguli M, et al. Practice parameter: early detection of dementia: mild cognitive impairment (an evidence based review). Neurology 2001;56:1133–1142.
26. Gauthier S. Advances in the pharmacotherapy of Alzheimer's disease. Can Med Assoc J 2002;166(5): 616–626.
27. Zgola JM. Care That Works: A Relationship Approach to Persons with Dementia. Baltimore: The John Hopkins University Press, 1999.
28. Kovach CR. Late-Stage Dementia Care: A Basic Guide. Milwaukee: Taylor & Francis, 1997.
29. Liu C, McDowd J, Lin K. Visuospatial inattention and daily life performance in people with Alzheimer's disease. Am J Occup Ther 2004;58(2): 202–210.
30. Folstein MF, Folstein SE, McHugh PR. Mini-mental state: a practice method for grading the cognitive

state of patients for the clinician. J Psychiatr Res 1975;12:198.
31. Herrmann N. Cognitive pharmacotherapy of Alzheimer's disease and other dementias. Can J Psychiatry 2002;47(8):715–722.
32. Family Caregiver Alliance. Dementia & driving: Fact Sheet. San Francisco: National Center on Caregiving, 2002.
33. Alzheimer's Disease Education & Referral Center. Multi-Infarct Dementia Fact Sheet. National Institutes of Health (publication no. 02–3433), 2003.
34. Kertesz A. Frontotemporal dementia/Pick disease. Arch Neurol 2004;61:969–971.
35. Kertesz A. Pick complex: an integrative approach to Frontotemporal dementia: primary progressive aphasia, corticobasal degeneration, and progressive supranuclear palsy. Neurologist 2003;9(6): 311–317.
36. Snowden JS, Neary D, Mann DM. Frontotemporal dementia. Br J Psychiatry 2002;180:140–143.
37. Kertesz A, Munoz DG. Frontotemporal dementia. Med Clin N Am 2002;86(3):501–513.
38. Knopman D, Jankowiak J. Recovery from dementia: an interesting case. Neurology 2005;64: E18–E19.
39. Burke D, Sengoz A, Schwartz R. Potentially reversible cognitive impairment in patients presenting to a memory disorders clinic. J Clin Neurosci 2000;7(2):120–123.
40. Hejl A, Hogh P, Waldemar G. Potentially reversible conditions in 1000 consecutive memory clinic patients. J Neurol Neurosurg Psychiatry 2002;73: 390–394.

Recommended Learning Resources

Kuhn D. Alzheimer's Early Stages: First Steps in Caring and Treatment. 2nd Ed. Berkeley, CA: Publishers Group West, 2003.

Mace NL, Rabins PV. The 36-Hour Day: A Family Guide to Caring for Persons with Alzheimer's Disease. Baltimore: Johns Hopkins University Press, 1999.

Peterson R. Mayo Clinic on Alzheimer's Disease. Rochester, MN: Mayo Clinic Health Information, 2002.

Restak R. The Secret Life of the Brain. Washington, DC: Joseph Henry Press, 2001.

Robinson A, Spencer B, White L. Understanding Difficult Behaviors: Some Practical Suggestions for Coping with Alzheimer's Disease and Related Illnesses. Ypsilanti, MI: Eastern Michigan University Alzheimer's Education Program, 1996.

Cerebrovascular Accident

Paula W. Jamison and David P. Orchanian

Key Terms

Agnosia
Aneurysm
Apraxia
Arteriovenous
Associated reactions
Ataxia
Atheromas
Atherosclerosis
Brain attack
Cerebrovascular accident
Collateral circulation
Decussation
Deep vein thrombosis
Dysarthria
Dysphagia
Embolism
Endarterectomy
Flaccidity
Hematoma
Hemianopsia (hemianopia)
Hemiplegia
Hemorrhagic stroke
Ischemia
Spasticity
Thrombus
Transient ischemic attacks
Unilateral neglect

E.C. is a 57-year-old Maine lobsterman, born and raised in Ogunquit, Maine. E.C. was born of Irish and Italian parents who taught him the value of hard work. His father was a lobsterman also and died at age 65 from heart disease and hypertension. His mother is still living in a nursing facility in a nearby community. Her health is failing, and E.C. is the nearest of three siblings, with his brothers all living outside of the state. E.C. has smoked tobacco in the form of pipes, cigarettes, and/or cigars since he was in the Army in Vietnam from 1966 to 1968. He now only chews tobacco when he is out fishing. He is about 30 pounds overweight for his 5-foot 10-inch frame, and over the past several months he has been experiencing shortness of breath when exerting himself. Other than surgery for a left inguinal hernia repair several years ago, E.C. does not visit physicians. He is unaware of his own blood pressure but has experienced periods of light-headedness when working. E.C. plays softball in the spring and summer with the volunteer fire department in Ogunquit. Usually he enjoys several beers every day. Last week when E.C. was out hauling lobster pots with his first mate he noticed that suddenly he was unable to grip the line firmly with his right hand. Additionally, he felt that the right side of his face and head was warm and tingling. He became sick to his stomach and his first mate decided to end the trip and head for port. By the time they docked, approximately an hour later, E.C. had vomited once and now complained of a throbbing headache.

What is happening to E.C.? Is there enough evidence to suspect that a stroke may be evolving? What should he and his first mate do? This chapter offers insight into E.C.'s condition and helps provide answers to these questions.

As life expectancy increases and the population ages, public awareness about stroke has increased dramatically. Stroke is the third leading cause of death in the United States and accounts for one out of 14 deaths (1). It is the number one cause of disability, which ranges from profound loss of function to subtle deficits (2). According to the Centers for Disease Control and Prevention (CDC), about 50% of stroke deaths occur before the person reaches the hospital, although survival rates continue to increase (1,2). Additionally, the financial and social impact of stroke is enormous and includes both direct costs for medical and professional services as well as indirect costs such as lost productivity from work (3). Much is currently being done to emphasize prevention and recognition of symptoms. For example, recent terminology that refers to stroke as a **brain attack** reflects an attempt to educate the public about the suddenness and potential severity of this condition (4,5). Outcomes for someone who has a stroke are highly variable and depend on many physical and socioeconomic factors, which will be addressed in this chapter.

Etiology

A stroke, or brain attack, results from an interruption in the blood flow to the brain, either because a blood vessel is blocked or ruptures. The consequence is an inadequate supply of oxygen and nutrients to this vital organ. Even a brief disruption of this blood flow can lead to brain damage. Medical practitioners use the term "**cerebrovascular accident**," often abbreviated as CVA, for stroke. A stroke can occur in any part of the brain, the cerebral hemispheres, the cerebellum, or the brainstem. The site and extent of the affected area, or infarct, determines loss of function.

Strokes are divided into two main types: ischemic and hemorrhagic. Ischemic strokes are characterized by blockages (the term **ischemia** refers to the lack of blood supply) and include atherothrombotic, lacunar, and embolic infarctions, in that order of frequency (6). **Hemorrhagic strokes** include intracerebral and subarachnoid hemorrhages (5,6). Both types of stroke lead to the death, or infarction, of brain tissue. These two groups of strokes can be differentiated further by the location of the insult and the precise causes of the ischemia or hemorrhage (6). In most cases, a loss of blood supply is the result of long-standing degeneration of the body's blood vessels. Less commonly, a CVA occurs because of an inborn abnormality or weakness of the brain's vascular supply (4). A brief review of cerebral circulation will help understand the impact of each type of stroke.

Cerebral Circulatory System

The blood supply of the brain is extremely important because the brain is one of the most metabolically active organs of the body. Although it comprises only 2% of the body's weight, the brain receives approximately 17% of the cardiac output and consumes about 20% of the oxygen used by the entire body (7).

In the brain, the arteries of the anterior circulation supply the front, top, and side portions of the cerebral hemispheres. The brainstem and cerebellum, as well as the back and undersurface of the cerebral hemispheres, are supplied by the posterior circulation. These two areas of circulation are further categorized into the extracranial portions (arising from outside the skull and traveling toward the brain) and the intracranial portions (arising from within the skull) (7).

Extracranial Vessels

Extracranial anterior circulation consists of the two carotid arteries, which travel in the front of the neck on each side of the trachea and esophagus (7). The word "carotid" is derived from the Greek word "karos" meaning "to stupefy," or render unconscious, indicating the significance of this main artery in maintaining consciousness and brain function (8). The right common carotid artery arises from the innominate artery. The left common carotid artery originates directly from the aortic arch. Around the fifth or sixth vertebrae, these common carotid arteries divide into external carotid arteries, whose branches supply the face and its structures, and the internal carotid arteries, which supply the eyes and the cerebral hemispheres (8).

The vertebral arteries arise from the subclavian arteries and make up the extracranial posterior circulation. They remain within the vertebral column for part of their course from about C6 to C2. The vertebral arteries enter the cranium through the foramen magnum (7).

Intracranial Vessels

The internal carotid arteries enter the skull through the carotid canal and form an S-shaped curve called the carotid siphon (8). The artery then enters the subarachnoid space by piercing the dura mater. It gives rise to the ophthalmic arteries, which supply the eyes; the posterior communicating arteries, which join with the posterior circulation; and the anterior cerebral arteries, which supply the orbital and medial surfaces of the frontal lobes and part of the basal frontal lobe white matter and caudate nucleus. The internal carotid artery also gives off the middle cerebral arteries, which supply almost the entire lateral surface of the frontal, parietal, and temporal lobes, as well as the underlying white matter and basal ganglia (7). The middle cerebral artery is the largest of the terminal branches of the internal carotid artery and is the direct continuation of this vessel.

The vertebral arteries enter the cranium within the posterior fossa and travel along the side of the medulla, where they give off their longest branch, the posterior inferior cerebellar artery. This artery supplies the lateral medulla and the back of the undersurface of the cerebellum (6). The two vertebral arteries then join at the junction between the medulla and pons to form the single midline basilar artery (7). The basilar artery gives off penetrating arteries to the base of the pons and two vessels (the anterior inferior and superior cerebellar arteries) that supply the upper and anterior undersurfaces of the cerebellum (6). At the level of the midbrain, the basilar artery bifurcates into the two posterior cerebral arteries (7). As they circle the brainstem, these two arteries give off penetrating branches to the midbrain and thalamus and then divide into branches that supply the occipital lobes as well as the medial and undersurfaces of the temporal lobes (6). One of the branches of the posterior cerebral artery, the calcarine artery, is of special significance because it is the main supplier of blood for the visual area of the cortex (7).

Communicating Arteries

The right and left carotid vessels connect with each other when they enter the brain, each sending out a small lateral branch that meets in the space between them. These are the anterior communicating arteries. They also branch backward to join with the right and left posterior cerebral arteries, called the posterior communicating arteries. This communicating vascular interchange is known as the circle of Willis, which is pictured in Figure 9.1. It protects the brain should one of the four major supplying arteries coming up through the neck be blocked (7). This important anatomical feature is named for Dr. Thomas Willis and was first described in the mid-17th century (7). Starting from the midline anteriorly, the circle consists of the anterior communicating, anterior cerebral, internal carotid, posterior communicating, and posterior cerebral arteries, from which it continues to the starting point in reverse order (6). When one major vessel supplying the brain is slowly occluded, either within the circle of Willis or proximal to it, the normally small communicating arteries may slowly enlarge to compensate for the occlusion (7). This system is imperfect, however, and it often fails to prevent strokes. In many individuals, the same atherosclerotic processes that caused a stroke also may damage communicating arteries. In addition, only about one fourth of strokes are caused by a blockage of the major neck vessels (2). For approximately one third of the population, the communicating artery may be insufficient or even absent (6). Such anomalies are more common in those who have strokes than in the general population and may be linked to increased risk of stroke in persons who also have **atherosclerosis** (8).

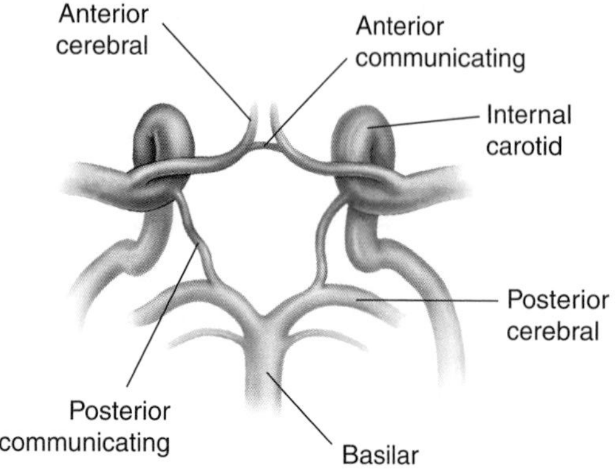

Figure 9.1 Circle of Willis in the human brain.

Types of Strokes

Ischemic Stroke

This is the most common type of stroke accounting for 80% of cases (2). Cerebral infarction, or brain tissue death, results when circulation to an area of the brain is obstructed, resulting in ischemia. Ischemic strokes are classified as thrombotic, embolic, or lacunar strokes. The damaged area has two components: the tissues that have died as a result of blood supply loss and the peripheral area in which there may be temporary dysfunction as a result of edema. Edematous brain tissue sometimes recovers slowly and gradually, resulting in a reappearance of function after a period of 4 to 5 months (2). In the past, prognoses for functional recovery have been limited to this time frame. However, recent research offers promising evidence that recovery is possible months and even years poststroke (9). Explanations focus on the brain's ability to reroute neural pathways, a phenomenon known as neural plasticity (9).

The actual physiologic events that follow an ischemic stroke occur in characteristic steps.

First, the membrane surrounding each affected neuron leaks potassium (a mineral necessary for producing electrical impulses) and adenosine triphosphate (ATP, an energy-producing biochemical found in the body). Fluid quickly accumulates between the blood vessel and neuron, making it difficult for oxygen and nutrients to pass from the bloodstream into the damaged neuron. The initial injury produces a vicious circle in which more cellular injury results. Irreversible cell death will occur in 5 to 10 minutes if oxygen and nutrients are unable to reach them from the bloodstream or in a slightly longer period if blood flow is only partially interrupted. These dead cells form a zone of infarction that will not regenerate (6).

Downstream from the infarcted zone is a zone of injury (penumbra) (6). This area may be served by collateral blood vessels and is capable of returning to normal functioning. A third area that reacts differently to the stroke process may also exist. In this area of hyperemia, the blood vessels are congested and swollen and also may have the potential for recovery.

The presence of these two zones, the regions of penumbra and hyperemia, may serve to minimize the total area of infarction. However, they do present problems for treatment because interventions that benefit one region may not help the other (10).

Thrombosis

Cerebral thrombosis occurs when a blood clot forms in one of the arteries supplying the brain, causing vascular obstruction at the point of its formation. The size and location of the infarct depends on which vessel is occluded and the amount of **collateral circulation**. Thrombosis occurs most frequently in blood vessels that have already been damaged by atherosclerosis (5).

Atherosclerosis is a gradual degenerative disease of the blood vessel walls. It is a pathologic process rather than a normal effect of human aging (8). Rough, irregular fatty deposits form within the intima and inner media of the arteries and often lead to the generation of a **thrombus**, or blood clot. This is the most common cause of stroke, with stenosis, or narrowing of the blood vessels, resulting in much fewer cases (2). Large-vessel atherosclerosis accounts for 60% of ischemic stroke (2). Because the body's blood vessels have a significant reserve capacity, ischemic strokes do not usually occur until the vessel is two-thirds blocked (11). The impact of atherosclerosis on the vascular system is considerable; it is also a major risk factor for heart disease.

To understand the process that produces a mass of degenerated, thickened material (plaque) called **atheromas**, imagine a glue bottle that has been allowed to collect the residuals of dried glue. The more clogged the cap of the bottle becomes, the more difficult it is for the glue to flow through. Squeezing the glue through the opening can push already dried glue more firmly against the opening. The opening will become smaller and smaller until it closes completely or bursts from the increased pressure.

In the cerebral circulation, atherosclerosis and thrombus formation are most likely to occur in areas where blood vessels turn or divide, such as the origins of the internal carotid artery and the middle cerebral artery and the junction of the vertebral and basilar arteries (12).

Cerebral thrombosis often causes stuttering or progressive symptoms that occur over several hours or days. Onset during sleep is common. Often a patient notices mild arm numbness at night and then awakens the next morning with paralysis. **Transient ischemic attacks** precede actual infarction about half the time (2).

Lacunar Strokes, or Penetrating Artery Disease

Lacunar strokes are small infarcts, usually lying in the deep brain structures, such as the basal ganglia, thalamus, pons, internal capsule, and deep white matter (2). Approximately 25% of ischemic strokes are the result of damage to these deep structures (13). Within a few months of onset of a lacunar stroke, a small cavity ("lacune" in French) is left (2).

Lacunar strokes result from an occlusion of small branches of larger cerebral arteries—middle cerebral, posterior cerebral, basilar, and, to a lesser extent, anterior cerebral and vertebral arteries (13). Lacunar infarcts range in size from 2 to 15 mm (13). Because of their small size, minimal neurological symptoms are often present, and many such strokes go undetected. Recent findings indicate, however, that long-term prognosis is not good for lacunar strokes, and the recovery rate is similar to that for other types of stroke (13). Typically, lacunar strokes produce purely motor deficits (weakness or **ataxia**), purely sensory deficits, or a combination of sensory and motor deficits (14). Symptoms do not usually include aphasia, changes in cognition or personality, loss of consciousness, homonymous **hemianopsia**, or seizures (14). The most consistently identified risk factor for lacunar infarction is hypertension, and treatment is aimed at controlling it (2).

Embolism

Embolism occurs when a clot that has formed elsewhere (thrombus) breaks off (embolus), travels up the blood stream until it reaches an artery too small to pass through, and blocks the artery (12). At this point, the effects of the embolus are similar to those produced by thrombosis. Embolic materials that travel to the arteries of the brain can originate from many sources, including the aortic arch and arteries arising from it, the extracranial carotid and vertebral arteries, and thrombi in the heart. Cardiac-source emboli occur in approximately 20% of ischemic strokes and are referred to as cardiogenic (3). Many cardiac abnormalities can give rise to a cerebral embolism, including atrial fibrillation, coronary artery disease, valvular heart disease, and arrhythmias. Cardiac surgery is also a cause (3). The middle cerebral artery is by far the most common destination of cardiac emboli, followed by the posterior cerebral artery (12).

In contrast to thrombotic strokes, embolic strokes typically occur during daytime activity (2). The embolism can be precipitated by a sudden movement, or even a sneeze, which raises blood pressure and dislodges the clot. Clinical symptoms are usually maximal at onset, but in some cases the neurological symptoms improve or stabilize somewhat, then worsen as the embolus moves and blocks a more distal artery. A history of transient ischemic attacks (TIAs) is rare. Seizures are often associated with embolic strokes (15,16).

Hemorrhagic Stroke

Approximately 20% of strokes are hemorrhagic (2). Hemorrhagic strokes are caused by a rupture in a blood vessel or an **aneurysm**, with resultant bleeding into or around cerebral tissue. An aneurysm is a bulging or outpouching of a wall of an artery as a result of weakness in the vessel wall; it is prone to rupture at any time. While fatality rates for hemorrhagic strokes are higher than for ischemic strokes, recent findings indicate that patients often make a better recovery after a hemorrhagic stroke (4). Hemorrhagic strokes are more common in young people than ischemic strokes as the vessel wall anomaly is often congenital. There are two types of hemorrhagic strokes. An intracerebral hemorrhage refers to bleeding directly into brain substance, whereas a subarachnoid hemorrhage is bleeding occurring within the brain's surrounding membranes and cerebrospinal fluid (CSF) (12). These two types of hemorrhage differ in incidence, etiology, clinical signs, and treatment.

Intracerebral Hemorrhages

Intracerebral hemorrhage results in bleeding directly into the brain and accounts for a high percentage of deaths because of stroke (4). It may occur in any part of the brain and is most commonly linked to hypertension. Other causes include blood vessel abnormalities, such as **arteriovenous** malformations or aneurysms, or trauma (17). Release of blood into brain tissue and surrounding edema will then disrupt the function of that particular brain region (18). Blood irritates the brain tissue and causes swelling, or it may form a mass called a **hematoma**. In either case the increased pressure on brain tissue can rapidly destroy them. Factors that increase the risk of intracerebral hemorrhage include blood and bleeding disorders such as hemophilia, sickle cell anemia, and leukemia; use of anticoagulants; and liver disease (17).

Clinical signs of intracerebral hemorrhage are usually focal, that is, unlike cerebral infarcts, hemorrhagic bleeds do not follow the anatomic distribution of blood vessels but move spherically through the tissue planes (19). Typically they develop suddenly, often during activity (17). While extremely small hemorrhages may go undetected, a large hematoma causes headache, vomiting, convulsions, and decreased levels of alertness (2,20).

Stupor and coma are common signs of very large hemorrhages and indicate a poor prognosis, especially among individuals over 85 (21,22). Nevertheless, recovery is possible.

Cerebral injury caused by intracerebral bleeding is a result of the damaging effect that the abnormal presence of blood has on the neurons. In addition to the irritant of the blood, abnormal pressure on neurons distorts their normal architecture. It also prevents oxygen and nutrients from passing to the cells from the blood stream. Eventually, bleeding will stop and a hard clot will form. During a period of months, the clot slowly recedes, breaks down, and is absorbed by the body's white blood cells (12). If not damaged by increased pressure, the tissues irritated by the blood may heal, leading to a positive outcome, perhaps even full recovery (4).

Subarachnoid Hemorrhages

Subarachnoid hemorrhages account for about 5% to 10% of all strokes and are slightly more common in women (23). About 95% are caused by the leakage of blood from aneurysms (23). A combination of congenital and degenerative factors, usually at the points of origin or bifurcations of arteries, can precipitate formation of an aneurysm (6). Blood may break through the weak point of the aneurysm at any time and, because of the force of arterial pressure, spread quickly into the CSF surrounding the brain. A subarachnoid hemorrhage also may be caused by bleeding from an arteriovenous malformation, which is an abnormal collection of vessels near the surface of the brain. Other less common causes of subarachnoid hemorrhages are hemophilia, excessive anticoagulation therapy, and trauma to the skull and brain (6).

The extravasated, or escaped, blood irritates the meninges, and intracranial pressure is increased owing to extra fluid in the closed cranial cavity. This can lead to headache, vomiting, and an altered state of consciousness. Sleepiness, stupor, agitation, restlessness, and actual coma are various manifestations of reduced consciousness. Headaches are usually severe and are described as the worst in the patient's life (23). Because the bleeding takes place around the brain and not in the actual brain substance, motor, sensory, or visual abnormalities on one side of the body usually are not seen. CT scans (see below) are the most reliable tool for detecting subarachnoid hemorrhage (6). If results are inconclusive, lumbar puncture with analysis of the CSF is the most reliable method of diagnosing subarachnoid hemorrhage (6).

Risk Factors

A number of risk factors are associated with the likelihood of stroke and resemble those for heart disease. This is not surprising, considering that atherosclerosis is an underlying cause for both conditions. While some of these risk factors are inborn or otherwise unavoidable, many are related to lifestyle and behavioral choices. Adopting healthy eating and exercise patterns early in life is especially important for individuals who are genetically at risk, although everyone can benefit. Regular visits to a family physician are important.

- Ethnicity—although all minority groups are at risk, stroke death rates are much higher for African Americans than for whites: data from 2000 indicated that out of 100,000 population, there were 87 deaths from stroke for black males and 78 for black females, compared to 59 for white males and 58 for white females (1). Recent data also indicate that blacks living in the South have a greater risk of dying from stroke than those who live in the northern states (24).
- Age—risk for stroke increases with age, especially after age 65. People with high blood pressure and who exhibit the other risk factors listed in this chapter are increasingly vulnerable as they age. Younger people are not immune, either: approximately 28% of strokes occur in individuals younger than age 65 (25).
- Heredity—a family history of stroke, particular on the father's side, increases one's risk (26). Genetic factors account for 7% to 20% of cases of subarachnoid hemorrhage, and some researchers recommend that people with more than one close relative who suffered a hemorrhagic stroke be screened for aneurysms (27).
- Obesity—being overweight is a known risk factor for hypertension and diabetes mellitus and also is associated with stroke. Weight that is centered in the abdomen (so-called apple shape) has a particularly high association with stroke as well as heart disease, while individuals whose weight is distributed around the hips are less at risk (27,28). A sedentary lifestyle is associated with rising levels of obesity and has been implicated in occurrence of strokes, as well as, hypertension (3).
- Hypertension—called the "silent disease," hypertension has long been acknowledged as the most significant controllable risk factor for both stroke and heart attack (3). Hypertension occurs in 25% to 40% of the U.S. population (6). Symptoms of hypertension are not clearly identifiable: an occasional headache, dizziness, or lightheadedness, which may indicate hypertension, can easily be attributed to other factors. Chronically elevated blood pressure exerts pressure on cerebral vessels, often resulting in lacunar infarctions or intracerebral hemorrhage (3). Hypertension also has been implicated in the atherosclerotic process because it drives fatty substances into the arterial walls, making them brittle, narrowed, and hardened (6,8). The impact of hypertension increases with age, moreover (3). For these reasons it is crucial to have regular blood pressure checks. Hypertension can be controlled through drug therapy, stress reduction, dietary control, and regular exercise, treatments that all require patient compliance for maximum effectiveness.
- Smoking—smoking doubles the risk of stroke (4,29). Quitting smoking reduces the likelihood of stroke, and there is some evidence to suggest that 5 years after quitting smoking, individuals lower their risk of having a stroke to nearly that of people of who have never smoked (6).
- TIAs—a TIA is considered an important risk factor for an impending stroke. Approximately 30% of all patients who

have had a TIA are at risk of having a stroke within 2 years. This risk is greatest in the first month, so it is important to seek medical intervention quickly (31).

- Geographic location—the highest death rates from strokes in the United States are in North and South Carolina, Georgia, northern Florida, Alabama, Mississippi, and Tennessee. Specific pockets of high death rates in Texas, Oklahoma, and all of the Hawaiian Islands have been noted (1,3). This geographical strip, often termed the "stroke belt," is the source of numerous studies on environmental, cultural, or other geographically determined risk factors. A person who grows up in a high-risk area and then moves to a lower-risk area as an adult continues to carry the greater likelihood of having a stroke. This has led to speculation that the causes may be diet related, cultural, or possibly even related to water supply or altitude (3).
- Diabetes mellitus—this disease is more common in stroke patients than in a normal population of similar age (3). Having diabetes increases the risk of stroke by two to three times, as diabetics have a tendency to form blood clots (4). Men are more vulnerable than women (6, 3).
- Oral contraceptives—women who have taken birth control pills, especially those with a high estrogen content, have an increased risk for stroke as they become older. Smoking while taking the pill further increases the risk (27).
- Hyperlipidemia—including elevated triglycerides and "bad" cholesterol, has long been suspected to be a risk factor for stroke (4). Its role in CVA has been confirmed by several recent studies (3). Cholesterol levels should be monitored and adults are encouraged to know their cholesterol counts. Dietary changes are effective in lowering cholesterol levels in some individuals; a class of drugs known as statins is also effective but may have side effects (8).
- Asymptomatic carotid bruits—bruit is an abnormal sound or murmur heard when a stethoscope is placed over the carotid artery. This slushing noise indicates turbulent blood, often caused by a significant degree of stenosis. Carotid bruit clearly indicates increased stroke risk. Complete occlusion of the carotid artery sometimes follows, resulting in stroke (8).
- Prior stroke—risk of stroke for a person who has already suffered a stroke is increased four to eight times (3).
- Heart disease—diseased heart (whether it be chronic disease, acute heart attacks, or prosthetic heart valves) increases the risk of stroke. Independent of hypertension, people with heart disease have more than twice the risk of stroke than people with normally functioning hearts (3,6). Atrial fibrillation, a condition in which the heart produces an irregular rhythm, is also a known risk factor for stroke (3,29).
- Infections and Inflammation—inflammation occurring with various infections, often mild, has been associated with stroke. A major study in 2003 indicated that periodontal (gum) disease is associated with a 20% high risk for ischemic stroke and heart disease, and that the risk may be even greater in adults under the age of 65 (3,27). Research is underway to determine whether other infections that produce arterial inflammation can lead to stroke or heart disease. For example, chronic infection with *Chlamydia pneumoniae*, which causes mild pneumonia in adults, has been linked with higher risk for stroke (27).
- Alcohol and Drug Abuse—numerous studies indicate that moderate consumption of alcohol decreases the risk of stroke and heart disease; however, excessive consumption and total abstinence are associated with higher risk (6). Cocaine and methamphetamine abuse are major factors in the incidence of stroke in young adults (27). Use of anabolic steroids for

body-building is also associated with increased risk of stroke (27).

- Sleep apnea—is a common disorder in which the throat becomes obstructed during sleep, interfering with normal breathing and sleep. Sleep apnea is worsened by obesity and may contribute to the narrowing of the carotid artery. Sleep apnea is currently thought to increase the risk of stroke three- to sixfold (27).

Of these many risk factors, several can be controlled by changes in lifestyle, including elevated blood cholesterol and lipids, cigarette smoking, use of oral contraceptives, excessive drinking of alcohol, and obesity. Some, such as hypertension, heart disease, TIAs, carotid bruits, and polycythemia, can be controlled by medical intervention. Factors that cannot be changed are age, sex, race, family history, diabetes mellitus, and a prior stroke. The potential benefits of all medical and surgical interventions currently available for cerebrovascular disease pale in comparison to what can be achieved through risk factor control (3). Understanding and awareness of these risk factors for stroke is an important first step in reducing the likelihood of having stroke.

Incidence and Prevalence

Stroke is the third leading cause of death in the United States, surpassed only by heart disease and cancer (3). The most common cause of disability, stroke, is the most widespread diagnosis among clients seen by occupational therapists for the treatment of physically disabled adults (18,26). An estimated 600,000 to 730,000 people in the United States suffer an episode each year, and about 4.5 million stroke survivors are alive today (3,26). Approximately 50% to 70% of people regain functional independence after a stroke; however, 15% to 30% of those who survive an ischemic or hemorrhagic stroke suffer some permanent disability (27). Of the two main types, hemorrhagic strokes occur much less frequently (20% of all strokes) than ischemic strokes, which account for about 80% of all strokes (6). Depression affects approximately one third of stroke survivors (3). Impact on family and caregivers is also enormous. If adequate social services and support are not available, caregivers assume the burden for functional tasks that the patient is unable to perform (3).

Despite these grim statistics, there is some good news. With the exception of subarachnoid hemorrhage, between 1950 and 1990 all types of strokes have shown a significantly decreased incidence (3,30). This may be partly the result of increased control of risk factors such as hypertension, diabetes mellitus, and heart disease (3). Individuals who have had a stroke now live almost twice as long; interestingly, one study even reported that long-term survivors appeared to be less depressed than the comparison group (27). Fewer people now die of stroke, notwithstanding the continuing debate as to whether this decline is the result of the occurrence of fewer strokes or better medical treatment (3). However, it should be noted that the absolute number of strokes occurring in the United States is rising, probably a result of the aging of the population (3). Moreover, dramatic increases in obesity, among children as well as adults, offer grave cause for concern, given the close links determined between obesity and vascular disease (28) (see Risk Factors, above).

Stroke in young children occurs in about 2.5 cases per 100,000 children per year as compared to 100 cases per 100,000 in the adult population (25). It is more frequent in children younger than 2 years of age. The effects of stroke among children are similar to those described in adults. Although the etiology of pediatric stroke is often unknown, the most common known cause is a congenital defect affecting the structure of the heart (25). Sickle-cell disease, which affects blood-clotting mechanisms, and genetic disorders are the next most common known causes. Forty-five percent of pediatric stroke patients experience neurological defects throughout their lives; however, one third of children with strokes display no symptoms afterward (25).

Signs and Symptoms

Stroke Warning Signs

To educate the public, the American Heart Association and National Stroke Association distribute pamphlets listing the warning signs of an impending serious stroke (5). Many hospitals and community clinics also distribute this information. These include

- Sudden numbness or weakness of the face, arm or leg; especially on one side of the body.
- Sudden confusion, trouble speaking or understanding.
- Sudden trouble seeing in one or both eyes.
- Sudden trouble walking, dizziness, loss of balance or coordination.
- Sudden severe headache with no known cause (5).

Some general medical symptoms related to type of stroke were discussed under Etiology. Signs and symptoms also depend on the size and location of the injury, and neurologists can often predict location by the symptoms the individual displays. However, it is important to remember that a stroke is complex, and each individual may experience a unique constellation of symptoms. Relying on stereotypical models of stroke leads to generalized and often inappropriate therapy.

In addition to the above list, it is important to be aware that symptoms resulting from a partial reduction or temporary change in the blood flow to the brain are extremely important warning signs for stroke (31). Several of these conditions are discussed below.

Transient Ischemic Attacks

TIAs result from a temporary blockage of the blood supply to the brain. The symptoms occur rapidly and last for less than 24 hours. Seventy-five percent of TIAs last less than 5 minutes. The specific signs and symptoms depend on the portion of the brain affected but may include fleeting blindness in one eye, hemiparesis, **hemiplegia**, aphasia, dizziness, double vision, and staggering. Carotid artery disease and vertebral basilar artery disease may lead to TIAs (2,8). The main distinction between TIAs and stroke is the short duration of the symptoms and the lack of permanent neurological damage. People who have had TIAs are 9 1/2 times more likely to have a stroke than those of the same age and sex who have never had a TIA (2). Without preventive treatment, a third of those who suffer TIAs will go on to have a stroke within 5 years (31). Thus, it is crucial to detect the cause of a TIA and begin appropriate intervention promptly (4).

Small Strokes (RINDs)

In some cases, the symptoms of a TIA may last longer than 24 hours. If they last a day or more and then completely resolve, or if they leave only minor neurological deficits, they are called *small strokes*, or *lengthy TIAs* (4). Often the remaining neurological deficits are barely noticeable. Like TIAs, however, these small strokes are important warning signs that a more serious CVA may occur (4). A small stroke that completely resolves is called a reversible ischemic neurologic deficit (RIND). An episode that lasts more than 72 hours and leaves some minor neurological impairments is called a partially reversible ischemic neurologic deficit (PRIND). The mechanism of injury in RIND and PRIND is the same as that for a stroke or TIA. Like ischemic strokes, RINDs typically occur in the morning; since blood pressure is low during sleep, sudden increases in blood pressure upon arising may cause problems (4).

Many small strokes are not reported to a medical practitioner, which makes the exact frequency of occurrence of these strokes difficult to determine. It is important to recognize the symptoms of a small stroke so that it can be treated early, reducing the risk of more permanent injury.

Subclavian Steal Syndrome

This is a rare condition caused by a narrowing of the subclavian artery that runs under the clavicle. Symptoms occur when the arm on the side of the narrowed vessel is exercised. Usually, movement of the arm produces light-headedness, numbness, and weakness. Other neurological symptoms also may be present. In this syndrome, blood is "stolen" from the brain and instead is delivered to the exercised arm. It is a warning sign that advanced atherosclerosis may be present in the arteries throughout the body, including the cerebral arteries (32).

Course and Prognosis

Strokes result in anoxic damage to nervous tissue that causes various neurological deficits, depending on where the blood supply was lost. If neuronal cell death occurs, it is considered irreparable and permanent, as no way has yet been found to regenerate nerve cells (6). However, the nervous system has a high level of plasticity, especially during early development, and individual differences in neural connections and learned behaviors play a major role in functional recovery. No two brains can be expected to be structurally or functionally identical (9). Spontaneous recovery may occur as edema subsides or viable neurons reactivate. Recovery also may occur with physiologic reorganization of neural connections or developmental strategies. Any injury brings different factors into play, affecting axonal and dendritic sprouting or collateral rearrangement, synaptic formation, the excitability of neurons, "substitution of parallel channels," and "mobilization of redundant capacity" (9). Recovery from neurological deficits thus depends on the etiology and size of the infarct (2). Approximately 90% of neurological recovery occurs within 3 months, with the rest occurring over a more extended time (2). It should be noted that recovery from hemorrhagic strokes proceeds more slowly, however (2).

Accuracy in the prediction of function or rate of return in a given stroke patient is difficult because of individual variability of anatomy and extent of brain damage, as well as differences in types of CVA, learning ability, premorbid personality and intelligence, and motivation (9,18). Generally, the prognosis for recovery of function is greater in young clients, possibly because the young brain is more plastic or because the young are generally in better physical condition.

Secondary complications are important to recovery and rehabilitation and may actually be more disabling than the stroke itself (33,34). These complications are discussed in this chapter and include depression, seizures, infection, bowel/bladder incontinence, thromboembolism, shoulder subluxation, painful shoulder, shoulder-hand syndrome, abnormal muscle tone, and **associated reactions** and movements.

Individuals with good sensation, minimal **spasticity**, some selective motor control, and no fixed contractures seem to make the greatest improvements in functional abilities. If an individual has no concept of the affected side and cannot localize stimuli to the affected side, or if he or she has fecal or urinary incontinence, the outlook for independence is generally poor. Some individuals may continue to have strokes, complicating recovery (33).

Neurological Effects of Stroke

An occlusion that causes a serious stroke can occur anywhere in the extracranial or intracranial system, but the most common site is in the distribution of the middle cerebral artery and its branches in the cerebrum. The majority of cerebral strokes occur in one or the other cerebral hemisphere, but not both (2). It is important to note that even in individuals with the same neurological deficit, the impact of disability is different, depending on the individual's life situation.

Left-Sided Cerebral Injuries: Middle Cerebral Artery

The left cerebral hemisphere controls most functions on the right side of the body because of the **decussation** of motor fibers (decussation of the pyramids) in the medulla. These fibers that cross, or decussate to the opposite side, form the lateral corticospinal tract. The rest of the fibers descend ipsilaterally, forming the anterior corticospinal tract (7). The proportion of crossing fibers varies from person to person, averaging about 85% (7).

A CVA in the region of the middle cerebral artery in the left cerebral hemisphere may produce the following symptoms:

1. Loss of voluntary movement and coordination on the right side of the face, trunk, and extremities.
2. Impaired sensation, including temperature discrimination, pain, and proprioception on the right side (hemianesthesia).
3. Language deficits, called aphasia, in which the patient may be unable to speak or understand speech, writing, or gestures. The breakdown of language function is complex; the many types of aphasia will be discussed later in this chapter.
4. Problems with articulation of speech because of disturbances in muscle control of the lips, mouth, tongue, and vocal cords **(dysarthria)**.
5. Blind spots in the visual field, usually on the right side.
6. Slow and cautious personality.
7. Memory deficits for recent or past events (18).

Right-Sided Cerebral Injuries: Middle Cerebral Artery

The right cerebral hemisphere controls most of the functions on the left side of the body and also is responsible for spatial sensation, perception, and judgment. Injury to the middle cerebral artery of the right cerebral hemisphere may produce a combination of the following deficits:

1. Weakness (hemiparesis) or paralysis (hemiplegia) on the left side of the body (face, arm, trunk, and leg).
2. Impairment of sensation (touch, pain, temperature, and proprioception) on the left side of the body.
3. Spatial and perceptual deficits.
4. **Unilateral neglect**, in which the patient neglects the left side of the body or the left side of the environment.
5. Dressing **apraxia**, in which the patient is unable to relate the articles of clothes to the body (18).
6. Defective vision in the left halves of visual fields or left homonymous hemianopsia in which there is defective vision in each eye

(the temporal half of the left eye and the nasal half of the right eye).

7. Impulsive behavior, quick and imprecise movements, and errors of judgment (2,18).

Anterior Cerebral Artery Stroke

The territory of the anterior cerebral artery is rarely infarcted because of the side-to-side communication provided by the anterior communicating artery in the circle of Willis (7). Symptoms of an anterior cerebral artery stroke include:

1. Paralysis of the lower extremity, usually more severe than the upper extremity, contralateral to the occluded vessel.
2. Loss of sensation in the contralateral toes, foot, and leg.
3. Loss of conscious control of bowel or bladder.
4. Balance problems in sitting, standing, and walking.
5. Lack of spontaneity of emotion, whispered speech, or loss of all communication.
6. Memory impairment or loss (18).

Vertebrobasilar Stroke

The vertebrobasilar system of arteries supplies blood primarily to the posterior portions of the brain, including the brainstem, cerebellum, thalamus, and parts of the occipital and temporal lobes. This posterior circulation is not divided into right and left halves, as in the anterior circulation (7). An occlusion here might produce:

1. A variety of visual disturbances, including impaired coordination of the eyes.
2. Impaired temperature sensation.
3. Impaired ability to read and/or name objects.
4. Vertigo, dizziness.
5. Disturbances in balance when standing or walking (ataxia).
6. Paralysis of the face, limbs, or tongue.
7. Clumsy movements of the hands.
8. Difficulty judging distance when trying to coordinate limb movements (dysmetria).
9. Drooling and difficulty swallowing (**dysphagia**).
10. Localized numbness.
11. Loss of memory (2).
12. Drop attacks in which there is a sudden loss of motor and postural control resulting in collapse, but the individual remains conscious (35).

TIAs in this area are common in the elderly. The vertebral arteries travel up to the brainstem through a bony channel in the cervical vertebrae. In older adults, osteoarthritis may develop in the cervical bones, causing narrowing of the cervical canal, especially when the head is extended or rotated (2).

Wallenberg's Syndrome

Wallenberg's syndrome is a classic brainstem stroke that also is referred to as lateral medullary syndrome (36). It occurs as the result of an occlusion of a vertebral or cerebellar artery. Strokes in this area may produce contralateral pain and temperature loss, ipsilateral Horner's syndrome (sinking of the eyeball, ptosis of the upper eyelid, and a dry, cool face on the affected side), ataxia, and facial sensory loss. Ischemia to ipsilateral cranial nerve fibers VIII, IX, and X results in palatal paralysis, hoarseness, dysphagia, and vertigo (7). There is no significant weakness in this syndrome (36).

Brainstem strokes often result in coma because of damage to the centers involved with alertness and wakefulness (reticular system) (7). A hemorrhage into the brainstem area is rare, quickly accompanied by loss of consciousness, and usually fatal. Among patients who survive brainstem stroke, however, recovery is often good (2).

Other Complications of Stroke

Secondary conditions may occur in addition to these deficits. These are important manifestations of the patient's recovery and rehabilitation and may actually be more disabling than the stroke itself (3). It is necessary to be aware of these complications so that they may be prevented.

Seizures

Brain scars that result from stroke may irritate the cortex and cause a spontaneous discharge of nerve impulses that may generalize to a full grand mal convulsion (16). Seizures develop in up to 10% of stroke patients and are more common with embolic than thrombotic infarcts (15). Anticonvulsant drugs are sometimes used in patients with early seizures, but their use is controversial (37).

Infection

Alteration of swallowing function, aspiration, hypoventilation, and immobility in the stroke patient often lead to pneumonia (27). Changes in bladder function may lead to bladder distention and urinary tract infection (3,18). Impaired sensation and inadequate position changes may result in pressure sores (decubitus) and consequent infection of these areas (18).

Thromboembolism. Immobility of the legs and prolonged bed rest often lead to thrombosis of dependent leg veins (38). In **deep vein thrombosis** (DVT), local pain and tenderness may develop in the calf, with some swelling and a slight increase in temperature. If the thrombosis is confined to the calf, it may not be serious. However, if the thrombosis spreads up toward the groin to involve the veins in the pelvis, there is a very real possibility of a clot breaking off into the blood stream. The clot will then travel through the right side of the heart and enter the lungs through the pulmonary arteries, resulting in sudden collapse and death owing to obstruction of the pulmonary arteries (38). Early mobilization of the patient is of utmost importance in preventing deep vein thrombosis and subsequent pulmonary embolism.

Medications and surgery may make a difference in the prognosis of an individual at risk for, or having had, a CVA.

Diagnosis

The diagnosis of stroke requires knowledge of the incidence of the different types of stroke and awareness of the presence of the risk factors mentioned above. Symptoms must be carefully noted from the patient or, if the patient is too ill, frightened, or confused, from the family (34). Neurologists, neurosurgeons, and some internists are the specialists usually involved in this acute diagnostic phase of treatment (34). A number of diagnostic techniques are utilized to distinguish stroke from other potential causes of observed symptoms and to assist in determining the location of lesions (6).

The physical examination of the patient with a suspected stroke or TIA includes a search for possible cardiac sources of emboli by listening to the heart and arteries of the neck. Also useful in the determination of cardiac-source emboli are electrocardiography (ECG), echocardiography, and monitoring for arrhythmias. In addition to cardiac testing, various neuroimaging techniques (see below) and analysis of blood and CSF may be performed (6). A neurological examination assists in determining the neurological disability and usually includes evaluation of higher cortical function (memory and language), level of alertness, reflexes, visual and oculomotor system, behavior, and gait (12).

Other diagnostic methods include noninvasive studies of blood vessels and invasive techniques requiring injection of dye into the arterial system, for example.

Neuroimaging Techniques

Computed tomography (CT) and magnetic resonance imaging (MRI) are invaluable noninvasive tools that depict pathological changes in the brain in patients with stroke (3,6). One or the other of these is almost always used at some point for every patient with a suspected stroke. CT and MRI are also capable of showing zones of edema and the shifting of intracranial material (2). Negative results of these tests may indicate that the ischemia is reversible (2).

Computed Tomography. CT is a type of radiographic examination that is widely used for analysis of cerebral injury (3,6). CT scans are employed to differentiate between a hemorrhagic stroke and an ischemic stroke (2). While they are useful in clarifying the location and the mechanism and severity of stroke, they are not particularly sensitive to subtle ischemic changes (6). It is most useful in the diagnosis of stroke caused by hemorrhage; CT findings may even be normal in patients with recent infarction. It is often not diagnostic in patients with TIAs and is not useful for imaging brainstem infarcts (6).

Magnetic Resonance Imaging. MRI is more sensitive than a CT scan and does not expose the patient to radiation. It provides detailed pictures of the brain by using a magnetic field. MRI is particularly helpful in revealing arteriovenous malformations (AVMs) (12). It is superior to CT in imaging the cerebellum, brainstem, thalamus, and spinal cord. It also provides better anatomical definition of the injury, but it does not distinguish hemorrhage, tumor, and infarction as well as CT (6).

Positron Emission Tomography. Positron emission tomography, or PET scan, is being used experimentally. This scan shows how the brain uses oxygen, glucose, and other nutrients and has increased understanding of the effects of stroke on the brain (3). Because these imaging techniques are not commonly available, PET scans are seldom used in the management of acute stroke (3).

Noninvasive Study of Blood Vessels

Noninvasive procedures used to evaluate both extracranial and intracranial blood flow include duplex ultrasonography as well as color-flow and transcranial Doppler ultrasound. These techniques can localize and determine the approximate size of the lesions within the arteries (2).

Duplex ultrasonography is useful in detecting the presence and severity of disease in the common and internal carotid arteries and in the subclavian and vertebral arteries in the neck. This scan can reliably differentiate between minor plaque disease, stenosis, and occlusive lesions. It is an excellent method of monitoring the progression or regression of atherosclerotic disease in the neck (2).

Color-flow Doppler ultrasound is used because it is effective in showing lesions of the carotid and vertebral arteries (2).

Transcranial Doppler ultrasound gives information about pressure and flow in the intracranial arteries. This procedure is useful in monitoring changes in arterial flow later in the course of the patient's disease (2,3).

Invasive Techniques

Cerebral angiography involves radiography of the vascular system of the brain after injecting a dye or other contrast medium into the arterial blood system. Computer-generated images are then produced that can show the entire visible length of cerebral arteries, as well as, the nature, location, and extent of pathological changes. This technique is now safer than before (less than 1% incidence of mortality and serious morbidity); however, it is recommended when noninvasive techniques have failed to yield a conclusive diagnosis or when surgery is being planned or considered (2,3).

Analysis of CSF is helpful in diagnosing subarachnoid hemorrhage. In a lumbar puncture, the subarachnoid space (usually between the third and fourth lumbar vertebrae) is tapped and CSF is withdrawn. Analysis of the pigments in the spinal fluid also can help in estimating the age of the hemorrhage and detecting rebleeding (12).

Other Techniques

Other diagnostic techniques used for stroke include electroencephalography (EEG), single-photon emission tomography (SPET), and special cardiac and coagulation tests that are useful in detecting unusual heart and blood disorders that can bring on a stroke (3). After this diagnostic phase of evaluation, a neurologist will evaluate the brain-damaged person's ability to function. Rehabilitation often will begin at that point to return the patient to the highest possible level of independent functioning (34,39).

Medical/Surgical Management

At present, the treatment of acute stroke is limited to management of the results of the primary event and preventive measures against further injury or occurrence (2). Much is still unclear about the effectiveness of the routine use of agents to reverse the cause or decrease the effects of stroke (2,3,6). Before the stroke can be treated, it must be accurately identified as either cerebral infarction or cerebral hemorrhage, since interventions that are beneficial with one type of stroke may be potentially dangerous to the other (6). Therefore, careful and exact diagnosis must be made first.

Drug management of CVA is constantly evolving. Common categories of drugs used to minimize the damage of cerebral infarction are described in the following sections.

Antiplatelet Therapy

Aspirin is often prescribed to patients when the vascular lesion is not severely stenotic (2). Aspirin has been shown to reduce risk of further stroke in patients who had suffered TIAs by 15% to 58% (6). It also benefits patients who have had a mild stroke but is not as effective in those with moderate or severe strokes (6,40). Aspirin is clearly not suitable for patients with cerebral hemorrhage or those at risk of bleeding. It is less successful when used by women as compared with men. Aspirin is relatively safe and inexpensive. Recently published studies have recommended a lower dose of aspirin to reduce harmful side effects (40).

Anticoagulants

These drugs inhibit clotting by interfering with the activity of chemicals in the liquid portion of blood that are essential for the coagulation process (6). Short-term (2 to 3 weeks) heparin therapy is prescribed for patients with complete blockages of large arteries, as heparin is effective in preventing the formation of emboli (6). For longer-term treatment (1 to 3 months), the drug warfarin may be used to prevent blockages in areas that cannot be treated by surgery (2,6).

Thrombolytics (t-PA)

Thrombolytic therapy (t-PA), used for dissolution of an occluding thrombus, is frequently applied in the acute treatment of myocardial infarction as well as in the treatment of stroke. It is effective before extensive brain infarction has occurred, so it is only appropriate in stroke patients whose arterial damage has been identified early (2). The potential benefit must be weighed against reperfusion damage, a bleeding tendency, and the possibility of re-occlusion. The Food and Drug Administra-tion (FDA) has approved the use of thrombolytic therapy, or t-PA, for treatment of acute stroke within 3 hours of onset (4). One study reported that patients treated with t-PA were 30% to 50% more likely to have minimal or no disability 3 months after onset of symptoms (4).

Surgical Interventions

In some cases, surgical treatment may be the best choice for the patient. The neurosurgeon must carefully consider many factors before surgery is performed, including the patient's overall health and life expectancy. Carotid **endarterectomy** is among the most commonly performed vascular surgeries in the United States (3,6). During the procedure, the diseased vessel is opened, the clot is removed, and an artificial graft put in place (3). Carotid endarterectomy is a treatment option for patients with more than 50% stenosis of the carotid artery ipsilateral to the affected hemisphere (6).

Subarachnoid hemorrhages are often caused by ruptured aneurysms or AVMs. Surgical clipping or lesion removal is the most effective treatment of these anomalies. If the patient survives the initial bleeding, the goal of surgery is to correct the problem before bleeding recurs. In intracerebral hemorrhage, small hematomas usually resolve spontaneously (2). Large hematomas, however, often produce death. Some lesions may expand, causing gradually increasing neurological signs. These expanding lesions can be drained surgically if they are near the surface of the brain, especially in the cerebral or cerebellar white matter. Generally, hemorrhages are evacuated only if they are large and life threatening or when surgery is necessary to treat an aneurysm, tumor, or AVM (2,41).

Superficial temporal artery bypass is a new, more delicate surgical therapy for preventing future strokes (41). The procedure begins with craniotomy to expose the brain; then a scalp artery is connected to an intracranial artery microsurgically. This operation is extremely challenging to perform and is thus performed less frequently than carotid endarterectomy. Surgeons who do the procedure, however, are enthusiastic about the results and claim that it revascularizes the brain better than endarterectomy (41).

Treatment of Secondary Effects

Specific pathophysiologic sequelae, or outcomes, follow the occurrence of any type of stroke. Treating these secondary effects is crucial to medical and functional recovery. Two of these are cerebral edema and ischemia. Oxygen therapy to reduce hypoxia, vasodilation to improve blood flow through ischemic areas, therapeutic hypertension, and hemodilution therapy are some of the treatments used for ischemia. Hemodilution results in a significant rise in cerebral blood flow and increased oxygen transfer (2,6).

Edema often complicates ischemic strokes and must be controlled, because most deaths during the first week after a massive stroke are caused by extensive cerebral edema and increased intracranial pressure (2,6). This pressure can displace the cerebrum downward and interfere with the functioning of the midbrain and lower brainstem, which control such basic vital functions as respiration and heart action (6).

Corticosteroid therapy can cause a significant reduction in interstitial cerebral edema, reducing swelling and improving outcomes after stroke (6,8). However, a review of the literature in 2001 indicates that there is no clear basis for evaluating the effect of corticosteroid treatment for people with acute ischemic strokes (42).

Impact of Conditions on Client Factors

The impact of stroke on an individual is unique and may affect any number of client factors. Deficits in motor, process, and communication skills, as well as impaired sensory functions and problems with perceptual processing, may be compounded by secondary complications, such as infection or depression. Together, these profoundly affect an individual's performance in all areas of occupation: activities of daily living (both basic and instrumental), work, play, leisure, and social participation.

Sensory Functions

Sensory functions can be affected at the very basic level of awareness and at the point of processing and modulation of sensory input. Loss of protective tactile functions, such as diminished awareness of temperature and pain, are common concerns for those with a CVA. Loss of these functions poses a safety risk. Individuals with proprioceptive dysfunction may show asymmetrical posture, have difficulty maintaining balance, appear to forget affected body parts, be unable to describe position or movement of limbs, and be susceptible to joint damage (19). Individuals with a loss of tactile sensation may demonstrate a lack of awareness of body parts simply because they forget what they cannot feel. They are also vulnerable to damage of affected body parts, particularly skin breakdown. Moreover, diminished tactile function hinders resumption of motor activities. Depending on the location of the infarct, individuals may experience diminished vestibular function, which will limit mobility efficiency and safety. Impaired balance may cause difficulties in assuming and maintaining a vertical posture and in automatic adjustments to changes of position and antigravity movement. As a result, individuals demonstrate an asymmetrical posture at rest, leaning or falling to the hemiplegic side during mobility, or fail to use normal protective reactions when falling (19,34).

Defects in visual field functions may impair reading, even in the absence of language dysfunction. For example, patients with right cerebral lesions may find reading difficult or impossible, because visuospatial deficits hinder tracking, or following the line of print across the page. Patients with homonymous hemianopsia on either side are unable to respond to people, objects, or the environment on the affected side. They may bump into objects or be startled by their sudden appearance. Individuals experiencing visual inattention have difficulty scanning and shifting their gaze, particularly toward the affected side (34).

Perceptual deficits may be difficult to understand for patient and family alike, but their impact on the patient's ability to resume independent function may be profound. Depending on the location of the lesion, or infarct, such deficits include visual **agnosia** and visuospatial agnosia—difficulty in understanding the relationship between objects and between self and objects (19,34). Individuals affected in this manner are unable to find their way in a familiar environment; they cannot trace a route on a map, pick out objects from a cluttered environment, copy drawings or simple construction, and may have difficulty in functional (spatial) tasks, such as dressing and reading a newspaper. Agnosia for sounds may also occur, so that the individual cannot understand or confuses nonverbal sounds (19). Another important loss is astereognosis, which affects functional use of the affected hand whenever vision is occluded: tasks such as finding keys or coins in a pocket, or a glass on a bedside table when it is dark, may be difficult (19).

The location of the infarct determines which functions are lost and which remain intact. For example, somatagnosia, in which an individual has no awareness of his or her own body and its condition, is commonly seen in right parietal lobe lesions. Deficits that result from right cerebral injuries often cause unilateral perceptual problems of the left body side and space, such as unilateral inattention. Lesions in the left cerebral hemisphere, however, cause bilateral problems, such as right/left discrimination (18). Impairment of the left parietal lobe results in apraxia, whereby individuals are unable to adjust movement of their own body parts. Yet impairment of the right parietal lobe causes an inability to adjust the position of external objects. Frontal lobe lesions may result in apraxia, in which sequencing of movement becomes difficult. Apraxic individuals may be unable to carry out a verbal request (for even a simple task such as combing the hair), although often they can perform such tasks automatically (34). They may perseverate, i.e., persist in purposeless movement, or they may be unable to complete a required sequence of acts, copy gestures, drawings, or carry out simple spatial constructional tasks (19,34).

Motor Functions

Sensory loss seldom occurs in isolation but typically accompanies the loss of motor functions. Motor dysfunction because of stroke usually results in changes in muscle tone that render normal movement impossible. It has been commonly said that hypotonicity (flaccid hemiplegia) gives way to hypertonicity (spastic hemiplegia); occasionally there is progress into a final stage, in which normal movement patterns re-emerge (19,43).

The muscle tone of individuals with an intact central nervous system operates within a range that permits effective voluntary movement. Normal muscle tone is high enough to stabilize and maintain a person through an activity, while at the same time low enough to allow ease of movement. This variability of tone allows mobility to be superimposed on stability (19).

Abnormal tone may be termed either low or high. Hypotonus, or **flaccidity**, is felt as too little resistance, or floppiness. When released, the extremity will drop. At the other extreme, when there is too much resistance, hypertonus, or spasticity, is felt. Spasticity is the result of hyperactive reflexes and loss of moderating or inhibiting influences from higher brain centers (19,43). Spasticity may be aggravated by pain, emotional upset, or efforts to hurry. Spasticity is never isolated to one muscle group but is always a part of what is known as either an extensor or flexor synergy, that is, a grouping of stereotypical movements. These movement patterns usually consist of a flexion pattern in the arm (scapular retraction and depression, shoulder adduction and internal rotation, elbow flexion, forearm pronation, wrist flexion, finger and thumb flexion and adduction) and an extension pattern in the leg (pelvis rotated back and internal rotation, knee extension, foot plantar flexion and inversion, toe flexion and adduction).

Abnormal tone is not limited to the extremities, however, and is manifested in the head and trunk. The head is usually flexed toward the hemiplegic side and rotated so that the face is toward the unaffected side. The trunk is rotated back on the hemiplegic side with side flexion of the hemiplegic side (19). These typical patterns of spasticity interfere with the normal, smooth, efficient, and coordinated movement necessary for locomotion in and manipulation of the environment. If untreated, spasticity may lead to contractures.

Addressing the return of motor function is an important part of rehabilitation and a number of theories and treatment methods have been developed. In recent years, one approach that is being studied for its effectiveness is known as constraint-induced therapy, which is outlined in Table 9.1.

Table 9.1 AN OVERVIEW OF CONSTRAINT-INDUCED MOVEMENT THERAPY

Upper-limb hemiparesis following stroke can make bathing, dressing, and feeding a challenge for patient and caregiver. Between 30% and 66% of stroke survivors have limited use of their affected arm (1), making the impairment one of the most commonly treated by rehabilitation clinicians (2).

Forced use of the hemiplegic upper extremity and the subsequent emergence of constraint-induced movement therapy (CI therapy) have received considerable attention as a means of helping some stroke patients avoid or overcome learned nonuse and regain upper limb function.

Forced use refers to the restriction of a patient's stronger limb to encourage focused and frequent use of the impaired limb during daily activities.

The theory guiding forced use and CI therapy is based upon the principle of preventing or overcoming learned nonuse through intensive use of the affected limb.

Current health care trends have placed limitations on lengths of hospital and rehabilitation stays, as well as curtailing the amount of therapy a stroke survivor can receive (3).

Intensive training with CI therapy involves practicing functional task activities using repetitive task practice and shaping.

Overcoming learned nonuse and the improvements following CI therapy are thought to result from use-dependent cortical organization.

To be eligible for CI therapy, stroke patients must have adequate balance and remain safe while wearing the limb restraint. They also must be able to demonstrate active wrist extension of at least 10 degrees from neutral, abduction/extension of the thumb of 10 degrees, and movement in at least two additional digits in the affected extremity (4).

From van der Lee JH, Wagenaar RC, Lankhorst GJ, et al. Forced use of the upper extremity in chronic stroke patients: results from a single-blind randomized clinical trial. Stroke 1999;30:2369–2375, Page SJ, Sisto SA, Levine P, et al. Modified constraint induced therapy: a randomized feasibility and efficacy study. J Rehabil Res Dev 2001;38:583–590, Aycock DM, Blanton S, Clark PC, et al. What is constraint-induced therapy? Rehabil Nurs 2004;29:4,114–116, Wolf SL, Blanton S, Baer H, et al. Repetitive task practice: a critical review of constraint-induced movement therapy in stroke. Neurologist 2002;8:325–338.

The hemiplegic shoulder is also a common concern. Typical problems include shoulder subluxation, pain, and immobility. Because of the unstable nature of the glenohumeral joint, the anatomy of the shoulder is particularly vulnerable to problems. Normally this lack of stability is partly compensated for by a strong surrounding musculature. However, subluxation is inevitable once the surrounding musculature of the shoulder, especially the so-called rotator cuff muscles, has been damaged (19). A closer look at the biomechanics of the glenohumeral joint makes this clear.

Two thirds of the humeral head is not covered by the glenoid fossa. In the normal orientation of the scapula, the glenoid fossa slopes upward. This orientation plays an important role in preventing downward dislocation of the humerus, as the humeral head would have to move laterally to move downward (34). When the arm is adducted, the superior part of the capsule and the coracohumeral ligament are taut, which prevents lateral movement of the humeral head and guards against downward displacement. The rotator cuff muscles play a crucial role: the supraspinatus muscle reinforces the horizontal tension of the capsule, while the infraspinatus and the posterior portion of the deltoid, because of their horizontal fibers, also play an important role in preventing subluxation. When the humerus is adducted sideways or flexed forward, the superior capsule becomes lax, eliminating support, and joint stability must then be provided by muscle contraction. Thus the integrity of the joint depends almost exclusively on the rotator cuff muscles (19,34).

After a stroke, changes in muscle tone and movement, the position of the scapula, and joint capsule stability allow the pull of gravity to draw the head of the humerus out of the glenoid fossa of the scapula, resulting in shoulder subluxation (19,34). Patients with hemiplegia have lost voluntary movement in muscles such as the supraspinatus, infraspinatus, and posterior fibers of the deltoid. In addition, the muscles that support the scapula in its normal alignment are affected, which leads to a change in angulation of the glenoid fossa.

Another typical complication is "the painful shoulder." This condition may either develop quickly after a stroke or at a much later stage. It presents with flaccid or spastic muscle tone and with or without subluxation. In hemiplegia, the normal, coordinated, and timed movement of the scapula and humerus (scapulohumeral rhythm) has been disturbed by abnormal and unbalanced muscle tone. The typical hemiplegic postural components of depression and retraction of the scapula and internal rotation of the humerus are especially important to the mechanism of pain. Fear of pain during passive movement of the arm will further increase abnormal flexor tone, which can become a vicious circle (19).

A chronically painful shoulder can lead to shoulder-hand syndrome, also known as reflex sympathetic dystrophy (RSD). This complex condition produces severe pain, edema of the hand, and limitations in range of motion on the involved side (19). These complications not only interfere with movement, they may have profound emotional consequences.

Another motor dysfunction caused by stroke is the presence of associated reactions. Associated reactions in hemiplegia are abnormal reflex movements of the affected side that duplicate the synergy patterns of the arm and leg (19). These movements may be observed when the patient moves with effort, is trying to maintain balance, or is afraid of falling. A flexor pattern of involuntary movement in the arm is often observed when the individual yawns, coughs, or sneezes. Associated reactions also are seen when new activities, such as running or putting on socks, are attempted after a stroke. They are stereotyped reactions and may occur even if no active movement is present in the limb. The limb returns to its normal position only after cessation of the stimulus and usually does so gradually (19).

Unlike associated reactions, associated movements accompany voluntary movements and are normal, automatic postural adjustments. They reinforce precise movements of other parts of the body or occur when a great amount of strength is required. They are not pathological and can be stopped at will. Associated movements often can be observed in the unaffected extremities of stroke patients who are trying new activities (19).

Other motor dysfunctions include orofacial weakness, which may cause difficulties in expression, speech (dysarthria), mastication, and swallowing (dysphagia) (19). Additionally, bladder or bowel incontinence may result from a communication disorder or from disruption of normal routine and diet, lack of awareness of body function, or emotional disorder (12,19).

Mental Functions

Severe strokes often result in cognitive deficits that affect global and specific mental functions (19,34). Milder strokes may have a more subtle impact on mental function, however. Commonly used psychometrics are not always sensitive to the wide range of mental functions and process skills that may permit effective occupational performance: initiation, recognition, attention, orientation, sequencing, categorization, concept formation, spatial operations, problem solving, and learning abilities (12,34). Moreover, basic visual deficits also have an impact on cognitive performance. For example, visual attending and scanning deficits lead to a decrease in the efficiency required for cognitive performance (34,19).

Emotional Functions

Stroke patients may experience a number of psychological changes, including depression, irritability, low tolerance for stressful situations, fear and anxiety, anger, frustration, swearing, emotional lability, and catastrophic reactions. Significant depression has been recorded in 30% to 50% of stroke survivors (3). These changes often are a major cause of concern to relatives and the individual. While depression is often viewed as a natural and understandable consequence of reduced function caused by stroke, proper treatment can result in observable improvement. Depression is more frequent and severe with lesions in the left hemisphere, as compared with right hemisphere or brainstem strokes (3). Both organic and psychological factors are probably involved in poststroke depression (44).

Emotional lability, sudden and extreme shifts of mood, may be the result of a release of inhibition. The individual may switch from laughing to crying for no apparent reason. Excessive crying is the most common problem and is frequently the result of organic emotional lability rather than depression or sadness over perceived losses. Organic emotional lability is characterized by little or no obvious relation between the start of emotional expression and what is happening around the person (34,19).

Catastrophic reactions are outbursts in which frustration, anger, and depression are combined. When individuals cannot perform tasks that used to be very easy, they may be unable to inhibit emotional expression and may begin sobbing, expressing a sense of hopelessness (19). Outbursts and emotional difficulties are to be expected after stroke. Relatives and families should be told that a tendency to cry easily or get upset will improve with time. Families and therapists need to develop a positive, understanding attitude if the individual is to overcome psychological sequelae. The psychosocial impact of stroke on patients and families can be lessened with increased social support and access to services once the patient has been discharged to home and community (3,44).

CASE STUDY

Case Illustrations

■ CASE 1

Initial Presentation

Mr. Posti is an 80-year-old man brought into the emergency department (ED) by his wife, who reported that she heard him fall to the floor in the bathroom at about 4:30 in the morning when he got out of bed to urinate. She noticed that his right side was weak, his speech was slurred, and he was having difficulty finding the correct words for "coat" and "hat." He was reportedly in his usual state of health when he went to bed the night before. On examination in the ED, he was alert but could not articulate clearly. His speech was hesitant and he seemed frustrated. His right face drooped and there was drool coming from the right corner of his mouth. His right arm and hand were flaccid, and his right leg demonstrated only slight flexion and extension of the knee. His reflexes were hyperactive on the right and normal on the left side. He had a positive Babinski on the right.

Mr. Posti retired from the City of New York Police Department 30 years ago, at the rank of Detective First Grade. Since his retirement he worked on and off at odd carpentry jobs. He has smoked cigarettes since he was 14 years old, but when he turned 70 he quit "cold turkey." He had osteoarthritis in both knees but refused knee replacement surgery. He had recently been told that he had type II diabetes. He had a myocardial infarction when he was 54 years old and had a triple artery bypass graft done at that time. His wife is 8 years his junior and in generally good health. She continues to work part-time as a hairdresser in a senior center.

Hospital Course

Mr. Posti was admitted to a monitored bed in the intensive care unit (ICU). An intravenous solution of 5% dextrose in .45% normal saline was started. Laboratory tests were all normal except for a blood glucose level of 315 mg/dL and occasional unifocal premature ventricular contractions. A CT scan of the brain, taken the day of admission, was normal except for mild atrophy. Nursing began regular turning and positioning and range of motion exercises. The physician ordered physical, occupational, and speech therapy consultations on the third day of hospital admission. On day 6 of his hospital admission, Mr. Posti continued to demonstrate dysphagia to all consistencies of food and fluid, and his oral intake was low.

Rehabilitation

At the end of his first week of stay in the hospital, Mr. Posti began to demonstrate some active movement in his right hand and leg. His bed mobility skills were improving, and he was able to roll from side-to-side and relieve pressure on his back and buttocks when lying on the bed. He was able to wash his face with set-up, and he was attempting more tasks each day using his nondominant left hand. The speech therapist was concerned about Mr. Posti's swallowing and the fact that he was most likely at high risk for aspiration. He lost 4 pounds since admission, and if not for the IV fluids being administered, he would likely have become dehydrated. The speech therapist recommended a videofluoroscopic examination in order to observe Mr. Posti's functional swallow while ingesting a variety of consistencies of food and liquid.

The outcome of the "cookie swallow" assessment should facilitate a decision regarding placement of a feeding tube. Physical therapy decided to hold program until Mr. Posti's nutritional status stabilized and his physical energy level improved. The rehabilitation stroke team was in close communication on a daily basis about this patient's status, in order to be able to grade the intensity of interventions as indicated.

■ CASE 2

Initial Presentation

Mrs. Stella Rojo is 66 years old, from Puerto Rico, and a retired housekeeper. She was brought into the emergency room (ER) by paramedics after complaining of a severe headache that began earlier in the day while she was cleaning the windows in her small apartment. She was on a step stool and reportedly fell to the ground and was unable to move her left arm or leg. She was able to pull herself to a coffee table in her living room and reach the telephone to dial 911. Initially in the ER she seemed confused about her surroundings, and it was reported that in the ambulance she had a generalized tonic-clonic seizure.

Hospital Course

Mrs. Rojo was intubated, and IV phenytoin sodium (Dilantin) was started for the seizures. An emergency CT scan of the head revealed an intracerebral hemorrhage in the internal capsule and thalamus. There was no evidence of intracranial pressure. Her blood pressure on admission to the ER was 190/110 mm Hg, but decreased within the first hour to 170/95 mm Hg. She was admitted to the neurointensive care unit of the facility. On day 2 she was extubated and began to open her eyes but still seemed confused.

Rehabilitation

Mrs. Rojo was much more alert by day 5. Her blood pressure was now 160/90 mm Hg. She started occupational therapy. When feeding, she demonstrated difficulty locating food items on the left side of her meal tray, and she called out for the nurses to find her drink container for her. When the nurses would tell her that it was on the left side of her tray she seemed to become irritated and think that they were belittling her. When visitors came to call on her Mrs. Rojo tended to become teary and even broke down into sudden crying spells. Her physician recommended transfer from the hospital to a skilled nursing facility (SNF).

At the time of discharge from the hospital the physician believed that Mrs. Rojo should be sent to a nursing facility because she was not thought to be a good candidate for in patient rehabilitation. The rehabilitation therapy team in the hospital reached this decision because of her apparent cognitive deficits and severe left-sided neglect. Mrs. Rojo's daughter, Yvonne, was her patient advocate and durable power of attorney, and she also agreed with the team's decision.

The rehabilitation therapy team in the nursing facility received orders from the medical director for evaluation and treatment as indicated. All therapies initiated their respective assessments within 24 hours of her admission to the facility. These included occupational therapy, physical therapy, and speech-language pathology. Mrs. Rojo was assessed to be in need of skilled rehabilitative care and admitted to the rehabilitation wing of the facility. Her treatment would be covered by her Medicare part A. Her family and her physician were informed that her Medicare coverage under part A would continue as long as Mrs. Rojo continued to need skilled care, demonstrated functional progress, and that the care was reasonable and medically necessary.

Even though all these criteria were met, there were still limits to the length of care coverage, and these were also discussed with the client's health care advocate.

Mrs. Rojo made consistent functional gains in balance, mobility, self-care dressing, grooming, toileting, and feeding skills. After approximately 4 weeks of combined therapies she reached her maximum potential in functional performance and was recommended for discharge from the therapy programs. Prior to discharge from occupational therapy, a home safety assessment was done, equipment and adaptation recommendations were shared with the family, and preparatory plans were set in motion.

Thirty-six days postadmission to the nursing facility, Mrs. Rojo was discharged to her daughter's home. Home-care services were arranged by the discharge planner and social services and included occupational therapy, physical therapy, and speech therapy. Home safety equipment was to include a wheelchair for trips to appointments, a quad-cane, over-toilet commode, transfer tub bench, wall safety grab bars, and a shower sprayer and flexible hose.

References

1. Atlas of Stroke Mortality: Racial, Ethnic, and Geographic Disparities in the United States, January 2003. Centers for Disease Control and Prevention Cardiovascular Health Program. Available at http://www.cdc.gov/cvh/library/fs_stroke.htm. Accessed March 13, 2005.
2. Cerebrovascular disease. In: Beers M, Berkow R, eds. The Merck Manual of Geriatrics. 3rd Ed. Rahway, NJ: Merck Research Laboratories, 2000.
3. Absher JR. Cerebrovascular disease. In: Ramachandran VS, ed. Encyclopedia of the human brain, vol 1. Boston: Academic Press, 2002:733–757.
4. McCaffrey P. Medical Aspects: Types of Strokes. CMSD 336, Neuropathologies of Language and Cognition [online serial]. 1998–2003. Available at: http://www.csuchico.edu/pmccaff/syllabi/SPPA336/336unit1.html. Accessed April 2, 2005.
5. What is a stroke? National Stroke Association. 2004. Available at: http://www.stroke.org/HomePage. Accessed April 2, 2005.
6. Zazulia AR. Stroke. In: Ramachandran VS, ed. Encyclopedia of the human brain, vol 4. Boston: Academic Press, 2002:475–492.
7. Lundy-Ekman, L. Neuroscience: Fundamentals for Rehabilitation. 2nd Ed. Philadelphia: WB Saunders, 2002.
8. O'Donnell SD, Gillespie DL. Atherosclerotic disease of the carotid artery. [emedicine online serial]. November 17, 2004. Available at: http://www.emedicine.com/med/topic2964.htm. Accessed April 7, 2005.
9. Ploughman M. A review of brain neuroplasticity and implications for the physiotherapeutic management of stroke. Physiother Can 2002;Summer: 164–176, 185.
10. Felberg RA, Naidech A. The five Ps of acute ischemic stroke treatment: parenchyma, pipes, perfusion, penumbra, and prevention of complications. Ochsner J 2003;5(1):5–11.
11. Chambless LE, Heiss G, Shahar E, et al. Prediction of ischemic stroke risk in the Atherosclerosis risk in communities study. Am J Epidemiol 2004;160(3): 259–269.
12. Brookshire RH. Introduction to Neurogenic Communication Disorders. 6th Ed. St. Louis: Mosby, 2003.
13. Norrving B. Long-term prognosis after lacunar infarction. Lancet Neurol 2003;2(4):238–245.
14. Steinke W, Ley SC. Lacunar stroke is the major cause of progressive motor deficits. Stroke 2002;33(6):1510–1516.
15. Poststroke seizures and epilepsy [review]. Phys Med Rehabil State Art Rev 1998;12(3);405–422.
16. Camilo O, Goldstein B. Seizures and epilepsy after ischemic stroke. Stroke 2004;35(7): 1769–1775.
17. Medical Encyclopedia: Intracerebral Hemorrhage. National Library of Medicine and National Institutes of Health Medline Plus. July 2004. Available at: http://www.nim.nih.gov/medlineplus/ency/article/000796.htm. Accessed April 2, 2005.
18. Pulaski KH. Adult neurological dysfunction. In: Crepeau EB, Cohn ES, Boyt Schell BA, eds. Willard & Spackman's Occupational Therapy. 10th Ed. Philadelphia: Lippincott, Williams & Wilkins, 2003:767–788.
19. Gillen G, Burkhardt A. Stroke Rehabilitation: A Function-Based Approach. 2nd Ed. St. Louis: Mosby, 2004.
20. Godoy DA, Boccio A, Leira R, et al. Early neurologic deterioration in intracerebral hemorrhage: predictors and associated factors. Neurology 2005;64(5):931–932.
21. Vermeer SE, Algra A, Franke CL, et al. Long-term prognosis after recovery from primary intracerebral hemorrhage. Neurology 2002;59(2):205–209.
22. Arboix A, Vall-Llosera A, Garcia-Eroles L, et al. Clinical features and functional outcome of intracerebral hemorrhage in patients aged 85 and older. J Am Geriatr Soc 2002;50(3):449–454.

23. Medical encyclopedia: Subarachnoid Hemorrhage. National Library of Medicine and National Institutes of Health. January 2004. Available at http://www.nim.nih.gov/medlineplus/ency/article/000701.htm. Accessed April 8, 2005.
24. Blacks in the South have greater risk of dying from stroke [abstract 47]. International Stroke Conference 2005. Available at: http://www.strokeconference.americanheart.org/portal/strokeconference/sc/02.02.05A. Accessed March 11, 2005.
25. Carlin TM, Chanmugam A. Stroke in children. Emerg Med Clin N Am 2002;20:671–685.
26. Health Impact of Heart Disease and Stroke. Cardiovascular Health Partners Healthy People 2010. U.S. Department of Health and Human Services 2000. Available at: http://www.heartandstrokepartners.org/impact.htm. Accessed April 2, 2005.
27. Stroke: patient education handout [online encyclopedia article]. Mdconsult. A.D.A.M. 2003. Available at: http://www.stroke.org/homepage.aspx?p. http://home.mdconsult.com/das/patient/body/0/10041/9387/.html?preview=t&printing=true. Accessed July 9, 2004.
28. Keller KB, Lemberg L. Obesity and the metabolic syndrome. Am J Crit Care 2003;12(2):167–170.
29. Reducing Risk and Recognizing Symptoms. National Stroke Association. Available at: http://www.stroke.org. Accessed August 20, 2004.
30. Stroke in Perspective: Epidemiology of Stroke. Internet Stroke Center, 1997–2003. Available at: http:://www.strokecenter.org/education/ais_epidemiology/rates.htm. Accessed April 2, 2005.
31. TIA: A Warning Not To Be Ignored [webcast transcript, April 20, 2000]. American Stroke Association. Available at: http://asa.healthology.com/webcast_transcript.asp?f=stroke_tia&spg=FIP. Accessed March 18, 2005.
32. Brophy DP. Subclavian steal syndrome [emedicine online series]. December 2001. Available at: http://www.emedicine.com/radio/topic663.htm. Accessed April 2, 2005.
33. Bottomley J, Lewis C. Neurological treatment considerations. In: Bottomley J, Lewis C. Geriatric rehabilitation: a clinical approach. 2nd Ed. Upper Saddle River, NJ: Prentice Hall, 2003: 399–448.
34. Woodson AM. Stroke. In: Trombly CA, Radomski MV, eds. Occupational therapy for physical dysfunction. 5th Ed. Philadelphia: Lippincott, Williams & Wilkins, 2002:817–853.
35. Welsh LW, Welsh JJ, Lewin B, et al. Vascular analysis of individuals with drop attacks. Ann Otol Rhinol Laryngol 2004;113(3):245–251.
36. Wallenberg's Syndrome information page. Office of communications and public liaison. National Institute of Neurological Disorders and Stroke. February 2005. Available at: http://www.ninds.nih.gov/disorders/wallenbergs/wallenbergs_pr.htm. Accessed April 1, 2005.
37. Preventing stroke-related seizures: when should anticonvulsant drugs be started? [review]. Neurology 2003;60(3):365–366.
38. Harvey RL. Prevention of venous thromboembolism after stroke. Top Stroke Rehabil 2003;10(3): 61–69.
39. Pomeroy VM, Tallis RC. Restoring movement and functional ability after stroke. Physiotherapy 2002;88(1):3–14.
40. Does aspirin decrease morbidity for patients with acute ischemic stroke? Evid Based Pract 2004;7(6):6–7.
41. Brain Bypass Surgery. Department of Neurological Surgery. Cerebrovascular Surgery Section. University of Pittsburgh. 2005. Available at: http://www. neurosurgery.pttt.edu/cerebrovascular/brainbypass.htm. Accessed April 7, 2005.
42. Qizilbash N, Lewington SL, Lopez-Arrieta JM. Corticosteroids for acute ischaemic stroke [abstract]. Cochrane database syst rev 2001;4:CD00064. Available at: http://www.cochrane.org/cochrane/revabstr/ab000064.htm. Accessed April 9, 2005.
43. Luke C, Dodd KJ, Brock K. Outcomes of the Bobath concept on upper limb recovery following stroke. Clin Rehabil 2004;18(8):888–898.
44. Mathews M, Budur K. Post-stroke depression. Clin Geriatr 2004;12(10):35–38.

Recommended Learning Resources

National Stroke Association
www.stroke.org

American Stroke Association
www.strokeassociation.org

National Institute of Neurological Disorders and Stroke
www.ninds.nih.gov

Children's Hemiplegia and Stroke Association
www.chasa.org

Pediatric Stroke Network
www.pediatricstrokenetwork.com

American Heart Association
www.americanheart.org

Family Caregiver Alliance
www.caregiver.org

Survivor and Family References

Senelick MD, Doughtery K, Rossi P. Living with stroke: A Guide for Families. Chicago: NTC/Contemporary Books, 1999.

Mayer TK. One handed in a two-handed world. 2nd Ed. Boston: Prince-Gallison Press, 2000.

Hachinski V, Hachinski L. Stroke: A Comprehensive Guide to Brain Attack. Toronto: Key Porter Books, 2000.

Rao PR, Ozer MN, Toerge JE, eds. Managing stroke: A Guide to Living Well After Stroke. Washington, D.C.: National Rehabilitation Hospital Press, 2000.

Personal Stories

Berger PE, Mensh S. How to Conquer the World with One Hand . . . and an Attitude. 2nd Ed. Merrifield, VA: Positive Power Publishing, 2002.

Brady D. When I Learn . . . Surviving a Stroke with Pride. Bloomington, IN: Authorhouse, 2002.

Hutton C, Caplan LR. Striking Back at Stroke: A Doctor-Patient Journal. New York: Dana Press, 2003.

Caregiving Handbook

Carr S, Choron S. The caregiver's Essential Handbook: More Than 1200 Tips to Help You Care for and Comfort the Seniors in Your Life. New York: McGraw-Hill, 2003.

Professional Texts

Bogousslavsky J, ed. Long-Term Effects of Stroke (Neurological Disease and Therapy 54). New York: Marcel Dekker, 2002.

Adams HP, Del Zoppo GJ, Von Kummer R. Management of Stroke: A Practical Guide for the Prevention, Evaluation and Treatment of Acute Stroke. N.p.: Professional Communications, 1998.

Davies PM. Steps to Follow: The Comprehensive Treatment of Patients with Hemiplegia. 2nd Ed. New York: Springer-Verlag, 2000.

Calliet R. Shoulder Pain. 3rd Ed. Philadelphia: FA Davis, 1991.

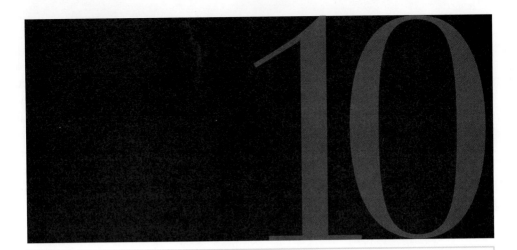

Cardiopulmonary Disorders

Jacqueline Eckert

Key Terms

Congestive heart failure
Cardiopulmonary
Chronic obstructive pulmonary disease
Diastolic
Dyspnea
Ecchymosis
Hypertension
Myocardial infarction
Pneumonia
Oxygen transport
Pulse oximetry
Sphygmomanometer
Spirometry
Systolic
Tuberculosis (TB)

Barbara was 87 years old and lived with her daughter. While she had successfully quit smoking at 70 years of age, the damage to her health was already in place after smoking for 49 years. As a result, she was diagnosed with emphysema, **congestive heart failure** and **hypertension.** With oxygen support required 24 hours per day, Barbara was limited in her basic activities of daily living as well as instrumental activities of daily living as a result of **dyspnea,** decreased mobility, strength, and endurance. Most of her day consisted of passive activity such as watching television, working on crossword puzzles and reading. Ultimately, Barbara developed an infection that she was unable to fight and gave up her will to live. This chapter is dedicated to my mother, Barbara, who was an inspiration for the content.

This chapter will review the etiology, incidence, pathophysiology, signs and symptoms, medical/surgical management, impact of the conditions on client factors, and case illustrations for **cardiopulmonary** conditions. Pulmonary conditions that will be covered include **chronic obstructive pulmonary disease**, **pneumonia**, and **tuberculosis**. Cardiac conditions that will be covered include **congestive heart failure**, **myocardial infarction**, and **hypertension**.

Respiratory System Anatomy

In order to understand the causes of cardiopulmonary diseases, it is helpful to have an understanding of the anatomy and physiology of the heart and lungs. The cardiopulmonary system is a combination of the cardiovascular and the respiratory systems. In basic terms, the cardiovascular system incorporates the blood vessels and the heart. The respiratory system includes the lungs and the upper and lower respiratory tract (5). The main purpose of the cardiopulmonary system is to deliver important gases and nutrients to all the cells in the body and carry away the waste products (6).

The respiratory system consists of the nasal cavity, the pharynx, the larynx, the trachea, and the bronchi and the lungs, which are made of smooth muscle tissue (Fig. 10.1). The upper respiratory tract is composed mainly of the nose and the pharynx. The lower respiratory tract involves the larynx, trachea, bronchi, and lungs. The muscles of the thoracic, abdominal walls and the diaphragm are responsible for respiration.

The main functions of the respiratory system includes gas exchange, which allows oxygen from the air to enter the blood and carbon dioxide to leave the blood and enter the air. In addition, the respiratory system regulates the blood pH factor, which is a measure of the acid or alkaline properties of blood circulation by changing blood carbon dioxide levels. Voice production and olfaction are also important associated functions of the respiratory system.

The primary functions of the nasal cavity are to serve as a passageway to humidify, warm, and clean the air we breathe. Additionally, it functions for smell and to provide resonating chambers for speech. The primary functions of the pharynx are to receive the air from the nasal cavity as well as to manage of the food and liquid arriving from the oral cavity. The primary functions of the larynx are to maintain an open passageway for air movement and serve as a primary source for sound production. The entrance of the larynx is covered with a small piece of tissue, called the epiglottis, which automatically closes during swallowing and prevents food or drink from entering the airway.

The trachea consists of a tube-like structure about 4 inches long and 1 inch in diameter. This structure moves downward from the larynx and branches into the left and right bronchi for each lung. With the appearance of an inverted tree, the bronchi branch out into smaller tubes called bronchioles and end up in thousands of small air sacs or alveoli. Within the alveolar walls are tiny blood vessels called capillaries, which diffuse the oxygen we breathe and return carbon dioxide back to the alveoli.

The lungs are soft, cone-shaped organs, located within the thoracic cavity. The left and right lungs are separated by the mediastinum, medially by the heart and enclosed by the diaphragm and thoracic cage. Each lung functions independently. If there is a perforation in one lung, the other lung remains intact. The right lung is larger, divided by fissures into three lobes, called the superior, middle and inferior lobes. The left lung is smaller, because it shares space on the left side with the heart and has two lobes. The sternum, ribs, and spine protect the lungs. Each lung is covered with two layers of

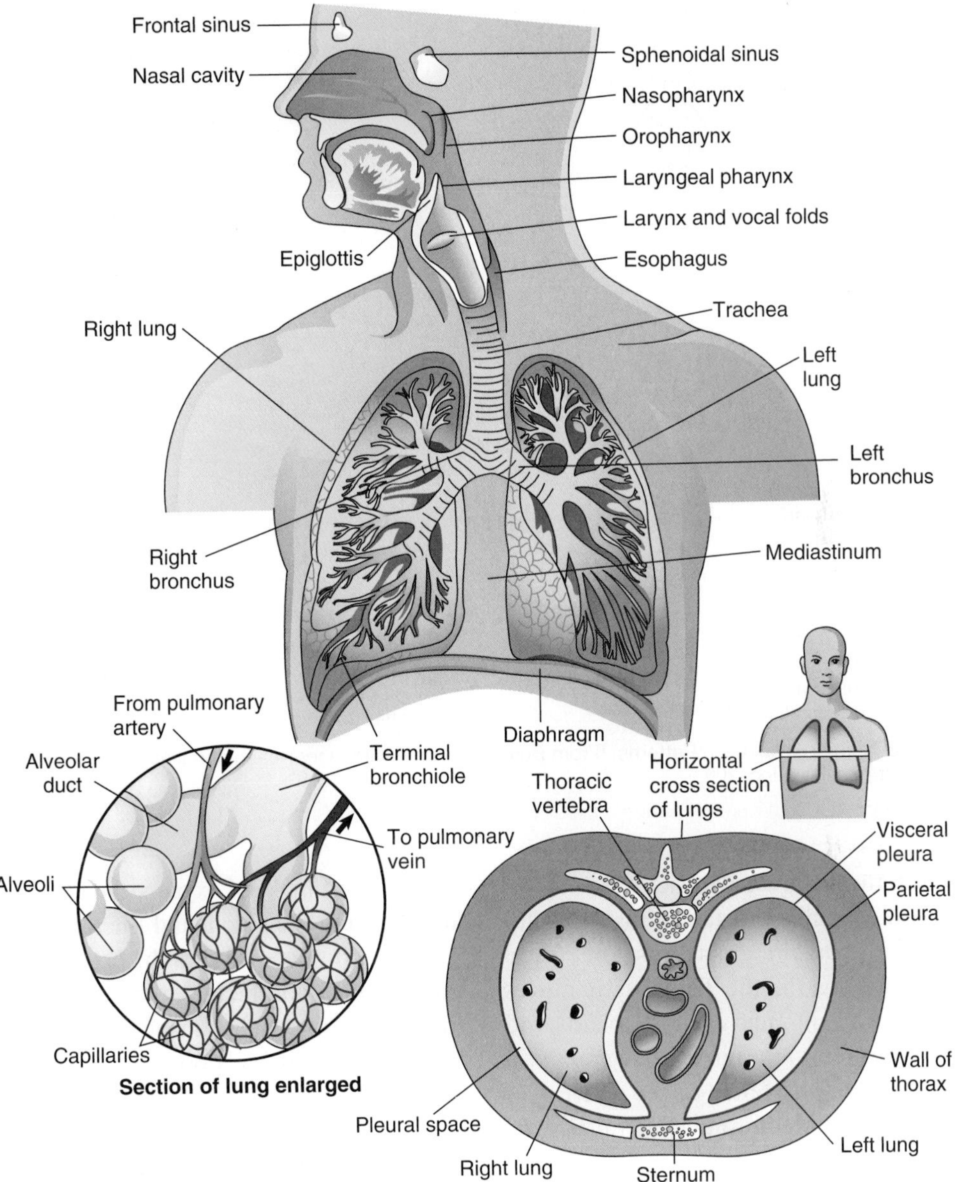

Figure 10.1 Respiratory system. (From Smelzter SC, Bare BG. Textbook of Medical-Surgical Nursing. 9th Ed. Philadelphia: Lippincott, Williams & Wilkins, 2000.)

pleura, which have a small amount of lubricating fluid that ensures smooth movements of the lung during breathing. One layer is called the parietal pleura, which lines the wall of the chest. The other layer is called the visceral pleura, which covers the surface of the lungs. The diaphragm, which is a bell-shaped sheet of muscle, is responsible for inspiration (expanding the lungs) and expiration (relaxing the lungs). The diaphragm is attached to the base of the sternum, the spine, and lower parts of the rib cage. All the muscles used in breathing contract only if the nerves connecting them to the brain are intact. This is why a person with a spinal cord injury may need to be ventilated for breathing. When breathing

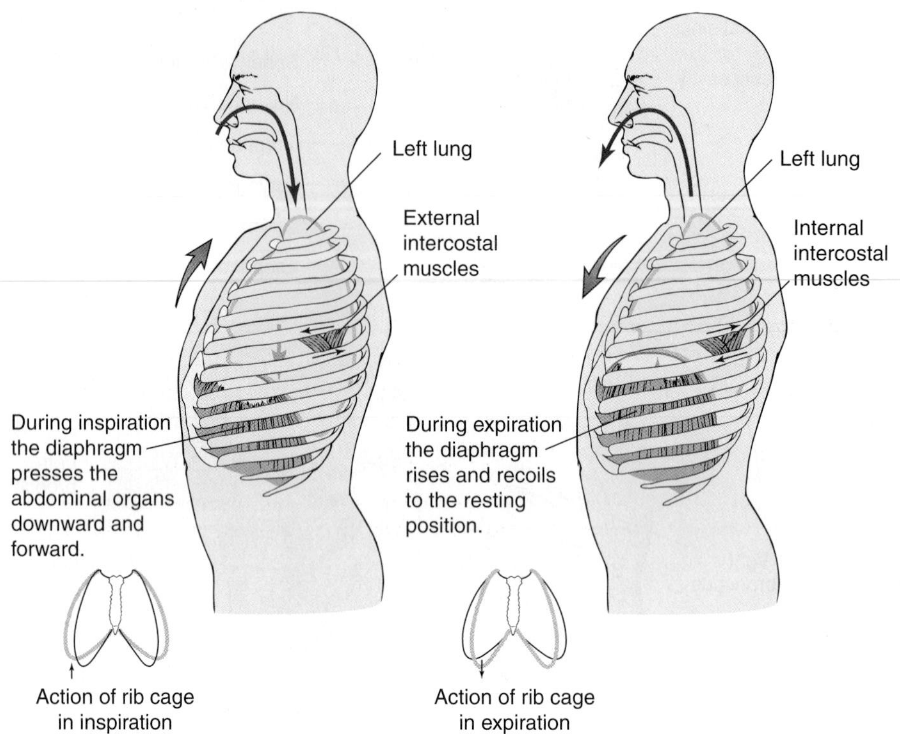

Figure 10.2 Normal Respiration Patterns. (From Burch S. Cardiopulmonary Health and Illness. Lawrence, Kansas: Health Positive, Inc. 2003)

out at rest, the respiratory muscles are passive but during exercise the abdominal muscles help push the diaphragm against the lungs. When breathing in, the diaphragm moves downward, the thoracic cavity expands and the air is forced into the airways (Fig 10.2) (7)

Oxygen transport refers to the delivery of fully oxygenated blood to peripheral tissues, the cellular uptake of oxygen, the utilization of oxygen from the blood, and the return of partially desaturated blood to the lungs (8,9). The most significant factors that interfere with **oxygen transport** are changes in gravitational stress, changes in body position, exercise stress, increased oxygen demand of working muscles, arousal, and emotional stress (Fig 10.3).

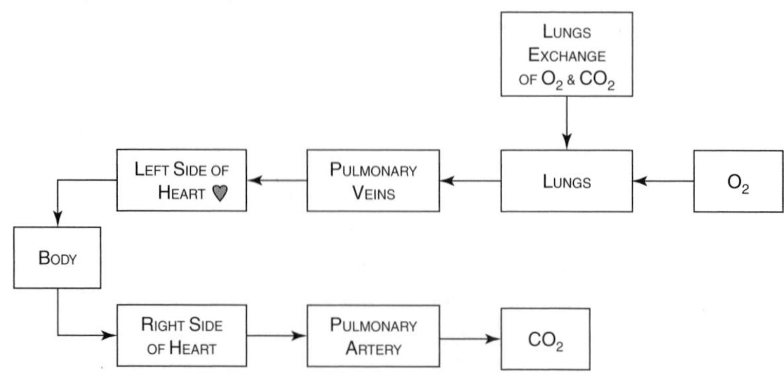

Figure 10.3 Oxygen transport

Chronic Obstructive Pulmonary Disease (COPD)

The fourth leading cause of death in the United States (10), chronic obstructive pulmonary disease (COPD), is a permanent and progressive airflow obstruction that interferes with the gas exchange and functional capacity in the lungs. This disease is usually associated with emphysema, which is an irreversible lung condition, and chronic bronchitis, which is an inflammatory disease of the lungs.

The primary dysfunction in COPD is a loss of lung function, with progressive reduction of airflow. The lung airways and alveoli lose their elasticity, the airway walls collapse, become clogged with mucus, and the air gets trapped in the lungs. The result is a decreased gas exchange, fatigue of the respiratory muscles, an increased oxygen need and flattening of the diaphragm due to hypoventilation (11). The person with COPD has to work harder to keep up with the need for increased oxygen during activity and experiences shortness of breath.

Etiology

Eighty percent to 90% of the causes for COPD are related to smoking and occupational exposure to certain industrial pollutants. A person who smokes is 10 times more likely to die of COPD than a nonsmoker. Other risk factors are second-hand smoke and a history of frequent childhood respiratory infections (11).

Incidence and Prevalence

The incidence of COPD has increased 17.5% in the past 10 years with a death rate of 43.2 per 100,000 (12) and takes the lives of 117,522 Americans every year (4). The incidence for COPD as a primary diagnosis was 5.3 per 100,000 in 2000. The annual cost for COPD is $32.1 billion, with health care expenditures of $18.0 billion and indirect costs, such as loss of income, estimated at $14.1 billion (4).

Signs and Symptoms

Signs and symptoms of COPD include dyspnea, fatigue, chronic cough, chest tightness, and sputum production. Maintaining adequate nutrition is a problem for 40% to 60% of the individuals with COPD (11). Individuals usually experience significant shortness of breath and reduced participation in activities of daily living, and social and leisure activities for many years before seeking medical advice. The symptoms are often mistakenly recognized as a typical effect of aging and lack of exercise rather than as a serious medical condition. The progressive loss of lung function results in a reduction in the performance of activities of daily living. A chronic cycle begins to develop and often damage is sustained before the person seeks medical advice. As the inactivity continues, the muscles atrophy, the individual develops feelings of inadequacy, a poor self-concept, and experiences further progression of the respiratory disability. (Fig. 10.4) (11)

Fifty one percent to 74% of persons with COPD suffer from depression, because of a change in life style, the fear of dyspnea and hopelessness.

Medical/Surgical Management

Medical management may include smoking cessation, avoiding exposure to secondhand smoke and air pollutants. A pneumonococcal

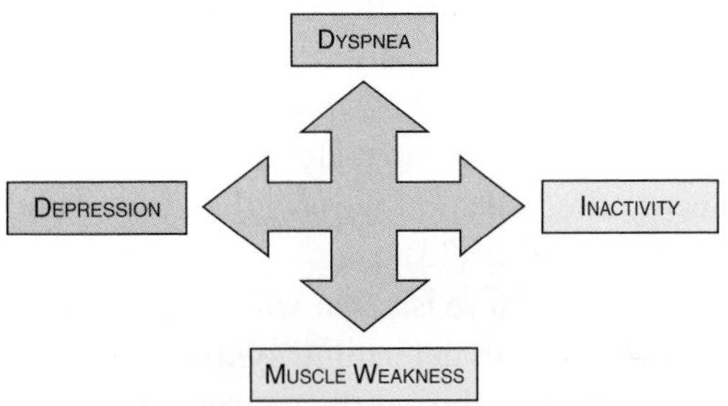

Figure 10.4 Dyspnea Cycle

vaccination is recommended every 5 years to avoid influenza or pneumonia. Other treatments may be oxygen therapy or advanced stages may require mechanical ventilation. Medications commonly used with COPD are bronchodilators, anti-inflammatory drugs, antihistamines, antileukotrienes, antibiotics, mucolytic drugs, antineoplastic drugs, anticoagulants, and immunizations.

Sixty percent of the people who have a lung transplant have COPD. Although 1,000 people in the United States underwent lung transplantations in 2002, there are approximately 4,000 people waiting for an organ (4). A lung transplant is considered only for an end-stage condition that typically includes a person whose medication regimen has failed and is expected to only live 1 to 3 years without a transplant.

Tests for diagnosing COPD include physical examination, pulmonary function testing, radiograph, arterial blood gases, computed tomography (CT), magnetic resonance imaging (MRI), bronchoscopy, and **pulse oximetry**. During assessment and intervention, physiologic monitoring is essential for heart rate, blood pressure, respiratory rate, and possibly pulse oximetry. A diagnosis should be confirmed by spirometry (13). COPD is classified by severity, from stage 0 to stage IV. In stage 0, the patient is at risk, with chronic cough and sputum production. Stage I is marked by mild airflow limitation and sometimes a cough and sputum production. Stage II includes moderate airflow limitation, shortness of breath with exertion and the progression of symptoms. Stage III is typified by a severe airflow limitation, increased shortness of breath, and repeated exacerbations of symptoms. In stage IV, the severe airflow limitation persists with an increasing loss of quality of life. Here, the patient is deeply affected and the exacerbations can be life-threatening (13).

Blood pressure is taken with a **sphygmomanometer** to determine **systolic** reading (the peak force during the contraction of the left ventricle) and **diastolic** pressure (the force when the heart is relaxed). Respiratory rate is determined by counting the number of times the chest moves for breathing for 30 seconds and multiplying by 2 and comparing that measure with normal values. Normal heart rate is 60–100 beats per minute and normal respiratory rate is 12 to 20 breaths per minute (5).

Levels of dyspnea are determined by various scales. One commonly used source is the American Thoracic Society Dyspnea Scale (5). The scale is numbered 0 to 4, with a rating of 0 indicating "no problems with breathing" to a rating of 4, which is noted as "very severe." Additionally, the Borg Category Scale for Rating Breathlessness (5) provides an indication of perceived exertion, both of which are helpful tools to measure breathlessness and effort. The scale is numbered 0 to 10, with a 0 rating indicating "no problems breathing "to a rating of 10, which indicates "maximum problem with breathing." Physical activity can be modified accordingly, or terminated, if oxygen saturation drops below 90% (10,11) or the client demonstrates signs of respiratory/cardiac stress. Additionally, the therapist should be aware of different postures to relieve dyspnea. Examples of these are sitting and leaning forward, arms supported on a surface or standing and leaning forward, or arms supported on a counter. These positions help expand the accessory breathing muscles for inspiration.

Team members include a physician, respiratory therapist, exercise physiologist, occupational therapist, physical therapist, psychologist, social worker, and a dietician. The respiratory therapist has an important role on the team, because of the progressive respiratory problems with this population. There is an increasing trend to transfer ventilator-dependent patients to extended care facilities or home, where they are assisted with home health services (14). As more dependent patients are sent home from shorter hospital stays, the occupational therapist should have a basic understanding of working around a ventilator and

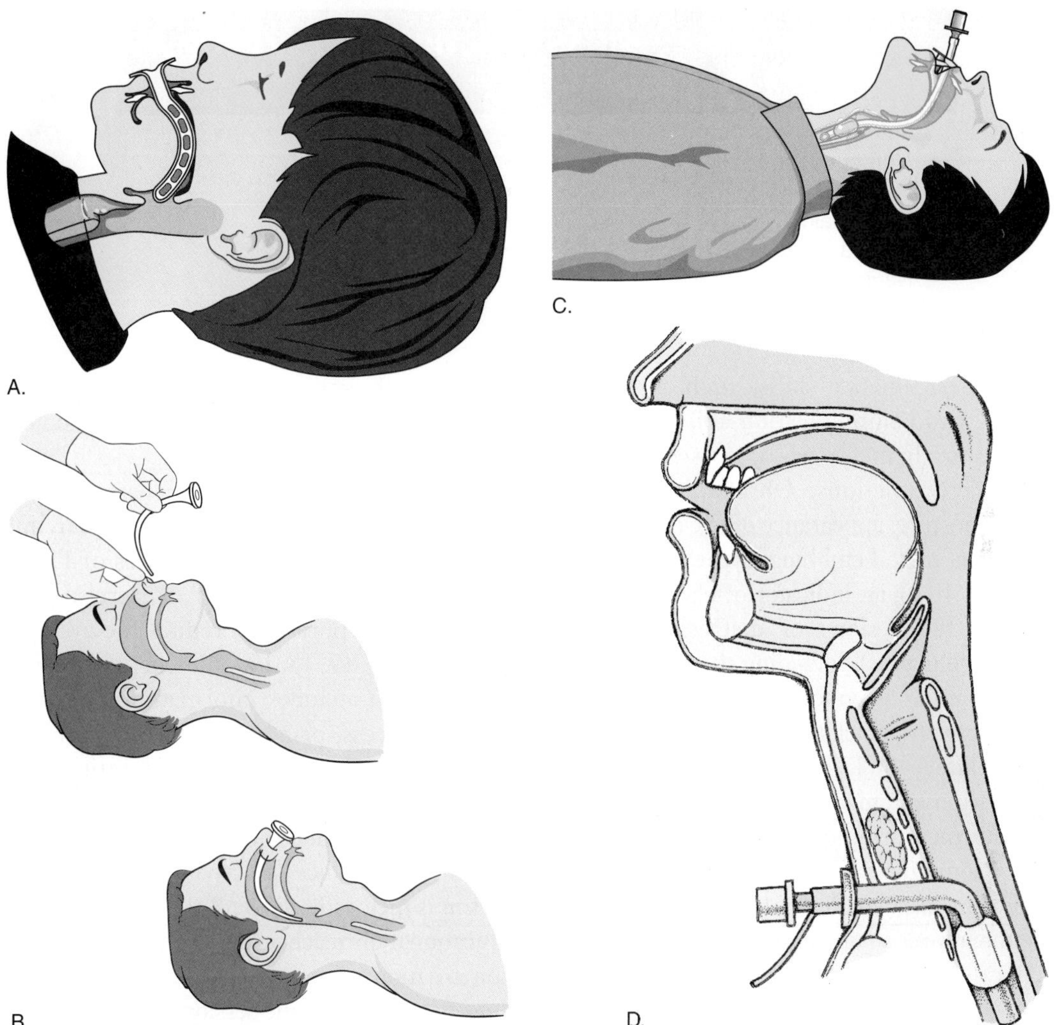

Figure 10.5 Artificial airways. **A,** Oropharyngeal airway. **B,** Nasopharyngeal airway. **C,** Endotracheal airway. **D,** Tracheostomy. (A–C From LifeART, copyright 2006, Lippincott Williams, & Wilkins; D from Neil O. Hardy, Westpoint, CT)

precautions associated with its use . If the patient is on life support, it is necessary to note the artificial airways (Fig. 10.5) and follow precautions for signs and symptoms of cardiopulmonary distress (Table 10.1).

Impact on Occupational Performance

An occupational profile and analysis of occupational performance are the main components of the evaluation process. An occupational profile includes an interview with the patient and family. The occupational therapy process emphasizes the importance of a client-centered approach, which means the client must be an active participant in the evaluation and interventions. The patient and family interview provides **the first** step in establishing a therapeutic relationship. The occupational therapist is able to gain an understanding of the patient roles, home and work responsibilities, culture, interests, leisure time activities, and goals for the future.

The analysis of the occupational performance is a process of gathering information

Table 10.1 SIGNS OF CARDIOPULMONARY DISTRESS

- Lightheadedness
- Fatigue
- Chest pain
- Altered breathing patterns
- Nausea
- Shortness of breath
- Perspiration
- Anxiety
- Cough
- Cyanosis

on the performance skills, such as motor, process, and communication abilities. More specific to client factors are assessment of pulmonary functions. Observation should include posture, appearance of the extremities for edema, digital clubbing of the fingers and toes (Fig. 10.6), an indicator of chronic tissue hypoxia, facial signs of distress and any cyanosis (blueness), including the nail beds. It is important to listen for phonation (interruption for breath), crackles, wheezes, dyspnea, or cough. The 6- or 12-minute walk test, a balance assessment, mental status and a questionnaire for measuring quality of life are examples of some tools available for assessment of cardiopulmonary conditions (15). A review of the literature reveals a number of Pulmonary assessments that can be utilized with this population (Table 10.2).

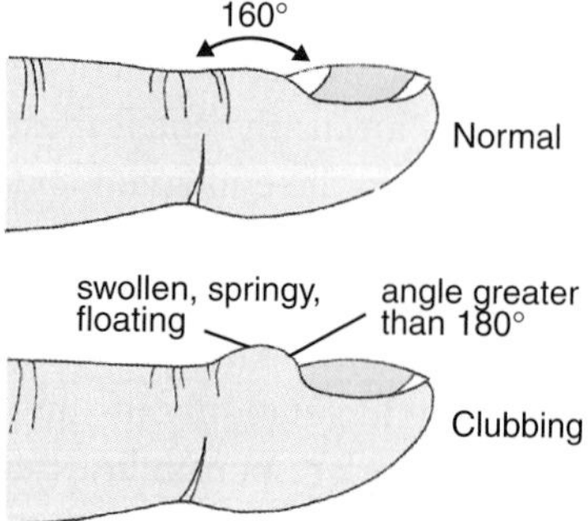

Figure 10.6 Digital clubbing of the fingers. (Reprinted with permission from Taylor C, Lillis C, LeMone P. Fundamentals of Nursing: The Art and Science of Nursing Care. 4th Ed. Philadelphia: Lippincott, Williams & Wilkins, 2001.)

Although specific treatment protocols are not within the scope of this text, it is noted that, in general. intervention includes graded activities to improve cardiopulmonary strength and endurance, activities of daily living (ADL) and Instrumental Activities of Daily Living (IADL) training and an exercise program are incorporated to reduce the cycle of inactivity (16, 17, 18, 19, 20). Client and family education includes information about the disease process, principles of work simplification, energy conservation, relaxation and self-management (21, 22).

The occupational therapist should emphasize the importance of activity as soon as the person is medically stable. Research has shown educational outreach visits and patient education are more effective over a longer period of time as opposed to one session. To avoid overloading the patient and assisting with the follow up process, dividing the information up will be of more benefit (23,24). Additionally, patient education materials should be developed according to reading level, cultural background, and age. Each client should receive a home program, for achieving maximal independence and a smooth transition back into the community. Cardiopulmonary rehabilitation has been shown to demonstrate an improvement in quality of life, muscle strength and endurance, a decrease in dyspnea, but no change in pulmonary lung status (25, 26, 27). An increase in the perception of effort affects muscular performance. The result of a greater tolerance to dyspnea may lead to an increase of activity with fewer symptoms.

Table 10.2 SUMMARY OF PULMONARY ASSESSMENTS

Assessment	Description	Reference
6-Minute Walk Test (6MWT)	Standardized, measures exercise tolerance for respiratory diseases: Adults	McGavin CR, Gupta SP, McHardy GJR. Twelve minute walking test for assessing disability in chronic bronchitis. BR Med J 1976;1:822–823
Chronic Respiratory Disease questionnaire (CRQ)	Measures items of change because of dyspnea and quality of life	Guyatt GH, Berman LB, Townsend M, et al. A measure of quality of life for clinical trials in chronic lung disease. Thorax 1987;42:773–778
Borg Scale of Perceived Exertion	Measures severity of dyspnea on a 1–10 category scale	Borg GA. Psychophysical bases of perceived exertion. Med Sci Sports Exerc 1982;14:377–381
COPD Self-Efficacy Scale	Confidence level	Wigel J, Creer T, Kotses H. The COPD Self-Efficacy scale. Chest 1991;99:1, 193–196
Summary of Human Activity Profile (HAP)	Activity level based on estimated measurement of exercise tolerance (METS)	Psychological Assessment Resources. Human Activity Profile. Psychological Assessment Resources, Inc
Summary of Pulmonary functional Status Scale (PFSS)	Questionnaire that covers ADL, IADL	Weaver TE, Narsavage GL. Physiological and psychological variables related to functional status in chronic obstructive pulmonary disease. Nursing Res 1992:41:286–291
Visual Analogue Scale (VAS)	Vertical line of 100 mm in length, to measure level of dyspnea	Mahler D: Dyspnea: diagnosis and management, Clin Chest Med 1987;8:2,215–230
Baseline Dyspnea Index and Transitional Dyspnea Index (BDI/TDI)	Measures baseline and transitional dyspnea	Mahler DA, Weinberg DH, Well CK, Feinstein AR. The measurement of dyspnea: contents, interobserver agreement and physiologic correlates of two new clinical indexes. Chest 1984;85:751–758
Health Knowledge Test	Measures what pulmonary rehabilitation patients have learned	Hopp JW, Lee JW, Hills R. Development and validation of a pulmonary rehabilitation test. J Cardiopulm Rehabil 1989;7:273–278

Impact on Client Factors

A survey by the American Lung Association (4) regarding the impact of COPD on the quality of life revealed that 51% of the respondents have limitations on their ability to work, 70% report an interference with normal physical exertion, 56% have difficulty with social activities, 50% have trouble sleeping, and 46% interference with family activities. Clearly, this condition affects all parts of the individual's life, including family participation.

The main objectives of an occupational therapy program for the person with COPD are to reinforce a diaphragmatic breathing control pattern, to teach "pursed lip breathing" during activities, to develop increased strength and endurance for exercise, and increased work tolerance for performance areas. In breath control, the client learns how to use the abdominal and lower thoracic muscles to exhale with exertion, and inhale during the nonresistant part of the activity. The movements should flow smoothly and not be performed in a hurry.

Raising the arms is a good position for inhalation and lowering the arms down to the side of the body is helpful for exhalation. The COPD client has to change the cycle of rushing through tasks in order to avoid dyspnea (27).

Pneumonia

Pneumonia, the seventh leading cause of death in 2000 within the United States, is defined as an inflammation of the lungs (4). Community-acquired pneumonia (CAP) is the most common infection faced in health care settings. In 2000, the diagnosis of pneumonia and pleurisy was the second most common condition with patients who received Medicare and were discharged after a short stay in the hospital (28).

The main types of pneumonia are bacterial, viral, and mycoplasmal. The most common routes for infection in the lower respiratory tract are inhalation and aspiration. Methods of transmission for bacteria or a virus are inhalation of droplets, having direct contact with infected respiratory secretions, or indirect contact with articles infected with the bacteria or virus. The air sacs in the lungs fill up with pus and other liquid. The result is a reduction in the amount of oxygen that is able to reaches the blood resulting in cellular damage (30).

Etiology

The main cause of pneumonia is an infection from bacteria, a virus, or mycoplasmas, which are a specific and unique species of bacteria. A virus causes an estimated 50% of pneumonia cases. Additional causes may be inhalation of food, liquid, gases, dust, or fungi. It is difficult to separate viral from bacterial cases, and at least 25% of CAP cases are without diagnostic findings (29). Most at risk are the elderly, the very young, individuals undergoing cancer treatment, organ transplant or persons who have additional health problems, such as COPD, diabetes mellitus, congestive heart failure, sickle cell anemia, or autoimmune diseases.

Incidence and Prevalence

In 2000, pneumonia and influenza ranked seventh in the leading cause of death (4). In 2002, the total number of deaths was 64, 954, an incidence rate of 22.5 per 100,000 individuals.

Signs/Symptoms

Streptococcus is the most common cause of bacterial pneumonia. Symptoms are shaking, chills, chattering teeth, severe chest pain, and a cough with rust- or green-colored mucus. Temperature may rise to 105°F, which may result in a confused or delirious mental state. Additional symptoms are increased breathing, pulse rate and sweating. Lips and nail beds may look blue, as a result of lack of oxygen in the blood.

Viral pneumonia symptoms are similar to the same as influenza such as a fever, dry cough, headache, muscle pain, and weakness. In a short period of time, there is increased breathing, the cough becomes worse and there may be blueness of the lips. Mycoplasma pneumonia symptoms include a violent cough, chills, fevers, some nausea, vomiting, and overall weakness (4).

Medical/Surgical Management

One of the problems in treating pneumonia is the identification of microbes resistant to antibiotics. The Pneumonia Severity Index (PSI) is a scale that is used for predicting pneumonia outcomes (30). This instrument is used for predicting mortality, length of stay, time to stability, intensive care unit admission and hospitalization. Drug therapy is the main form of treatment, specifically antibiotics for bacterial pneumonia. Additional medication is used to ease chest pain and provide relief from the coughing. The American Lung Association encourages the following high-risk people to receive a pneumonia vaccine: ages 65 and older, postoperative patients, individuals with a chronic illness, or those living in a nursing home environment.

Assessment for pneumonia may include the 6- or 12-minute walk test, a balance assessment, activities of daily living, range of motion, communication, observation, and muscle strength testing. Physiological monitoring needs to be included before, during, and upon completion of evaluation. Examples of interventions are graded activities to improve overall endurance and strength, increased tolerance for functional activity, and patient education. Work simplification and energy conservation are standard areas to focus for return to home and community re-entry (30).

Tuberculosis

Tuberculosis (TB) is an infectious chronic disease. TB testing has revealed a 50% increase of Mycobacterium tuberculosis among health care workers in New York for the past 8 years (31). In 1994, the Centers for Disease Control and Prevention (CDC) published the Guidelines for Preventing the Transmission of Mycobacterium tuberculosis in Health Care Facilities.

Transmitted by airborne particles, M. tuberculosis is inhaled through the air passages and 1 to 5 bacteria are transferred to the terminal alveolus. The lung is the main site for 80% to 85% of the infected population (33). The system, such as human immunodeficiency virus (HIV), from the aging process, or the use of corticosteroids. Extrapulmonary TB affects other parts of the body other than the lung, for example, the kidneys and lymph nodes.

Etiology

Tuberculosis is an infectious disease, caused by M. tuberculosis, which is airborne and transmitted by inhalation of contaminated droplets and dispersed through the air by coughing, sneezing, or talking.

Incidence

There are 1 billion individuals infected with TB worldwide (31). Every year, 8 million people develop TB and 3 million die of complications. Between 30% and 60% of adults in the developing countries are infected and this is the first cause of death for people older than 5 years of age. In 2000, the incidence rate in the United States was 5.8 cases per 100,000. According to the CDC, 22% were older than age 65 (32). The TB cases are often present in the urban, poor African-American, Native American, and immigrant populations (32, 33). In 2004, the incidence rate in the United States was 4.9 per 100,000 and the new goal for 2010, as part of a national strategic plan for TB elimination is <1 case per 1,000,000 (32).

Three types of infection are latent, active, and extrapulmonary. Ninety percent to 95% of the populations have a latent infection, where the bacteria remain dormant and the person does not develop any symptoms. Five percent to 10% of the people infected with TB move into an active stage, where symptoms and the ability to spread the disease occur (33). Activation of the dormant bacteria is often a result of an immunocompromised.

Signs and Symptoms

Signs and symptoms of TB are cough, hemoptysis (spitting up blood), fever, night sweats, and weight loss.

Medical/Surgical Management

Medication consists of chemotherapeutic agents, which are administered daily, and then 2 to 3 times a week under direct observation for 6 months. Directly observed therapy (DOT) is an important part of the treatment, for compliance reasons. More than 85% of the patients under this medication schedule have negative sputum cultures within 2 months after treatment has been initiated. A test to

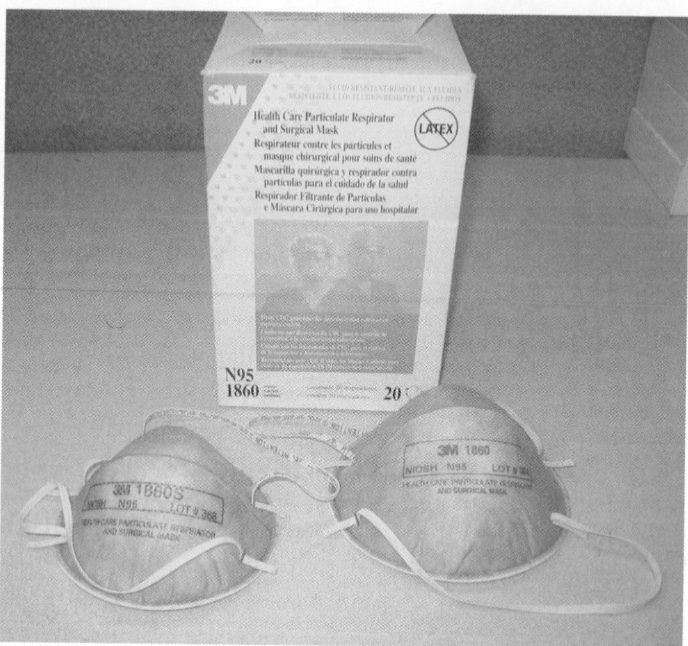

Figure 10.7 N95 disposable respirator mask.

verify previous exposure to the M. tuberculosis is the TB skin test. The most inexpensive way to identify TB is microscopic examination of sputum. Radiologic images have been determined to be the most useful diagnostic test (32, 33). Tests utilized for diagnosis are cultures of mucus, blood, bone, and tissue. If indicated, surgery to remove a portion of the lung is an alternative for drug-resistant infections. Early recognition and treatment of the active TB is a preferred way to stop transmission to others.

The Occupational Safety and Health Administration (OSHA), requires infection control procedures for all employees with exposure to blood and other body fluids. Personal protective equipment (PPE), such as gloves, masks, face shields, coats, gowns, caps, and shoe covers must be available to the employees. Clinical staff must be fit-tested for the N95 disposable respirator mask (Fig. 10.7) that is National Institute of Occupational Safety and Health (NIOSH)-approved and filters our the particles in the air we breathe. Employees, who have not been fit-tested, must use the powered air-purifying respirators (Fig. 10.8).

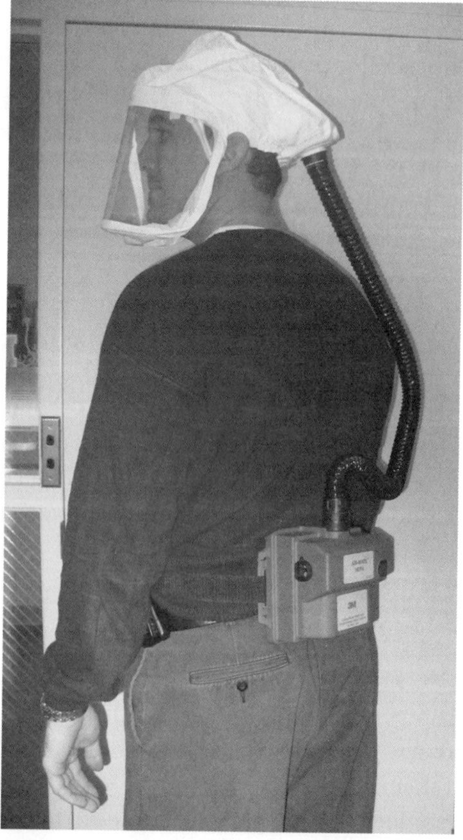

Figure 10.8 Powered air purifying respirator.

Assessment for TB may include participation in ADL and IADL, observation and muscle strength testing. Goals should include: principals of work simplification and energy conservation as well as graded activities to improve overall strength and endurance.

Coronary Artery Disease

The next section of this chapter describes common conditions specific to coronary artery disease. These include Myocardial Infarction, Congestive Heart Failure and Hypertension. As in pulmonary conditions, a review of the anatomy of relevant structures is helpful in understanding the conditions described.

Anatomy of the Cardiovascular System

The main functions of the cardiovascular system are:

1. Generating blood pressure through the blood vessels.
2. Routing blood to oxygenate the blood flowing to the tissues.
3. Ensuring one-way blood flow through the heart and blood vessels.
4. Regulation of the blood supply to help us during rest, exercise, and body position changes.

The cardiovascular system is made up of the blood, heart, and blood vessels (Fig. 10.9). The main responsibility of the cardiovascular system is transportation of blood to all parts of the body.

Our body contains 5 to 6 quarts of blood. Blood is made up of 22% solids, 78% water, and makes up 7% to 8% of the body's total weight (7). It takes 20 to 30 seconds for the blood to circulate through the body and return to the heart. The main functions of the blood are to transport gases, nutrients and waste products, processed and regulatory molecules, regulation of the pH (the body's acid-base balance) and osmosis, maintenance of body temperature, protection against foreign substances and clot formation. Blood is a mixture of plasma, red blood cells, white blood cells, and platelets. Red blood cells make up 40% of the blood's volume and the main function is to transport oxygen and carbon dioxide. There are fewer white blood cells than red blood cells and the main function is to protect the body against invading microorganisms, and to remove dead cells and debris from the body. Platelets are fewer in number than red blood cells. (a ratio of 1 platelet to 20 red blood cells) (33). The main function of platelets is to release chemicals necessary for blood clotting.

The heart is a muscle, which pumps blood to the tissues and cells. Shaped like a blunt cone, the heart is located in the middle to the lower part of the chest cavity between the lungs, on the left side. The blunt rounded point is called the apex and the larger, flat part on the opposite end of the cone is called the base. The size varies with body size and has three layers: the pericardium, which is the outer layer, the myocardium, which is the second layer and the endocardium, the inner layer. The heart of a healthy adult (70 kg) pumps approximately 1,900 gallons of blood each day (6). The right side of the heart pumps blood to the lungs, where oxygen is combined with the blood and carbon dioxide is removed. The left side pumps blood to the rest of the body, where oxygen and other nutrients are delivered to the tissues and waste products, including carbon dioxide are transferred to the blood and removed by other organs.

The heart has four chambers: the right and left upper and lower chambers. The upper chambers are thin walled and called the atria, forming the superior and posterior portions of the heart. The right atrium receives blood from the body tissues and the left atrium receives blood from the lungs. Lower chambers are called ventricles and

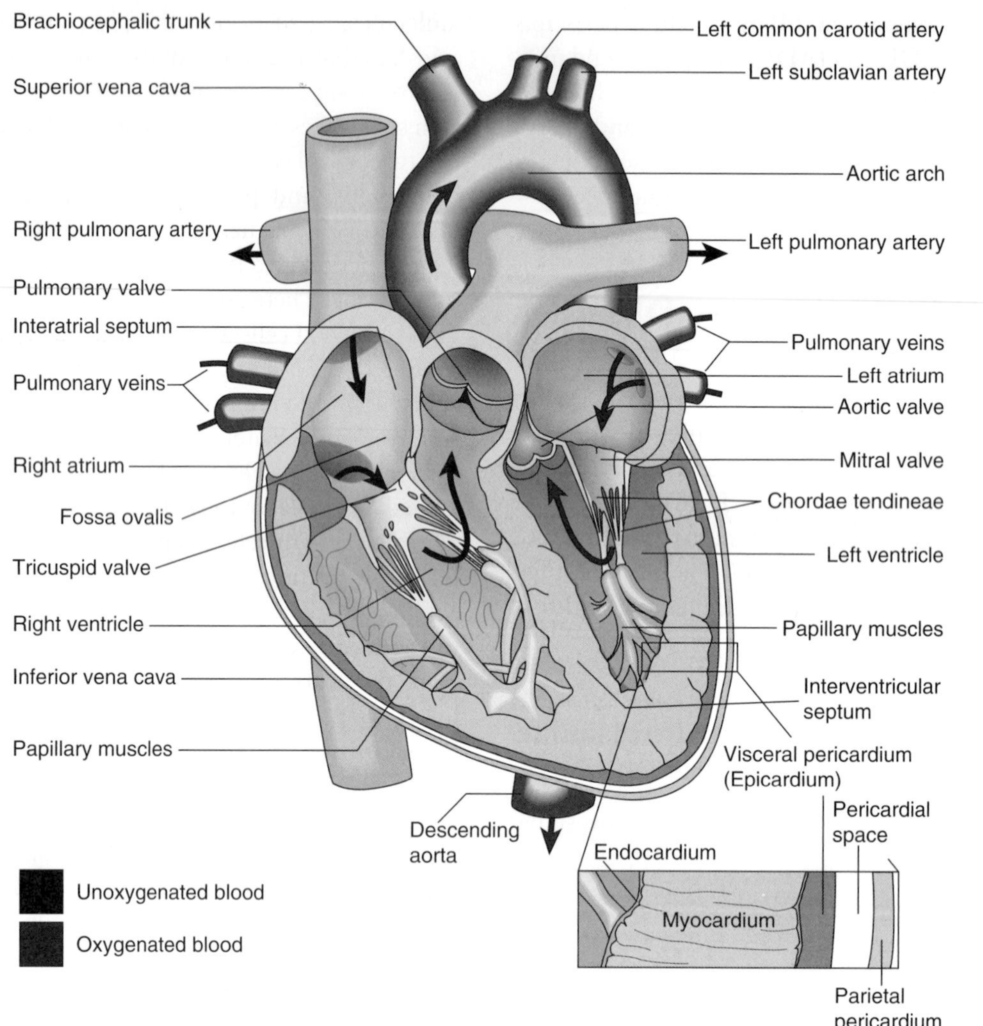

Figure 10.9 Anatomy of the cardiovascular system. (From Smeltzer SCO, Bare BG. Brunner and Suddarth's Textbook of Medical-Surgical Nursing. 9th Ed. Philadelphia: Lippincott, Williams & Williams, 2002.)

pump blood. The thick-walled ventricles form the anterior and inferior portions of the heart. The right ventricle pumps blood to the lungs for oxygen and the left ventricle pumps blood to all parts of the body. Valves are positioned between the atrium and the ventricles, which assist blood to flow in only one direction and prevent blood from flowing back into the atrium from the ventricles. The tricuspid valve is between the right atrium and ventricle. The mitral valve (bicuspid valve) is between the left atrium and ventricle (6).

The phases of heart action include the following steps:

1. During systole, the working phase, the heart contracts. As the heart contracts, blood is pumped through the blood vessels
2. During diastole, the resting phase, the heart chambers fill with blood.

There are three groups of blood vessels: the arteries, capillaries, and the veins. Arteries carry blood away from the heart. The aorta is the largest artery, rich in oxygen. The aorta receives blood directly from the left ventricle, branches into other arteries, which carry blood to all parts of the body. The smallest branch of an artery is called an arteriole. Arterioles connect with blood vessels called capillaries. Food, oxygen, and other nutrients pass from the capillaries into the cells of the body. Waste products, including carbon dioxide, are picked up from the cells to the arterioles. Veins return blood to the heart and are connected to capillaries by venules. Venules, small veins, branch together to form veins. The two main veins near the heart are the inferior vena cava and the superior vena cava, which empty into the right atrium. The inferior vena cava carries blood from the legs and trunk. The superior vena cava carries blood to the head and arms. Venous blood is dark red in color, because it has little oxygen with significant amounts of carbon dioxide (6).

Route of Blood Flow

Deoxygenated venous blood enters the heart through the right atrium from the tissues of the body and flows through the tricuspid valve into the right ventricle. The right ventricle pumps blood through the pulmonary semilunar valves into the pulmonary trunk to the pulmonary arteries on the way to the lungs. From the lungs, the pulmonary veins carry the oxygenated blood to the left atrium, through the bicuspid valve, and pump into the left ventricle. The blood flows through the aortic semilunar valves to the aorta and onto the body tissues (Fig.10.10)

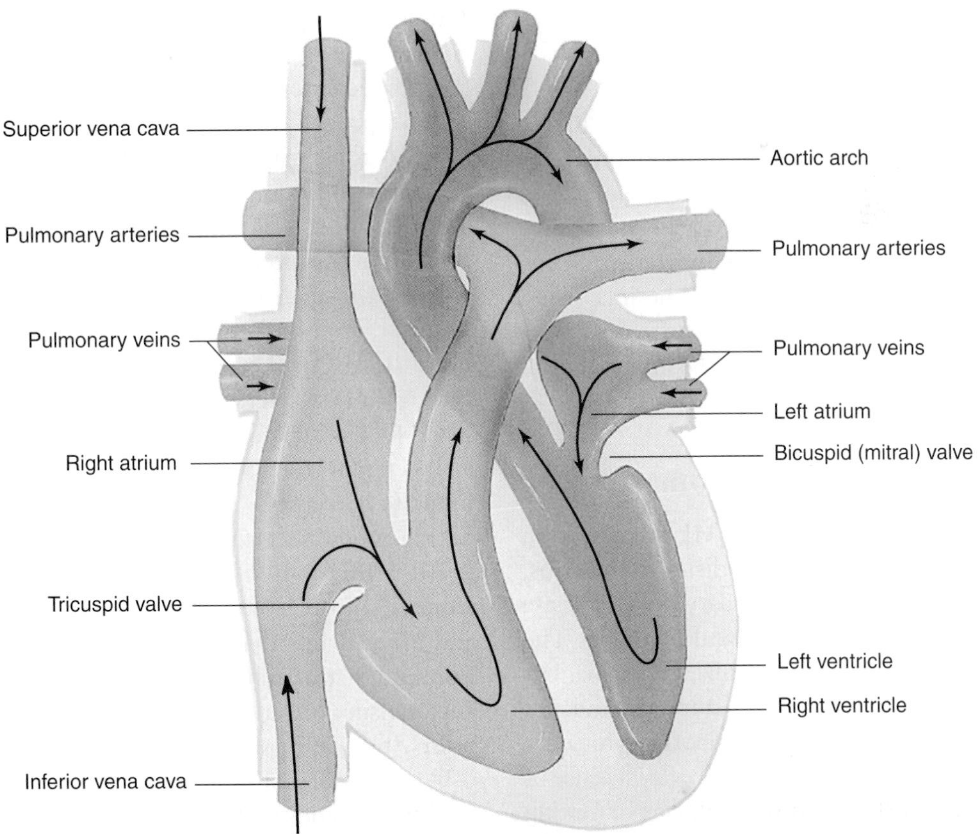

Figure 10.10 Blood flow through the heart. (From Anatomical Chart Co. Baltimore; Lippincott, Williams and Wilkins: 2004)

Myocardial Infarction

Etiology

Myocardial infarction (MI) is commonly referred to as a heart attack and is caused by a blockage of blood flow to a portion of heart muscle. This blockage is typically caused by atherosclerosis or by a thrombic/embolic occlusion. A sudden interruption of blood flow to the myocardium leads to ischemia (tissue damage). If the blood supply does not come back, then infarction (tissue death) develops. Some of the different risk factors are cigarette smoking, a family history of heart attack, diabetes, obesity, high blood pressure, high blood cholesterol, low high-density lipoprotein (HDL) cholesterol, age, stress, and a sedentary lifestyle (33).

Incidence

One of the most common diseases in the United States, MI affects 1.5 million Americans (34, 35), and has an incidence rate of 3.5 of the total population in 2001 (12). The average age is 65.8 for men and 70.4 for women, affecting more men than women. The increasing number of men and women, who have sustained a heart attack, lead to the importance of evidence-based therapies (33).

Signs/Symptoms

The primary symptoms of a MI are chest pain, located substernally, that radiates to the arms, back, or upper jaws. Secondary symptoms are dyspnea, nausea, vomiting, and confusion. The pain of a heart attack is similar to angina, but more intense, is longer in duration and not relieved by rest or nitroglycerin. Unfortunately, one in five people have mild or even absence of symptoms, which results in a delay of getting medical assistance (36). Some of the complications of a heart attack are myocardial rupture, scar tissue around the site of damage, ventricular aneurysm that may cause abnormal heart rhythms and reduced pumping of the heart, blood clots in the arteries supplying the heart, and heart failure from tissue death. Depression may play a role following a MI, as a result of life style changes and should be addressed in the plan of care (37).

Medical/Surgical Management

Medical assessment and intervention may include electrocardiography (ECG), which records the electrical activity in the heart and cardiac enzyme blood tests, which help to detect and diagnose a heart attack. The three enzymes are creatine phosphokinase (CPK), lactate dehydrogenase (LDH), and Troponin I. A cardiac catheterization test helps to determine a build-up of plague in the coronary arteries. The procedure involves injecting a contrast dye into the coronary arteries. If the coronary arteries are blocked, the doctor may order a procedure which is called percutaneous coronary intervention (PCI). Some of the interventions are angioplasty, where a small balloon is inflated inside a coronary artery or more often, stenting, which involves inserting a small wire tube into the artery. A surgical option is a coronary artery bypass graft (CABG). The blood flow is routed through a new artery or vein to increase the blood flow to the heart.

In a recent study, four classes of medications found to have a 90% reduction in their risk of having another heart attack or sudden cardiac death within 6 months of being discharged from the hospital are antiplatelets (aspirin and other drugs that keep blood clots from forming), statins, (cholesterol lowering drugs), angiotensin-converting enzyme (ACE) inhibitors (blood pressure-lowering drugs), and β-blockers (adrenaline-blocking drugs) (38).

While it is not within the scope of this text to describe specific cardiac rehabilitation protocols, an overview of the common approach is helpful to describe.

Table 10.3 SIGNS OF CARDIAC DISTRESS

- Change in pattern of angina or dyspnea
- Heart palpitations
- Feeling lightheaded, dizzy or confused
- Feeling more fatigue than expected
- Unusual pain or discomfort in muscles or joints after exercise
- Sweating
- If blood pressure falls >20 mm Hg or heart rate is >20 bpm over resting rate

Cardiac rehabilitation begins with inpatient status, progresses to outpatient treatment and to community based maintenance programming (28). The four stages of cardiac rehabilitation typically include the following:

Phase I: Acute hospitalization which will include monitored self care activities, progressive ambulation and limited transfers.

Phase II: Post acute phase which begins at discharge and continues for 12 weeks. A progressive program of endurance as tolerated is the focus of this phase.

Phase III: Continuation of endurance training along with a focus on risk reduction education and modification with preparation for return to work, if applicable.

Phase IV: Focus is on maintenance of a regular prescribed exercise program and continued monitoring of risk modification.

During each phase of cardiac rehabilitation, a unit of choice to measure energy expenditure, the metabolic equivalent (MET) is used to determine progression of activity. One MET is equal to 3.5 mL of oxygen per kilogram of body weight per minute. There are easily accessed MET charts that will illustrate various daily activities and corresponding MET values, which range from 1 to 5. As an example, 1 MET is sitting and reclining in a comfortable chair, whereas 5 MET's would be equal to ascending a flight of stairs.

Evaluation and treatment must include adherence to cardiac precautions and physiologic monitoring before, during and on completion of activities. Table 10.3 and Table 10.4 list some cardiac assessments that are commonly used.

Treatment is focused on maximum independence, with increased activity tolerance and re-integration in areas of occupation according to tolerance. An exercise program can improve endurance and the quality of life with mild to moderate heart failure clients (38, 39, 40). A walking program is a functional form of exercise, frequently accessible to patients and without cost. Return to work or a productive life leads to a better sense of self-worth and avoids the road of disability and depression (40, 41). Additionally, cardiac precautions need to be followed and a baseline established for setting an exercise goal. As indicated earlier in this chapter, the metabolic values are used to determine appropriate exercise, home, and leisure activity levels for improved functional status (28). The rate of perceived exertion (RPE) scale can assist with the person's perception of effort, strain, discomfort and/or fatigue before, during and after activity, targeting 11 and 14 (28). The maximum age-adjusted heart rate is used to calculate the patient's exercise heart rate range. To calculate, take the number 220, subtract the patient's age, and this gives you the MAHR. To determine the exercise heart rate range, multiply the maximum age-adjusted heart rate by 50% and 85% (27).

Table 10.4 SUMMARY OF CARDIOVASCULAR ASSESSMENTS

Assessment	Description	Reference
Borg Rated of Perceived Exertion Scale (RPE)	Measurement of tolerance with exercise, keeping intensity between 11 and 14	Borg, G. Borg's Perceived Exertion and Pain Scales. Human Kinetics. 1998.
Metabolic Equivalent Table (MET)	Units of measures for how much oxygen consumption is used with activity	Ainsworth BE, Haskell WL, Leon AS, et al. Compendium of physical activities: classification of energy costs of human physical activities. Medicine and Science in Sports and Exercise 1993;25(1):71–80.
Duke Health Profiles	Measures depression	Parkerson GR Jr, Broadhead WE, Tse CK. The Duke Health Profile. A 17-item measure of health and dysfunction. Med Care. 1990 Nov; 28(11):1056–72.

Congestive Heart Failure

Congestive heart failure (CHF) occurs when the heart looses the ability to pump blood through the body. Chronic heart failure is a progressive condition that usually has no cure and often requires many lifestyle changes.

Etiology

Some of the causes for CHF are coronary artery disease (CAD), a history of MI, hypertension, abnormal heart valves, heart muscle disease (cardiomyopathy), congenital heart defects, severe lung disease, and diabetes (30).

Incidence and Prevalence

CHF affects 10 out of 1,000 people older than age 65. Seventy five percent of cases have antecedent hypertension. The overall death rate in 2004 was 18.7 and affects 2 to 3 million Americans (45% of our population) with 400,000 new cases per year (41). Patients 65 years of age and older who are diagnosed with CHF are the largest population of hospital admissions. Direct and indirect costs associated with CHF are $25.8 billion and the increase of incidence and survival may result in greater disability costs for the future.

Pathophysiology

The two forms of heart failure are systolic dysfunction (more common) and diastolic dysfunction. CAD is the most common cause of systolic dysfunction. Systolic dysfunction occurs when the heart cannot pump out all the blood, a reduced amount is pumped to the body, lungs and the heart (left ventricle) usually enlarges. Diastolic dysfunction entails the reduction of heart contraction, because the walls of the heart cannot relax, blood backs up in the left atrium and the lung blood vessels, leading to congestion. Untreated hypertension is the most common cause of diastolic dysfunction.

Signs/Symptoms

Overall, symptoms of heart failure are dyspnea, persistent coughing or wheezing, edema, fatigue, lack of appetite, nausea, increased heart rate, confusion, and impaired thinking. One study refers to an increase in cognitive impairments with CHF in the elderly (42). There are four levels of severity for symptoms, used by the New York Heart Association. Class I is no symptoms and no limitations in ordinary physical activity; Class II is mild symptoms and slight limitation during ordinary activities; Class III is marked limitation in activity due to symptoms, comfortable only at rest; Class IV is severe limitations, experiencing symptoms even while at rest (42). Symptoms differ with right-sided and left-sided heart failure. The main symptoms of right-sided heart failure are edema in the feet, ankles, legs, liver, and abdomen. Left-sided heart failure leads to fluid accumulation in the lungs, causing shortness of breath. As the condition progresses, the person begins to experience feelings of restlessness, anxiety and suffocation (33).

Medical/Surgical Management

Diagnosis of CHF is completed with a chest radiograph, an ECG, an echocardiograph, radionuclide imaging, angiography, exercise stress test, and blood tests. An echocardiogram is an ultrasound test that evaluates the heart wall thickness and function of the heart valves with sound waves. Radionuclide imaging involves introducing radioactive materials into the patient's body, to view detailed images of different parts of the body. Common tests include positron emission tomography (PET) scan and single-photon emission computed tomography (SPECT) scans. An exercise stress test measures the heart's tolerance for exercise and can identify heart disease. The stress tests may be in combination with an ECG or with echocardiography.

Typical medication for heart failure are ACE inhibitors, angiotensin II receptor blockers, β-blockers, vasodilators, cardiac glycosides, loop diuretics, thiazide and thiazide-like diuretics, anticoagulants, opioids, and positive inotropic drugs. Surgical options include a coronary artery bypass surgery or in an end-stage case, a heart transplant.

The overall goal is to reduce and control the stress placed on the heart. Cardiac precautions must be followed, as described with a MI. One method of measuring exercise tolerance for patients with CHF is the New York Heart Association Functional Classification of Heart Disease, noted earlier in this chapter. Treatment includes lifestyle changes, medications and perhaps, surgery. Lifestyles changes may include weight loss, smoking cessation, exercise, and reducing stress, following a diet of low saturated fat and reduced sodium. ADL and IADL need to be graded, according to tolerance. Additionally, use of the RPE as well as education on the principles of work simplification and energy conservation assist with a safe community re-entry and return to work (33). An increase in physical training can improve the quality of life and exercise tolerance for men with CHF (43).

Hypertension

When blood pressure stays elevated for a period of time, it can be considered "high blood pressure" (HBP) or "hypertension." This condition results in excessive cardiac output and increases the risk for heart failure, heart attack, and kidney failure. Two thirds of people older than age of 65 have HBP. HBP can be a result of other conditions, such as CHF and kidney disease.

HBP is described as a systolic pressure of 140 mm Hg or above and a diastolic pressure of 90 mm Hg or above. Pressures between 120/80 mm Hg and 139/89 mm Hg can be categorized as "prehypertension." This disease can occur in children, but is usually associated with adults (45).

Etiology

In 90% to 95% of the cases of HPB, the cause is unknown. Factors that are linked to HBP are age, atherosclerosis, race (a high percent are African

Americans), obesity, family history, prehypertension, unhealthy diet, birth control pills, pregnancy, postmenopause, excessive alcohol use, diabetes mellitus, gout, or kidney disease (44).

Incidence

One in five Americans has HBP and 22% of American adults have "prehypertension." The mortality rate is 16.5 in 2001, with indirect and direct costs of $55.5 billion. There were 251,000 U.S. deaths in 2000 (12, 42).

Pathophysiology

Systolic pressure is the force of blood in the arteries as the heart beats and goes through the circulatory system and is the top number in a blood pressure reading. Diastolic pressure is the force of blood in the arteries as the heart relaxes between beats and is the bottom number in a blood pressure reading.

Under normal conditions, the heart beats 60 to 80 beats per minute. Blood pressure can change quickly with changes in posture, exercise or sleeping. The heart pumps blood through the arteries to arterioles and then to capillaries, to supply oxygen and the other nutrients to body organs. The blood then returns through the veins to the heart (42, 45).

Signs/Symptoms

Prehypertension is a systolic blood pressure of 120 to 139 mm Hg or a diastolic blood pressure of 80 to 89 mm Hg. Hypertension is divided into two stages. Stage I is a systolic pressure of 140 to 159 mm Hg or a diastolic pressure of 90 to 99 mm Hg. Stage II is a systolic pressure of 160 mm Hg or higher or a diastolic pressure of 100 mm Hg or higher. Potential risk of heart failure and stroke increases with patients in stage two. A person can have HBP for years and not even know it, since the condition usually has no symptoms. This is why the disease is called the "silent killer" (44).

Medical Management

If you have HBP, lifestyle modifications that may be recommended are reduced salt intake, weight loss and increased physical activity. Medications commonly used with HBP are antihypertensives such as diuretics, β-blockers, vasodilators and ACE inhibitors. Patient-centered counseling, self-monitoring of blood pressure and structured training courses have been found to be effective interventions for HPB. Counseling leads to BP improvement as well as structured training courses (42). The Surgeon General's Report reveals moderately intense aerobic exercise at 40% to 60% of maximum oxygen consumption, such as 30 to 45 minutes of brisk walking on most days of the week can lower blood pressure. A study has shown that progressive resistance exercise may slightly lower resting blood pressure, which can decrease the risk of stroke and coronary heart disease (46, 47, 48). Some of the literature reveals a sedentary lifestyle can lead to a higher risk of death in preretirement adults.

Assessments should include an interest checklist, examination of current lifestyle and functional abilities for activities of daily living, leisure and work. The overall goal is to reduce the blood pressure through modification of lifestyle and implementation of healthy behaviors. Examples of intervention include grading activities to increase tolerance for activities of daily living, patient education to assist in understanding the connection between exercise, functional activities, risk modification, and role performance.

Summary

In summary, with the main goal of increasing the quality and years of healthy life, as stated in Healthy People 2010 (1), one of the leading health indicators is regular physical activity. Engaging in occupation is a key to facilitating better health and overall well-being. The focus of occupational therapy is to enhance performance skills and performance patterns for maintaining as well as changing life roles. This philosophy is especially relevant to cardiopulmonary diseases as much of what has been presented here is preventable by way of better personal health management practices.

CASE STUDY

Case Illustration

■ CASE 1

The context is a long-term care facility. Mrs. X has a diagnosis of COPD, pneumonia and sinusitis. The medical information reveals a history of bronchospasms. Mrs. X was functioning independently with her ADL, living at home with her husband prior to re-admission to this facility. Discharge plans include return to home with her husband. Mrs. X wears corrective lenses. Pulse oximetry drops to below 90% with 30 second to 1 minute conversation and her pulse rate is 130 beats per minute with rest. Precautions are 4 liters of oxygen, 24 hours a day. Date of onset is 4/20/04, the date of OT evaluation is 4/26/04.

RESULTS OF OCCUPATIONAL THERAPY EVALUATION

Performance in Areas of Occupation
Activities of Daily Living (ADL)

SKILL	Prior Level Date: 4/16/04	Evaluation	STG	LTG	Comment on Current Status
Eating and Feeding	I	I	I	I	Device: No
Oral Hygiene	Mod I	Mod I	I	I	
Grooming	Mod I	Mod I	I	I	
Bathing UB	SBA/Min	Min	Mod I	I	Device: No, Bedside
Bathing LB	Min/Mod	Mod	Min	I	Device: No, Bedside
Dressing UB	SBA/Min	SBA/Min	Mod I	I	Device: No
Dressing LB	Mod A	Min	CGA	I	Device: No
Toileting	SBA	SBA	Mod I	I	Bedside Commode, Hygiene: WFL, Clothing Management: WFL
ADL Transfers	Min A	SBA	Mod I	I	Toilet/Commode
Bed Mobility	Mod I	Mod I	I	I	
Wheelchair Mobility	SBA/Min A	Mod I	I	I	Safety: WFL, W/C Set-up Safety, Brakes/Footrests, WFL

Homemaking	Max A	Max A	Mod A	Min A	Resident takes >30 min for basic AM self care; R/T need for frequent rest breaks

Assessment Rating Scale: I, Independent, WNL; MI, Modified Independence, extra time/device, WFL; S, Supervision Set-Up/Cueing; SBA, Stand By Assist; CGA, Contact Guard Assist; MIN, Minimal Assistance 25%; MOD, Moderate Assistance 50%; MAX, Maximum Assistance 75%; DEP, Dependent 100% Assistance; NT-Not Tested; NA, Not Applicable;
UB, Bilateral Upper Extremities; LB, Bilateral Lower Extremities; WFL: Within Functional Limits

Sitting is normal, standing is fair, and positioning in bed and the wheelchair are good. She is able to propel the wheelchair without assistance. She requires stand by assistance with walker-supported ambulation, and walks at a slow pace for 30 feet. Mrs. X is right hand dominant and fine motor coordination is WFL, bilaterally, with some tremors. Energy/endurance is poor; pulse oximetry drops with talking and pulse increases from 130 to 156 with 30 feet of walking slowly. Pulse oximetry decreased to 87% and it took 2 minutes to recover. Functional activity tolerance is poor. Edema is present in the left lower extremity and in the face from steroid use.

Cognitive assessment reveals intact alertness problem solving, sequencing, and safety awareness. She is able to follow four-step commands and memory and orientation are intact. Verbal and written communication skills are intact and Mrs. X is able to speak by blocking her tracheostomy site for whisper volume. Mrs. X has useful habits as indicated by independent level of functioning prior to admission to the facility. Routines and roles are acceptable for discharge.

Mrs. X has a strong Italian culture, is 58 years old, lives in own home with her spouse, and is an active church member in her community.

Acknowledgments

A note of thanks to Stacey Wolfe, OTR, who provided the case study for this chapter.

References

1. U.S. Department of Health and Human Services. (2000). *Healthy people 2010: Understanding and improving health* No. 017-001-001-00-550-9). Washington DC: U.S. Government Printing Office.
2. American Occupational Therapy Association. Occupational therapy practice framework: Domain and process. Am J Occup Ther 2002;56:609–639.
3. Jobin., Mattais F, Poirier P, et al. Advancing the frontiers of cardiopulmonary rehabilitation. Champaign, IL: Human Kinetics, 2002.
4. American Lung association. (2004). Available at: http://www.lungusa.org/site/pp.asp?c=dvLUK9O0E&b=33347. Accessed 6/8/04.
5. Hillegass E, Sadowsky SH. Essentials of cardiopulmonary physical therapy. Philadelphia: W.B. Saunders, 2001.
6. Seeley RR, Stephens TD, & Tate P. Anatomy and physiology. Dubuque, Iowa: McGraw-Hill/WCB, 1998.
7. Burch S. Cardiopulmonary Health and Illness. Health Positive, Inc., 2003.
8. Jones M, Moffatt F. Cardiopulmonary Physiotherapy. Oxford, UK: BIOS, 2002.
9. Hannon W, Hasson S: Cardiopulmonary pathophysiology. In: Principles and Practice of Cardiopulmonary Physical Therapy (3rd Edition) Frownfelter, Dean E (eds), Mosby, pp. 71–97, 1996.
10. US Department of Health & Human Services, National Institutes of Health, National Heart, Ling, and Blood Institute. Available at: http://www.nhlbi.nih.gov/health/public/lung/other/copd_fact.pdf_WhatIs.html. Accessed 6/8/04.
11. Chronic Obstructive Pulmonary Disease (2005). Available at: http://www.nhlbi.nih.gov/health/dci/

Diseases/Copd/Copd_WhatIs.html.asp/165. Accessed 6/8/04
12. Centers for Disease Control and Prevention. National Center for Health Statistics. (2004). Available at: http://www.cdc.gov/nchs/fastats. Accessed 6/2/04.
13. National Heart, Lung and Blood Institute, World Health Organization. Global Initiative for Chronic Obstructive Lung Disease. Pocket Guide to COPD, Diagnosis, Management, Prevention. New York: World Health Organization 2004.
14. Modawal A, Candadai NP, Mandell KM, et al. Weaning success among ventilator-dependent patients in a rehabilitation facility. Arch Phys Med Rehabil 2002;83(2):154–157.
15 Pratt RK, Fairbank JC, Virr A. The reliability of the shuttle walking test, the swiss spinal stenosis questionnaire, the oxford spinal stenosis score, and the Oswestry disability index in the assessment of patients with lumbar spinal stenosis. Spine 2002;27(1):84–91.
16 Vagaggini B, Taccola M, Severino S, et al. Shuttle walking test and 6-minute walking test induce a similar cardiorespiratory performance in patients recovering from an acute exacerbation of chronic obstructive pulmonary disease. Respiration 2003;70(6):579–584.
17 Booth S, Adams L. The shuttle walking test: a reproducible method for evaluating the impact of shortness of breath on functional capacity in patients with advanced cancer. Thorax 2001;56(2): 146–150.
18 Solway S, Brooks D, Lacasse Y, Thomas S. A qualitative systematic overview of the measurement properties of functional walk tests used in the cardiorespiratory domain. Chest 2001;119(1): 256–270.
19. Enright PL. The six-minute walk test. Respir Care Clin N Am, 2003;48(8):783–785.
20. Wijkstra PJ, TenVergert EM, et al. Long term benefits of rehabilitation at home on quality of life and exercise tolerance in patients with chronic obstructive pulmonary disease. 1995
21. Lacasse Y, Brosseau L, Milne S, Martin S, Wong E, et al. Pulmonary rehabilitation for chronic obstructive pulmonary disease (Cochrane Review). In: The Cochrane Library, Issue 3, 2004.
22. Berzins GF. An occupational therapy program for the chronic obstructive pulmonary disease patient. Am J Occup Ther 1970;24(3):181–186.
23. Smith B, Appleton S, Adams R, Southcott A, Ruffin R. Home Care by outreach nursing for chronic obstructive pulmonary disease (Cochrane Review). In: The Cochrane Library, Issue 3, 2004.
24. Thomson O'Brien MA, Oxman AD, Davis A D, et al. Educational outreach visits: Effects n professional practice and health care outcomes [Abstract]. The Cochrane Library, (3), 2004.
25. Strijbos JH, Postma DS, van Altena R, et al. A comparison between an outpatient hospital-based pulmonary rehabilitation program and a home-care pulmonary rehabilitation program in patients with COPDA follow-up of 18 months. Chest 1006;109(2): 366–372.
26. Monninkhof EM, Van der Valk PDLPM, Van der Palen J, et al. Self-management education for chronic obstructive pulmonary disease. The Cochrane Library, (3), 2004.
27. Trombly C, Radomski M. Occupational Therapy for Physical Dysfunction. Baltimore, Maryland: Lippincott, Williams & Wilkins, 2002.
28. Vecchiarino P, Bohannon RW, Ferullo J, et al. Short-term outcomes and their predictors for patients hospitalized with community-acquired pneumonia. Heart Lung 2004;33(5):301–307.
29. Korppi M. Non-specific host response markers in the differentiation between pneumococcal and viral pneumonia: what is the most accurate combination? Pediatr Int 2004;46(5):545–550.
30. Yepes JF, Sullivan J, Pinto A. Tuberculosis: medical management update. Oral Surgery, Oral Medicine, Oral Pathology, Oral Radiology, Endodontics 2004;98(3):267–273.
31. Centers for Disease Control. Guidelines for Preventing the Transmission of Mycobacterium tuberculosis in Health-Care Settings. 2005. Available at: http://www.cdc.gov/mmwr/preview/mmwrhtm1/rr5417a1.htm?s_cid=rr5417a1_e. Accessed 6/2/04.
32. Willard HS, Spackman CS. In: Crepeau B E, Cohn ES Schell BA, eds. Occupational Therapy. 10th Ed. Philadelphia: Lippincott, Williams & Wilkins, 2003.
33. Merck manual. 2nd Ed. Whitehouse Station, NJ: Merck Research Laboratories, 2003.
34. Mookadam F, Arthur HM. Social support and its relationship to morbidity and mortality after acute myocardial infarction: Systematic overview. Arch Int Med 2004;164(14):1514–1518.
35. Avezum A, Makdisse M, Spencer F, et al. Impact of age on management and outcome of acute coronary syndrome: Observations from the global registry of acute coronary events (GRACE). Am Heart J 2005;149(1):67–73.
36. Johansson I, Stromberg A, Swahn E. Factors related to delay times in patients with suspected acute myocardial infarction. Heart Lung 2004;33(5): 291–300.
37. Ellis JJ, Eagle KA, Kline-Rogers EM, et al. Depressive symptoms and treatment after acute coronary syndrome. Int J Cardiol 2005;99(3):443–447.
38. Mukherjee D, Fang J, Chetcuti S, et al. Impact of combination evidence-based medical therapy on mortality in patients with acute coronary syndromes. Circulation 2004;109(6):745–749.
39. Ellis JJ, Eagle KA, Kline-Rogers EM, et al. Perceived work performance of patients who experienced an acute coronary syndrome event. Cardiology 2005; 104(3):120–126.
40. McBurney CR, Eagle KA, Kline-Rogers EM, et al. Work-related outcomes after a myocardial infarction. Pharmacotherapy 2004;24(11):1515–1523.

41. American Association of Cardiovascular & Pulmonary Rehabilitation. Guidelines for cardiac rehabilitation and secondary prevention programs. Champaign, IL: Human Kinetics, 2004.
42. Acanfora D, Trojano L, Iannuzzi GL, Furgi G, Picone C, et al. The Brain in congestive heart failure. Archives of Gerontology and Geriatrics 1996;23:247–256.
43. Larsen A, Kristiansen M, Haugland A, et al. Assessing the effect of exercise training in men with heart failure. Eur Heart J 2001;22: 684–692.
44. American Heart Association. (2004). Available at http://www.americanheart.org/presenter.jhtml?identifier=2139, accessed 6/3/04.
45. Sorrentino S. Assisting with Patient Care. St. Louis: Mosby, 1999.
46. White W. Update on the drug treatment of hypertension in patients with cardiovascular disease. Am J Med 2005:118:695–705.
47. Boulware LE, Daumit GL, Frick KD, et al. An evidence-based review of patient-centered behavioral interventions for hypertension. Am J Prev Med 2001;21(3):221–232.
48. Kelley GA, Kelley KS. Progressive resistance exercise and resting blood pressure: a meta-analysis of randomized controlled trials. Hypertension 2000;35(3):838–843.

Recommended Learning Resources

American Association of Cardiovascular & Pulmonary Rehabilitation. (2004). Guidelines for Cardiac Rehabilitation and Secondary Prevention Programs. (4th ed.) Champaign, IL: Human Kinetics

American Association of Cardiovascular & Pulmonary Rehabilitation. (2004). Guidelines for Pulmonary Rehabilitation Programs. (2nd ed.) Champaign, IL: Human Kinetics

Hillegass, E., & Sadowsky, S.H. (2001) Essentials of Cardiopulmonary Physical Therapy. Philadelphia: W.B. Saunders

Journal of Cardiopulmonary Rehabilitation, the official journal of the American Association of Cardiovascular and Pulmonary Rehabilitation and the Canadian Association of Cardiac Rehabilitation. The publisher states that this is the only professional journal for the entire cardiovascular and pulmonary rehabilitation team. Published by Lippincott Williams and Wilkens.

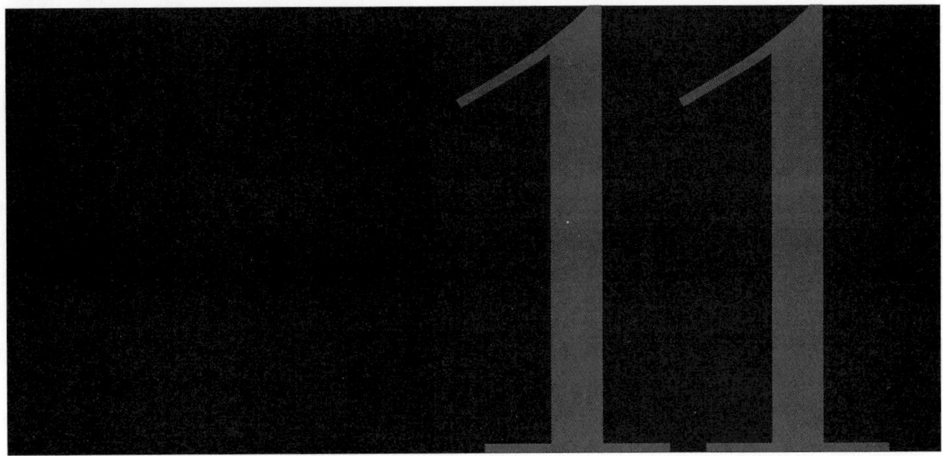

Diabetes

Joanne Phillips Estes

Key Terms

Diabetic foot
Diabetic ketoacidosis
Hyperglycemia
Hypoglycemia
Nephropathy
Neuropathy
Polydipsia
Polyphagia
Polyuria
Retinopathy
Type 1 diabetes
Type 2 diabetes

Sara is a 22-year-old female diagnosed as having **type 1 diabetes** at the age of 12. In order to control the disease, maintain health, and deal with the progression of potential complications, Sara must check her blood glucose levels and inject insulin four times per day. She also takes six additional medications daily. Although she is supposed to watch her nutritional intake and exercise, she lacks motivation to do so. She finds her regimen to be restrictive and subsequently becomes depressed, which further impedes the following of her prescribed treatment program. Sara is fearful of becoming blind or having a limb amputation, which further adds to her anxiety and depression.

Diabetes mellitus (DM) is a metabolic condition characterized by a deficiency of, or reduced sensitivity to insulin, a hormone produced by the pancreas, whose purpose is to regulate glucose metabolism. Insulin is required for the cellular uptake of glucose, which is required for energy. Without insulin, liver, muscles, and fat tissues cannot take up absorbed nutrients (1). This ultimately leads the body to use its own fat or lipids as an energy source, which produces toxic acid waste products in the blood called ketones. High concentrations in the blood are lethal. Until insulin was characterized and manufactured in the 1920s, the diagnosis of diabetes often was a death sentence. Although this is no longer so, diabetes does carry a significant risk for individuals to develop major impairments. In the United States, diabetes is the fourth most common reason for physician visits (2). It also is the leading cause of blindness among working-age people, end-stage renal disease (ESRD), and nontraumatic limb amputation (2). Furthermore, diabetes increases the risk of cardiac, cerebral, and peripheral vascular disease from twofold to sevenfold (2). Few diseases have the same potential for damaging as many organ systems.

Diabetes is classified according to etiology (3) as either type 1 or type 2. Type 1, formerly known as insulin-dependent DM or juvenile-onset DM, occurs predominantly in children. Type 2, formerly known as noninsulin-dependent DM or adult-onset DM, typically occurs with increasing age. However, the incidence of **type 2 diabetes** is increasing rapidly in younger age groups, particularly in minority adolescents who are obese (4).

Etiology

The exact cause of diabetes is unknown. In patients with **type 1 diabetes**, an autoimmune response occurs that produces antibodies against and destroys pancreatic beta cells that produce insulin (2). It is thought to involve some type of genetic disposition along with an environmentally based inciting event. The inciting event may be acute illness (2) or virus (5), diet (high in fat or nitrosamines), environmental toxins, or emotional or physical stress (5). The pancreas continues to produce insulin in type 2 diabetes. However, the amount may not be enough to meet bodily demands or there may be desensitization of insulin receptors (2). Genetic factors are thought to be involved, but little is known about specific genetic abnormalities (2).

Obesity also is associated with a risk for developing type 2 diabetes (5), as at least 85% of type 2 diabetics are obese (2). Finally, aging (40 and older) is believed to contribute to etiology (6).

Incidence and Prevalence

Diabetes is increasing worldwide (7). In the United States, the number of people with diabetes more than doubled between 1980 (5.8 million) and 2002 (13.3 million) (7). Each year 800,000 people in the United States develop diabetes (6). Overall, the incidence is similar for males and females throughout most age ranges but is slightly greater for males older than age 60 (6).

Type 1 diabetes occurs at a rate of 15/100,000 per year (5) and accounts for 5% to 10% of all diabetic cases (8). The mean age at onset is 8 to 12 years (5). It occurs equally among males and females; however, the mean onset age is 1.5 years earlier in females (5). Prevalence of type 1 diabetes is associated with ethnicity. African Americans and people of Asian descent have the lowest rates (2), whereas Caucasians and people of Finnish, Scandinavian, Scottish, and Sardinian descent have the highest (2). Prevalence rates differ among ethnic groups living in the same geographic region; Caucasian children in Allegheny, Pennsylvania, or Colorado are 50% to 70% more likely to develop type 1 diabetes than nonwhites living in the same area (2). Genetic factors associated with susceptibility are believed to explain these differences.

Type 2 diabetes occurs at an incidence of 300/100,000 per year and accounts for 90% of all diabetic cases (6). Among Caucasians it is more prevalent in females than males (5). Its prevalence is 10% to 15% among people older than age 50 (5). Type 2 diabetes is most prevalent among African-Americans (1.6 times as likely as the general population), Latinos (1.5 times as likely), and Native Americans (2.2 times as likely) (9). One tribe in Arizona has the highest rate of diabetes in the world: about 50% of people in this tribe between the ages of 20 and 64 have diabetes (10).

Signs and Symptoms

The signs and symptoms of type 1 diabetes are (5):

- **Polyuria** (increased frequency of urination)
- **Polydipsia** (excessive thirst)
- **Polyphagia** (extreme hunger), which is classic but not common
- Anorexia that results in a 10% to 30% weight loss
- Increased fatigue
- Decreased energy
- Chest pain and occasional difficulty breathing
- Nausea
- Muscle cramps
- Irritability
- Emotional lability
- Blurred vision
- Altered school and work behaviors
- Headaches
- Anxiety attacks
- Abdominal pain and discomfort
- Diarrhea or constipation

Some signs and symptoms of type 2 diabetes are the same as type 1. These are polyuria, polydipsia, polyphagia, unusual weight loss, extreme weakness and fatigue, and irritability. Additional symptoms include frequent skin, gum, or bladder infections, cuts or bruises that are slow to heal, and numbness or tingling in the hands or feet (9). Finally, symptoms related to **hyperglycemia** and complications can occur (**nephropathy, neuropathy, and, retinopathy**) (9). These complications may be present upon diagnosis if preceded by long periods of hyperglycemia (6).

Course and Prognosis

After initial diagnosis of type 1 diabetes, a temporary remission period usually occurs for 3 to 6 months. During this time, overall control of the disease is easier and insulin needs are less. Insulin production gradually regresses until levels are insignificant and a state of total diabetes is reached (5). Longevity and quality of life are currently better than in the past owing to improvements in insulin delivery regimens. Life expectancy is lower overall than for persons who do not have diabetes, however, in the past 20 years, the life expectancy of those with diabetes has increased dramatically (5). Quality of life depends on development of potential complications common to people who have type 1 diabetes. Whether the vascular and neuropathic complications of diabetes can be prevented or delayed by improved glycemic control has been debated for more than half a century (2). In 1993, the National Institutes of Health (NIH) completed a 9-year study called the Diabetes Control and Complications Trial. Its purpose was to learn if intensive insulin therapy could prevent diabetic complications or retard progression of mild retinopathy (2). Subjects were divided into intensive insulin and conventional care groups. The conclusion drawn from the results was that glucose control matters (2). The intensive insulin group showed significantly less development of retinopathies and neuropathies. However, it was noted that participants were highly motivated and more compliant than the average person with diabetes, which also may explain the results.

Complications

Following is a description of common complications that may occur during both types 1 and 2 diabetes disease processes. These complications can be either acute or chronic.

The major acute complication is **diabetic ketoacidosis** (DKA). This is an emergency state of metabolic imbalance that usually signals onset of type 1 diabetes (2). It occurs in patients with established disease because of illness (infection), inappropriate reduction in insulin intake, or missed injection (2). It can also occur in patients who are sick and who fail to increase insulin and consume extra fluids accordingly.

Chronic complications impact multiple organ systems. These are typically responsible for morbidity and mortality associated with DM (4). Risk of chronic complications increases with hyperglycemia (6).

Hyperglycemia is a condition of too-little insulin causing abnormally high blood glucose levels. Signs are thirst, heartburn, fast and deep breathing, excessive urination, headache, nausea, abdominal pain, blurred vision, and constipation (5). If untreated, the patient is at risk for entering into a diabetic coma. Mortality from hyperglycemia increases with age and is usually caused by the presence of a comorbid condition (myocardial infarction [MI], cerebral vascular accident, sepsis). Treatment depends on insulin to reverse metabolic abnormalities and on detection and successful treatment of the comorbid condition.

Hypoglycemia or insulin shock is a condition of too much insulin and not enough glucose in the blood stream (5). This is the most frequent complication of type 1 diabetes, affecting 10% to 25% of individuals per year (2). Symptoms are vague: fatigue, headache, drowsiness, lassitude, tremulousness, shallow breathing, and nausea (5). It may produce seizures, accidental injury, catecholamine response, or arrhythmia or cardiac ischemia in patients with underlying cardiac disease (2). The patient needs to ingest some form of sugar, such as orange juice, cola, candy, or jelly, if able to swallow. On an emotional level, this could become a great fear of the patient's leading to less-than-optimal blood sugar control (2).

Diabetic retinopathy is caused by many physiologic changes in the eye (microaneurysm, neurological changes, or vascular leakage). It typically occurs 15 years after onset of diabetes (2). Blindness occurs 20 times more frequently for those with diabetes than in the general population; 10% to 15% of patients with type 1 diabetes and 5% to 8% of those with type 2 become legally blind (2). At present, medical therapy is restricted to optimization of glycemic control, which delays and slows progression of nonproliferative retinopathy. Little evidence suggests that improving glycemic control benefits the more advanced stages of retinopathy (2).

Diabetic nephropathy affects 25% to 30% of persons with type 1 and 15% to 20% of those with type 2 diabetes. Diabetes is the leading cause of ESRD; one third of individuals with ESRD have diabetes (2). Gross protein in the urine appears about 15 years after diagnosis of diabetes. Subsequent development of renal failure is highly variable, especially among people with type 2 diabetes. Most patients develop ESRD approximately 10 years after creatinine in blood levels begins to rise. Initially, tight control of blood sugar levels and aggressive treatment of hypertension (HTN) may slow progression of renal failure. Once clinical nephropathy is present, blood sugar control is less effective.

People with diabetes tolerate uremia (toxic effects of waste products build up in blood owing to renal failure) less well than those who do not have diabetes. Retinopathy and neuropathies develop more quickly, HTN is more difficult to control, and generalized atherosclerosis increases. Treatment options are transplantation, hemodialysis, or continuous ambulatory peritoneal dialysis (CAPD).

Hemodialysis removes waste products from the patient's blood as it circulates through an artificial kidney. This requires the patient to be at a dialysis center and hooked up to a machine two or three times per week for 3 to 5 hours each treatment. Side effects of hemodialysis include weakness, fatigue, nausea, headaches, or hypotension.

CAPD is accomplished by infusing dialysis fluid into the abdomen through a catheter where waste products are collected by osmosis. These fluids are drained out to remove waste products from the body and the cycle is repeated. To do this, the patient must have sufficient grip, pinch, and peripheral sensation. CAPD patients are at risk for developing peritonitis (abdominal infection) because of the body's direct communication with the external environment. Hemodialysis is the most common intervention for persons with ESRD. However, often it is not tolerated well. Among individuals receiving dialysis, mortality is substantially higher for those with diabetes than for those who do not have diabetes. This is primarily because of the more rapid development of vascular insufficiency among persons with diabetes (2).

Diabetic neuropathy at symptomatic, potentially disabling levels affects nearly 60% to 70% of those with diabetes (8). Current treatment, which involves control of blood glucose, is primarily effective before clinical symptoms are present. Distal sensorimotor neuropathy is the most common form. Damage is typically more sensory than motor in nature. Symptoms include numbness and tingling in hands and feet, variable loss of distal reflexes, intrinsic muscle wasting in the hands and feet, and pain. Axonal loss encompasses both small (pain and temperature) and large (position and touch) fibers (2). The individual also could develop autonomic neuropathy, which carries a poor prognosis. This may result in abnormal cardiovascular, skin, gastrointestinal, bladder, and sexual functioning. There is no treatment intervention to reverse neuropathies once developed. Pain control, however, is an important part of management.

Diabetic foot is the cause of 60% of nontraumatic limb amputations (8). In this condition, foot ulcers result from insignificant trauma; they heal slowly and may lead to gangrene. Diabetic foot is characterized by:

- Chronic sensorimotor neuropathy
- Autonomic neuropathy
- Poor peripheral circulation
- Visual loss that compromises ability to care for feet
- Loss of sensation (inability to detect mild trauma)

Treatment aimed at prevention and education can reduce the risk of amputation by 50% (2).

Cardiovascular disease is also prevalent. HTN is more common and the onset of atherosclerosis is both earlier and more severe for those with diabetes. People with diabetes have a two to four times higher risk for heart disease and cerebral vascular accident than those without diabetes (8). In 2002, 38% of people with diabetes had a comorbid diagnosis of cardiovascular disease (7). The major cause of death among people with diabetes is atherosclerosis of cerebral, cardiac, and peripheral blood vessels (2). Smoking cigarettes compounds this risk.

Diagnosis

Diabetes is diagnosed based on laboratory results of blood tests. Type 1 diabetes has a sudden or rapid onset. Diagnosis is based on excessive amounts of glucose in the blood and excessive amounts of glucose and ketones in the urine. Often, the first indicator of type 1 diabetes is DKA. Pathological findings include inflammatory changes in pancreatic tissue (2).

Onset of type 2 diabetes is more gradual and the patient may have it without being aware. Fasting blood sugar (FBS) levels of ≥126 mg/dL (6) or random plasma glucose ≥200 mg/dL plus presence of classic symptoms (polydipsia, polyuria, polyphagia, weight loss) are indicators of the disease (5).

Medical/Surgical Management

Type 1 Diabetes

There is no known cure for diabetes. The primary focus of treatment is to replace insulin in the body, which is typically accomplished through subcutaneous injection. An alternate method is continuous subcutaneous insulin infusion (CSII), which is an external pump that delivers continuous basal rates of insulin (2). Recent studies have shown that inhaled insulin maintains glycemic control and provides greater user satisfaction as compared to subcutaneous injections (11). Oral hypoglycemics (to simultaneously lower blood glucose levels) are usually not indicated (5). Immunosuppressants (such as cyclosporine) may be given to reduce the rate of autoimmune destruction of pancreatic cells and must be started in the initial weeks after diagnosis is made.

Insulin regimens must be carefully designed and monitored for effectiveness. Commercial preparations differ in the amount of time before onset and length of effectiveness (2). Absorption depends on the site of injection. It occurs faster when (a) injected into the abdomen than into an extremity and (b) injected into an upper extremity than a lower extremity (2). Absorption is accelerated if injection is in an extremity that is either exercised or massaged or warmed. Finally, absorption is faster if injection is deep or intramuscular (2).

The secondary focus of treatment is to make lifestyle changes to facilitate insulin therapy and optimize health (2). Diet must consist of nutritionally sound meals and a careful balance between caloric intake and energy expenditure, adjusting for periods of increased activity by consuming more food (2). Long delays between meals should be avoided, as not eating in a predictable pattern according to insulin regimen may cause hypoglycemia. Frequent, small snacks at the time of peak insulin action should also be taken to avoid hypoglycemia.

Regular exercise is recommended to enhance general well being and decrease the likelihood of vascular complications. There is little evidence that exercise improves glycemic control for persons with type 1 diabetes (2). Exercise can, however, enhance insulin sensitivity and decrease overall insulin requirements (2).

Type 2 Diabetes

Lifestyle changes and dietary control are the key management interventions. Often, metabolic states can be normalized by these alone. The American Diabetes Association provides dietary recommendations for management of diabetes that include increased complex carbohydrates (soluble dietary fiber) (2), decreased saturated fat, and moderation in salt and alcohol intake (10). It is important to balance caloric intake with insulin and activity level or exercise (6).

Regular exercise is recommended as an adjunctive treatment. It can help weight reduction, improve insulin action, and decrease risk of cardiovascular complications. When diet and exercise are ineffective in controlling blood glucose level, oral glucose-lowering agents are indicated. These are used if hyperglycemia is mild, the patient is older, or obesity is pronounced. Individuals with type 2 diabetes may initially respond to oral hypoglycemics but then not respond well after years of this therapy. This could be the result of decreased compliance with diet and exercise, progression of pancreatic failure to produce insulin, complications from comorbid medical conditions or drugs, or development of tolerance to medication. Insulin therapy is indicated at this point. Insulin is also the first-line intervention for those who are younger, nonobese, severely hyperglycemic, pregnant, or require temporary treatment owing to increased stress (injury, infection, surgery) (2).

Self-monitored blood glucose (SMBG) levels are crucial for both type 1 and type 2 diabetes. Urine testing is unreliable and should be used when the only goal is prevention of symptomatic hyperglycemia (2). Self-monitoring requires that individuals with diabetes take active control of their own health and well-being, allows for more rapid treatment adjustments, and reinforces dietary guidelines.

Portable glucose meters are available that take blood for sampling, give a digital readout of glucose levels, and have a computerized memory for record keeping. People with type 1 diabetes should monitor glucose levels before each meal and at bedtime (2). People with type 2 who are insulin dependent should monitor before breakfast, dinner, and bedtime, with the goal of monitoring being to avoid hypoglycemia. Persons with type 2 who are noninsulin-dependent should learn to do SMBG for urgent situations.

Intensive insulin treatment rarely restores glucose homeostasis to levels achieved by those who do not have diabetes (2). In severe cases, and based on availability, a transplant of pancreatic (insulin-producing) tissue is performed. Most patients remain stabilized for many years postoperatively. However, transplantation is an option for only a small group of individuals because of the need for long-term immunosuppression (2). Individuals with type 1 diabetes who have received a kidney transplant benefit most from pancreatic tissue transplantation, as it may be effective in preventing nephropathy of the transplanted kidney.

Impact of Condition on Client Factors

Body Functions

Complications during the course of the disease have the potential to impact the majority of body functions (Table 11.1). The degree of impairment may range from minimal impact to very severe and extremely debilitating. The course is variable for each individual and depends only in part on patient compliance and successful self-management. Often medical

Table 11.1 POTENTIAL COMPLICATIONS OF DIABETES

Complication	Symptom
Hyperglycemia	Too little insulin with high blood glucose
Hypoglycemia	Too much insulin with low levels of blood glucose
Retinopathy	Visual impairment that may result in blindness
Nephropathy	Renal impairment that may result in kidney failure
Neuropathy	Neurological damage resulting in sensorimotor symptoms
Diabetic Foot	Distal neuropathy, poor circulation, and lack of sensation, resulting in ulcers that are slow to heal which may lead to gangrene
Cardiovascular Disease	Hypertension and atherosclerosis

intervention can do little to slow or prevent these impairments.

Acute and chronic complications impact mental functioning. Acutely, insulin and blood glucose levels influences level of arousal. Symptoms of hypoglycemia include drowsiness and fatigue. Hyperglycemia can lead to coma if not treated. Chronic complications include cognitive impairment. Studies have shown that verbal memory deficiencies are associated with type 2 diabetes (12).

Emotional functioning may be impacted as depression and eating disorders (in women) are more common in type 1 and type 2 diabetes (6). Variations in blood glucose levels can cause mood swings and irritability. A person with diabetes must also cope with having an "invisible disability"; to others, their strict dietary and medication regimens may appear hypochondriacal in nature. Often, there is anger and frustration over lifestyle and body image changes. They must also adjust to progressive impairment and feelings of lack of control over their health and well-being.

The remaining effects of complications impacting body functions are the result of motor, sensory, or autonomic peripheral neuropathies. For sensory function and pain, visual perception is reduced to varying degrees in the presence of retinopathies which may ultimately lead to blindness. Touch sensation may be impaired with resultant numbness, tingling, or loss of sensation especially in the distal extremities (6). A sharp or shooting pain is also present. As the neuropathy progresses, pain subsides and is replaced by a sensory deficit (6). Neuromusculoskeletal function is also impacted via decreased muscle strength resulting from the presence of sensorimotor neuropathies.

Complications resulting in autonomic nerve dysfunction to internal organs also impact body functions. As noted above, cardiovascular system involvement results in increased risk of hypertension and accelerated atherosclerosis. Fatigability is a symptom of diabetes and must be managed throughout the course of the disease. Hypoglycemia also leads to fatigue. Digestive system function is compromised when impacted by autonomic neuropathy. Symptoms include constipation, diarrhea, and gastroparesis. Gastroparesis leads to nausea, vomiting, feelings of bloating after eating (2), and delayed emptying of the stomach (6).

Genitourinary function can be affected resulting in bladder dysfunction. Symptoms include infrequent urination, incomplete emptying of the bladder, dribbling, incontinence, and frequent urinary tract infection (2). Sexual dysfunction is also common. Up to 50% of males with diabetes experience erectile dysfunction (2) and retrograde ejaculation. Females experience vaginal dryness and loss of desire (13).

Skin is impacted by complications of the disease with the primary manifestations being prolonged wound healing and skin ulcerations (6). The skin is also more prone to bacterial infections and is often dry and cracked, secondary to decreased sweating. These are of particular concern with the diabetic foot as healing is impaired, which could lead to gangrene and ultimately limb amputation.

Impact of Condition on Occupational Performance

Performance in all areas of occupation may be affected by complications of diabetes. Common motor skill involvement includes impaired walking, manipulation, and grip strength secondary to neuropathies. These impairments result in difficulty performing activities of daily living (ADL) tasks such as dressing, grooming, and functional mobility. Effective personal hygiene and grooming care is critical in preventing diabetic foot complications. Sexual activity may also be impaired by fatigue, comorbid conditions, decreased sensation, and emotional issues (anxiety, fear, guilt, anger, or shame) (1). Furthermore, sexual dysfunction leads to decreased quality of life for people with diabetes (13,14).

Function in instrumental activities of daily living (IADL) tasks is also affected by diabetes. Meal preparation must meet dietary guidelines. Effective health management and maintenance related to SMBG levels and managing insulin regimen is vital to well-being and control of potential complications. Likewise, people with diabetes must demonstrate ability to respond to emergencies related to hyperglycemia or hypoglycemia.

CASE STUDY

Case Illustrations

■ CASE 1

Mrs. D. is a 44-year-old Caucasian female with a diagnosis of type 1 diabetes mellitus. Onset of her disease was at the age of 12 years. Mrs. D.'s medical history includes diagnoses of HTN 5 years ago and diabetic retinopathy 10 years ago. She has had peripheral neuropathies in four extremities for 7 years. She has ESRD and is receiving hemodialysis three times a week, as she has been for 2.5 years. She will be undergoing bilateral nephrectomies in 1 week because of her history of chronic pyelonephritis (infected kidneys). She has been on a list for a kidney-pancreas transplantation for 2 years.

Mrs. D.'s medication routine is extensive. She takes 20 units of Humulin N (insulin) subcutaneously twice a day; Catapres TTS#3 change weekly (once per week blood pressure patch); one Nephrocaps (multivitamin) by mouth each day; 325 mg of ferrous sulfate twice a day for anemia; three 667 PhosLo tablets by mouth three times a day with meals (calcium binds phosphorus with foods eaten to prevent phosphorus from going into the body, normal kidneys eliminate extra phosphorus in body, secondary hyperparathyroidism can occur); Kayexalate 1T in diet soda pop by mouth daily (binds potassium so it can be eliminated with bowel movement); and 100 mg of Colace orally each day for constipation.

Mrs. D. has been married to a veterinarian for 19 years. They have two daughters, ages 12 and 14. She has a bachelor of arts degree in education and worked as an elementary school teacher for 4 years before having children. She has been a full-time homemaker and mother since then. Her hobbies include travel, gardening, and listening to recorded books.

Mrs. D. is right-hand dominant and receives dialysis through her left upper extremity (LUE). She has pain and numbness in her LUE because of an ischemic neuropathy that is the result of decreased blood flow because blood is diverted to her dialysis access site. She is legally blind as a result of diabetic retinopathy. She has full bilateral upper extremity active range of motion but decreased peripheral sensation (tactile, pain, and temperature). Mrs. D. recently stepped on a tack, did not feel it, and subsequently developed an infection that has been slow to heal. A moderate decrease in bilateral grip and pinch strength has been noted, with her left side weaker than her right. Her physician notes chronic flat affect that may be an indication of mild depression.

She communicates little information to the physician during hemodialysis visits.

Transportation services bring her to and from dialysis, as blindness prevents driving. She ambulates independently with guidance owing to her decreased vision. Mrs. D. is independent in all transfers, feeding, dressing, bathing, and hygiene. Her laboratory results show poor compliance with fluid restriction (1,800 mL fluid/day) and noncompliance with dietary restrictions. Her husband contacted the physician with concerns about her lack of interest in caring for their daughters, in gardening, and in sexual activity. Her husband seems supportive but notes recent marital tension.

Mrs. D. is moderately disabled by the physical and emotional ramifications of diabetes, retinopathy, neuropathies, and renal failure. This is affecting her role of wife and mother. Her physical environment must be adapted to accommodate her disabilities. Socially, she is becoming withdrawn. The context of her occupational performance further reflects the impact that diabetes has on decreasing the quality of her life.

■ CASE 2

S. is a 9-year-old boy who attends third grade at the local public school. He is the middle child, having an older brother and younger sister, and lives with both parents. S. is an extremely bright and athletic child. He enjoys playing sports and is especially competitive with his older brother. He has several good friends and typically enjoys spending time with them and his siblings.

He was in good health until 8 months ago when his parents found him in bed, lethargic, confused, weak, complaining of being very thirsty and cold, and vomiting. They also noticed that his breath was "sweet-smelling." After ambulance transportation to the local emergency room, S. was diagnosed as being in a state of DKA and having type 1 diabetes. Initially, management of his disease was easy. His parents monitored blood glucose levels four times per day and little insulin was needed for control. After this "honeymoon period" ended, S.'s blood glucose levels became more difficult to manage.

S. says he's embarrassed and does not want his friends to know that he has diabetes. Consequently, he often does not follow dietary restrictions. He becomes irritable and combative with his parents regarding SMBG and insulin injections. He avoids socializing with friends and his teachers report a significant decline in his academic performance. S. refuses to do homework and spends most of his time alone in his bedroom. He often says that he doesn't care what could happen to him if he doesn't follow dietary and medication requirements.

Sensorimotor and cognitive functioning are currently intact except level of arousal. As his glucose levels fluctuate, S. becomes drowsy and fatigued. This often occurs during school, when he lays his head on his desk and sleeps. These fluctuations obviously impair his ability to learn.

At this point, psychosocial skills and psychological functioning are challenged. S. is having difficulty adjusting to the fact that he is *different* from his friends and often refuses to follow dietary restrictions in their presence. Recently he refused to attend his best friend's birthday party because he could not have the cake, ice cream, and candy the other kids would be enjoying. S.'s mother notes increased arguing and fighting between S. and his siblings and friends.

S.'s mother also is having difficulty coping with her son's diagnosis because her father died of complications from diabetes when she was 14. She is distressed that S. is not enjoying his friends and school like a *typical* 9-year-old boy would. She is also concerned that his physical, social, emotional, and intellectual development will lag because of his diabetes. S.'s father is spending more time at work than he used to. There are many extended family members living in the area who have voiced concern and support.

References

1. Tilton M. Diabetes and amputation. In: Sipski M, Alexander C, eds. Sexual Function in People With Disability and Chronic Illness: A Health Professional's Guide. Gaithersburg, MD: Aspen, Inc. 1997:279–302.
2. Sherwin R. Endocrine and reproductive diseases. In: Bennett J, Plumb F, eds. Cecil Textbook of Medicine, vol 2. 20th Ed. Philadelphia: WB Saunders, 1996:1258–1277.
3. Gavin JR, Alberti KGMM, Davidson MB, et al. Report of the expert committee on the diagnosis and classification of diabetes mellitus. Diabetes Care 1997;7:1183–1197.
4. Rosenbloom AL, Joe JR, Young RS, et al. Emerging epidemic of type 2 diabetes in youth. Diabetes Care 1999;22:345–354.
5. Dambro M. Griffith's Five Minute Clinical Consult. Baltimore: Williams & Wilkins, 1995:306–311.
6. Powers AC. Diabetes mellitus. In: Braunwald E, Fauci AS, Kasper DL, et al., eds. Harrison's Principles of Internal Medicine. 15th Ed. New York: McGraw-Hill, 2001:2109–2137.
7. Center for Disease Control's Diabetes Program-Data and Trends. Available at: http://www.cdc.gov/diabetes.statistics/cvd. Accessed January 16, 2005.
8. National Diabetes Information Clearinghouse (NDIC): A service of the National Institute of Diabetes, Digestive, and Kidney Diseases. Available at: http://diabetes.niddk.nih.gov/dm/pubs/statistics/index.htm. Accessed August 25, 2004.
9. 2003 National Diabetes Fact Sheet: Department of Health and Human Services; Centers for Disease Control and Prevention. Available at: http://www.cdc.gov/diabetes/pubs/factsheet.htm.Accessed August 23, 2004.
10. Diabetes is a major health problem for Native American Indians. American Diabetes Association. Available at http://aihc1998.tripod.com/diabetes.html. Accessed August 23, 2004.
11. Gerber RA, Cappelleri JC, Kourides IA, et al. Treatment satisfaction with inhaled insulin in patients with type 1 diabetes. Diabetes Care 2001;24:1556–1559.
12. Strachen MWJ, Deary IJ, Ewing FME, et al. Is type II diabetes associated with an increased risk of cognitive dysfunction? Diabetes Care 1997;20:438–445.
13. Enzlin P, Mathiew C, Van den Bruel A. Sexual dysfunction in women with type 1 Diabetes. Diabetes Care 2002;25:672–677.
14. De Barardis G, Franciosi M, Belfiglio M. Erectile dysfunction and quality of life in type 2 diabetic patients. Diabetes Care 2002;25:284–291.

Recommended Learning Resources

Brown DW, Balluz LS, Giles WH, et al. Diabetes mellitus and health-related quality of life among older adults: Findings from the behavioral risk factor surveillance system (BRFSS). Diabetes Res Clin Pract 2004;65:105–115.

Cate Y, Baker SS, Gilbert MP. Occupational therapy and the person with diabetes and vision impairment. Am J Occup Ther 1995;49:905–911.

Gregg EW, Brown A. Cognitive and physical disabilities and aging-related complications of diabetes. Clin Diabetes 2003;21:113–118.

Handevidt F. Peripheral neuropathy in persons with diabetes. Clin Excell Nurse Pract 2001;5:17–20.

Karlsen B, Bru E, Hanestad BR. Self-reported psychological well-being and disease-related strains among adults with diabetes. Psychology and Health 2002;17:459–473.

Koch T, Kralik D, Sonnack D. Women living with type II diabetes: the intrusion of illness. J Clin Nurs 1999;8:712–722.

American Diabetes Association
1701 North Beuregard Street
Alexandria, VA 22311
Tel: 1–800-DIABETES
http://www.diabetes.org

Center for Disease Control Public Health Resource
www.cdc.gov/diabetes

Juvenile Diabetes Research Foundation International
www.jdrf.org

National Diabetes Education Program, a joint program of NIH and CDC
www.ndep.nih.gov

National Institute of Diabetes and Digestive and Kidney Diseases of the National Institutes of Health
www.niddk.nih.gov

Consumer Resource

American Diabetes Association complete guide to diabetes. 3rd ed. Alexandria, VA: American Diabetes Association, 2003.

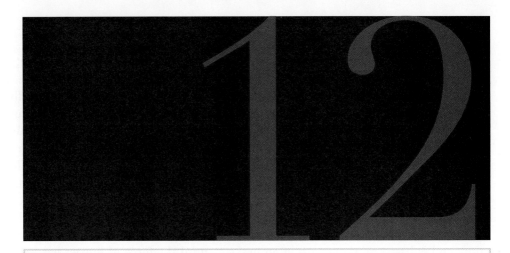

Traumatic Brain Injury

Gerry E. Conti

Key Terms

Mild traumatic brain injury (TBI)
Moderate traumatic brain injury
Severe traumatic brain injury
Coma
Decerebrate rigidity
Decorticate rigidity
Aspiration
Retrograde amnesia
Anterograde amnesia
Procedural learning
Executive functions
Hydrocephalus
Physiatrist

It had been a hot summer day, the work was hard, and the boss kept hanging around the garage. At last it was over. J.D. picked up Kathy, his girlfriend of 4 years, and headed for the beach. Five hours and many beers later, they sped home on familiar secondary roads. John negotiated the first part of an S-curve fine, but his reflexes were too slow to manage the second. Overcompensating, he lost control of the car, slamming it up against a tree. Kathy was killed. J.D., age 20, survived, with a moderate TBI (see Case Study 1).

Traumatic brain injury (TBI) is defined by the Brain Injury Association of America (1) as "an insult to the brain, not of degenerative or congenital nature caused by an external physical force that may produce a diminished or altered state of consciousness, which results in impairment of cognitive abilities or physical functions. It can also result in the disturbance of behavioral or emotional functioning."

TBI involves a complex matrix of physical, cognitive, and neurobehavioral changes that may have a lifetime effect on a person's ability to participate in occupations. Many functions are compromised, including the ability to produce coordinated movement, speak, remember, reason, and alter behavior (2). The combination of these changes makes the total disability far greater than any single deficit (3). The extent of the disability is identified within 48 hours of medical evaluation, and is based on the length of amnesia and/or **coma** and ratings using the Glasgow Coma Scale (GCS), which will be discussed in the prognosis section. The following definitions will be used throughout this chapter:

Mild TBI: clinically identified as a loss of consciousness <10 minutes, or amnesia, GCS rating of 13 to 15, no skull fracture on physical examination, and a nonfocal neurological examination (4).

Moderate TBI: hospitalization of at least 48 hours, an initial GCS rating of 9 to 12 or higher (5).

Severe TBI: loss of consciousness and/or posttraumatic amnesia greater than 24 hours, and a GCS rating of 1 to 8 (5).

Etiology

Primary brain damage, which may be focal or diffuse, is created by acceleration, deceleration and rotation, or the possible intrusion of a penetrating object. Focal lesions are limited in scope and are associated with direct impact of short duration such as occurs with a bullet or knife. Diffuse lesions occur throughout multiple brain areas. Diffuse axonal injuries (DAIs) occur as a result of collisions with the head at a velocity of approximately 15 miles per hour or greater (6). DAI therefore can occur with high-speed running collisions with others, as in football, soccer, or hockey, as well as, with motor vehicle accidents. Motor vehicle accidents typically occur at high speeds and result in both coup and contrecoup injuries. With these injuries, direct damage is incurred as the cerebrum rotates on the more stable brainstem while accelerating from the force of impact. The cerebrum strikes the skull (coup), then reaccelerates in the opposite direction to strike the skull at a distant location (contrecoup). This continues until the force of impact has been absorbed (7,8). The mechanism for DAI is stretching and shearing of brain cell axons, and is associated with immediate coma following brain injury. Injury to the tracts leading from the hypothalamus and/or pituitary stalk result in medical complications of hormonal changes, disorders of salt and water metabolism, altered temperature regulation, and dysfunctional control of satiety (6). Structures sensitive to diffuse axonal injury include the parasagittal white matter of the cerebral cortex, corpus callosum, brainstem, and the cerebellum (6–8). Common cognitive deficits associated with these structures include difficulty with memory for new information, a decreased ability to process information and limited **executive functions** (6).

Secondary damage occurs shortly after impact and is mainly a result of limited oxygenation of the brain or DAI. Factors causing secondary damage include increased intracranial pressure, ischemia or cerebral hypoxia, and intracranial hemorrhage. Increased intracranial pressure results in swelling, which cannot be accommodated within the rigid structure of the skull. Swelling, in turn, may lead to herniation of brain tissue (9). Ischemia occurs when blood vessels rupture and can no longer provide sufficient blood to the brain. Intracranial hemorrhage is an additional source of hypoxia, leading to cell death within minutes after injury. Physiologic changes from DAI, already discussed, include hyperthermia, electrolyte disturbances, hyperventilation, and abnormal responses of the autonomic nervous system (6,9).

Medical complications are frequent and impair recovery following TBI. Following a high-impact TBI, such as occurs with a motor vehicle accident, 70% of victims have single or multiple seizures (10), **hydrocephalus** (11), extremity injuries including lacerations and fractures (12), and/or cardiovascular complications (13). Respiratory function is often impaired, requiring nasal intubation or tracheostomy, and pneumonia may occur. Neurogenic bowel and bladder disorders require catheterization and close monitoring. Deeply comatose patients must be repositioned routinely to avoid the development of decubiti.

Incidence and Prevalence

An estimated 5.3 million Americans, or 2% of the U.S. population, live with a TBI-related disability, and approximately 1.5 million U.S. residents sustain a TBI in the United States each year (14). Of these, about 50,000 will die, 230,000 will be hospitalized, and between 80,000 and 90,000 persons will experience lifetime disability. Age, gender, environment, and ethnicity affect this incidence rate. At greatest risk are young men between the ages of 15 and 24, a group that is twice as likely as women to sustain a head injury (15). Other age groups that show an increased incidence of traumatic brain injury include adults older than 75 years and children below the age of five (15). Inner-city environments have high incidence rates (16), with persons of African American ethnicity having the highest death rates from TBI of all races (17,18).

The three leading causes of TBI are vehicular crashes, violence, and falls. Vehicular crashes are still the leading cause of TBI for survivors. Persons involved in vehicle-related accidents tend to be both male and female adults, white, and employed. Among children involved in vehicular crashes resulting in moderate to severe injury, half were unrestrained at the time of the accident (19). In the United States, survivors of violence, the second major cause of TBI, are more likely to have a racial heritage other than white, to be unemployed, and to have been arrested previously (20,21). Falls caused the greatest number of TBI deaths among elderly persons and children younger than age 5 (17).

Severity of injury is related to cause. Approximately 90% of firearm TBIs result in death, of which two thirds may be suicidal in intent (15). Surviving vehicle crash victims tend to be injured more severely than survivors of either falls or violence, and to have additional injuries such as long-bone fractures and plexopathies; falls are more often associated with mild injury. Intoxication, which is present in one third to one half of individuals at the time of injury (22) is significantly negatively correlated with outcome. Persons who were intoxicated when injured tend to be hospitalized longer and have greater severity of injury, greater incidence of death, and a lower cognitive status at the time of discharge, as well as greater periods of posttraumatic amnesia (23). When all head injuries are considered, approximately 75% result in mild injury, 20% in moderate or severe injury, and 5% are fatal (24).

The costs of TBI, both individually and for society, are staggering. Direct and indirect costs of TBI totaled an estimated $56.5 billion in the United States in 1995 (25). Direct costs for acute medical and rehabilitation services for new cases are over $25 billion annually (26), or more than $117,000 for each person seen in the Traumatic Brain Injury Model Systems (27). The average lifetime cost of health care for each person with severe TBI is between $600,000 and $1,875,000 (28). As only 20% to 50% of TBI survivors are employed (2), an additional $1 billion annually may be incurred due to lost wages, lost income taxes, and increased public assistance (29).

Signs and Symptoms

Level of Consciousness

Brain injury involves associated cerebral and brainstem depression or destruction that, in turn, affects the person's level of consciousness. Mild brain injury may result in a relatively short loss of consciousness, with no or minimal **retrograde amnesia**, or memory of events prior to the trauma. Coma, defined as a nonsleep loss of consciousness associated with unresponsiveness to touch, pain, sound, or movement that lasts for an extended period (30), is typically present following moderate to severe brain injury. During coma, cerebral function is minimal.

Diffuse cerebral hypoxia or extensive cortical damage, with minimal to no impairment of the brainstem, may result in a vegetative state. In this state, the individual's eyes may be open and follow a moving object, and the limbs may move but without apparent purpose. However, there is no response to pain or simple verbal requests, and there is no evidence of cortical function (3). Persons in a vegetative state may live only a short time or for years.

Those who recover from coma typically progress through multiple stages of recovery over a wide range of time from days to months. These stages have been identified in the Rancho Los Amigos Level of Cognitive Functioning Scale (LCFS) (Fig. 12.1). This scale classifies the admitted patient into one of eight levels of cognitive functioning, and has been shown to have good inter-rater and test-retest reliability (31). While this scale does not adequately reflect small changes in recovery, may not accurately place a patient with characteristics of two or more categories, and is less accurate at higher levels, it is the accepted tool for general classification.

Level I of the LCFS is a period of dense unresponsiveness to all external stimuli. In level II, an inconsistent, nonpurposeful and often delayed response to external stimuli is seen. Responses may be gross body movements, vocalizations, or physiologic changes such as sweating. Visual tracking of large objects is present, but the eyes do not appear focused. In level III, or localized response, there is an inconsistent but specific response to a strong stimulus such as pain or a bright object. Vague body awareness may be present, as may be shown in pulling at nasogastric or catheter tubing. At level III, deficits of vision and visual perception, somatosensation, movement, and cognition may become apparent.

Level IV is a highly variable stage, which may last for shorter or longer periods of time for the individual person. In level IV, the confused-agitated level, the person is confused and agitated and primarily responsive to internal stimuli. Behavior is frequently aggressive, explosive, and/or nonpurposeful, with incoherent verbalization. As this behavior is often significantly out of character for the patient, it can be quite upsetting for family and friends. However, the patient has severely limited awareness of these inappropriate behaviors and, similarly, the impact of these behaviors on others. Disorientation to person, place, time, and circumstance is also evident. Attention is severely limited, and is frequently driven by visual stimuli. In the absence of motor deficits, sitting, standing, reaching, and ambulating are possible but do not occur purposefully or consistently on request (32,33).

During Level V, or the confused-inappropriate-nonagitated level, more consistent motor response to requests becomes possible. Agitated and exaggerated behavior may still occur, more frequently in response to external stimuli. An inability to maintain selective attention is present, and frequent redirection is needed for any task completion. Simple social and automatic communication is possible but only for short periods of time. Memory is severely impaired, and initiation is often limited. While the person may be

RANCHO LOS AMIGOS SCALE
AKA level of cognitive functioning scale (LCFS)

___(1) **Level I** - *No response.*
Patient does not respond to external stimuli and appears asleep.

___(2) **Level II** - *Generalized response.*
Patient reacts to external stimuli in nonspecific, inconsistent, and nonpurposeful manner with stereotypic and limited responses.

___(3) **Level III** - *Localized response.*
Patient responds specifically and inconsistently with delays to stimuli, but may follow simple commands for motor action.

___(4) **Level IV** - *Confused, agitated response.*
Patient exhibits bizarre, nonpurposeful, incoherent or inappropriate behaviors, has no short-term recall, attention is short and nonselective.

___(5) **Level V** - *Confused, inappropriate, nonagitated response.*
Patient gives random, fragmented, and nonpurposeful responses to complex or unstructured stimuli - simple commands are followed consistently, memory and selective attention are impaired, and new information is not retained.

___(6) **Level VI** - *Confused, appropriate, response.*
Patient gives context appropriate, goal-directed responses, dependent upon external input for direction. There is carry-over for relearned, but not for new tasks, and recent memory problems persist.

___(7) **Level VII** - *Automatic, appropriate response.*
Patient behaves appropriately in familiar settings, performs daily routines automatically, and shows carry-over for new learning at lower than normal rates. Patient initiates social interactions, but judgment remains impaired.

___(8) **Level VIII** - *Purposeful, appropriate response.*
Patient oriented and responds to the environment but abstract reasoning abilities are decreased relative to premorbid levels.

Figure 12.1 Rancho Los Amigos AKA Level of Cognitive Functioning Scale (LCFS). (From Rehabilitation Institute of Chicago. Brain Injury Team. The Rancho Levels of Cognitive Functioning: A Clinical Case Management Tool. Available online http://lifecenter.ric.org/ Accessed July 4, 2006).

physically able to complete simple self-care and feeding, verbal supervision is needed to accomplish tasks. The use of selected formal or standardized assessments may become possible at level V.

In stages VI through VIII, the injured person becomes increasingly more aware of the external environment and other persons and is able to intentionally plan movement sequences. Responses to request become consistently more appropriate, and the supervision level decreases for previously learned tasks. New learning is still impaired until level VIII (32,33).

Motor Deficits

Damage to the brain stem between the vestibular nuclei and the red nucleus produces **decerebrate rigidity**, defined as an extensor posture of all limbs and/or the trunk. When the brainstem is intact despite severe brain cortical damage, **decorticate rigidity** is present, with flexion of the upper but extension of the lower limbs. Abnormal reflexes complicate movement patterns. During deep coma, brainstem reflexes may result in grimacing to noxious stimuli, which may be accompanied by a change in postural tone in the extremities.

These deficits decline as coma lightens, and motor disturbances reflecting neural damage become apparent. These deficits may include quadriparesis, hemiplegia, or monoplegia, with or without fluctuating muscle tone, as well as disorders of coordination.

Coordination deficits include tremor and ataxia. Tremor types include cerebellar, resting, essential, and physiologic. Cerebellar tremors are associated with ataxia, hypotonia, and balance disorders. They tend to occur in trunk and proximal muscles with intentional movement, at a frequency of approximately 4 to 6 per second. Resting tremors are correlated with striatal damage and involve pill-rolling movement at rest, occurring at a similar rate. Essential tremors affect more distal musculature, occur at a frequency of 8 to 12 per second, and increase with anxiety and maintained positions. Physiologic tremor, commonly seen with aging, occurs at the same rate and is exacerbated by fatigue and stress (34). Posttraumatic ataxia is a result of damage to the sensory, equilibrium, or cerebellar systems and has been shown in 20% to 30% of persons sustaining DAI (34).

Cranial Nerve Dysfunction

As the cranial nerves originate from the brain stem, TBI typically results in damage to both the sensory and motor functions of these nerves. Pupillary reflexes are important early indicators of brain damage. The absence of a pupillary reflex in response to light by an unconscious patient is an indication of damage to the midbrain, from which the oculomotor nerve (III) originates (30). A fixed dilated pupil, indicative of pressure on the oculomotor nerve, is frequently seen following moderate to severe traumatic brain injury (35).

As coma lightens, significant visual deficits typically become apparent, because of damage to the oculomotor (III), trochlear (IV), and abducens (VI) nerves. These deficits include binocular, oculomotor, accommodative, refractive, visual field, lid-movement dysfunction, as well as nystagmus, ptosis, and diplopia (36). Indeed, the composite of diplopia, blurred vision, visual-field loss, decreased oculomotor skills, and seeing movement in the stable external environment has been termed posttrauma vision syndrome (37,38). Double vision has been called the hallmark of visual deficits for persons with TBI, and often results in the individual closing one eye for greater clarity. In addition to sensory deficits, visual perceptual disorders may also occur including unilateral neglect or inattention, spatial relations, and figure-ground disorders. However, perceptual disorders are less often seen than in persons following a stroke.

Loss of the sense of smell occurs in 7% to 20% of the brain-injured population, as a result of damage to the olfactory nerve (cranial nerve I), and is often the only cranial nerve damaged in mild brain injury (37). Anosmia, or the absence of smell, is especially common following frontal or occipital blows, as nerve endings cross through the thin and easily fractured cribriform plate of the ethmoid bone in the nose. Recovery of smell is not universal and often incomplete. A study of persons with TBI by Costanzo and Becker found that only 33% of TBI victims improved in smell function. If recovery occurs, it typically occurs between 6 and 12 months postinjury (37).

The ear is the most commonly damaged sensory organ following TBI (39). Eighty percent to 90% of individuals with TBI who receive a longitudinal fracture of the temporal bone will experience a conductive hearing loss as a result of damage to the vestibulocochlear nerve (VIII). Additional problems with disruption of this nerve include nystagmus, ataxia, and balance deficits.

Damage to the glossopharyngeal (IX) and vagus (X) nerves in the medulla result in an absent or depressed gag reflex and decreased movement of the palate and uvula, making swallowing hazardous and necessitating the initial use of nasogastric or gastrostomy feeding tubes. In a study of swallowing disorders in brain-injured patients, Lazarus and Logemann (40) found that 81% of patients had a delayed or absent swallowing reflex, 50% demonstrated limited tongue control, and 33% had slowed peristalsis. **Aspiration**, or pathologic inhalation of food or mucus into the respiratory tract, was found in one third of all persons with TBI. The presence of aspiration is highly correlated with the development of pneumonia. In later stages of recovery, there may be hypotonia of the oral musculature, resulting in drooling, limited lip closure and tongue control, pocketing of food in the cheek, and a delayed swallow trigger (41,42).

Course and Prognosis

Response to and recovery from TBI tends to be highly individual, despite known neuropathological effects. Even so, identifying early factors that are predictive of recovery has been a major focus of research. Numerous methodological and theoretical problems, however, make the identification of predictive factors difficult (32).

Persons with mild TBI typically report symptoms such as headaches, dizziness, fatigue, visual disturbance, and memory and executive-thinking difficulties during the first week following injury. For most persons, these symptoms resolve over the next 3 months. However, for some individuals, these difficulties persist from 3 months to the lifetime, causing significant distress and disruption of daily activities (43).

Assessing potential outcome for those with moderate and severe TBI is difficult. The GCS was the first scale developed to predict both mortality and outcome for the comatose patient (44,45). The Disability Rating Scale (DRS) (Fig. 12.2) has expanded on this information to provide a quantitative assessment of the disability of patients with severe brain injury. The DRS (Fig. 12.2) includes four categories, arousal, awareness, and responsivity; cognitive abilities for self care activities; dependence on others; and psychosocial adaptability (46). The DRS has demonstrated high inter-rater and test-retest reliability (46,47), as well as concurrent and predictive validity (46,48,49).

Other factors, such as memory loss, age, and intracranial pressure are also associated with outcome. Posttraumatic amnesia of less than 1 day suggests a mild injury, whereas amnesia lasting more than 1 day is indicative of a more severe injury. A younger age at injury improves both the chance of survival and overall outcome. Prolonged increased intracranial pressure is associated with death and severe disability (44,45).

Cognitive and Behavioral Deficits

Cognitive and behavioral problems are among the most common, difficult, and long-lasting consequences of TBI. The effects of cognitive dysfunction are apparent in delayed and inconsistent cognitive function, impairment in routine activities of daily living (ADL), difficulty learning new motor routines, and adapting to new or cognitively challenging situations (50). Retrograde and **anterograde amnesia** inhibit learning and cognitive rehabilitation. Retrograde amnesia, or memory loss prior to the accident, may gradually but incompletely improve. Anterograde amnesia, defined as the inability to learn new long-term declarative information, is typically the last to improve. **Procedural learning**, or the ability to learn new motor, perceptual, or basic cognitive behaviors, often becomes functional during the rehabilitation process despite amnesia and declarative memory loss.

Following initial agitation, confusion, and disorientation, cognitive deficits appear. These may include difficulties with sustained

Patient Name ____________
Rater ____________
Date Completed ____________

Disability rating scale (DRS)

Arousability, awareness, & responsivity

Eye opening
- ❑ 0 Spontaneous
- ❑ 1 To speech
- ❑ 2 To Pain
- ❑ 3 None

Communication ability
- ❑ 0 Oriented
- ❑ 1 Confused
- ❑ 2 Inappropriate
- ❑ 3 Incomprehensible
- ❑ 4 None

Motor response
- ❑ 0 Obeying
- ❑ 1 Localizing
- ❑ 2 Withdrawing
- ❑ 3 Flexing
- ❑ 4 Extending
- ❑ 5 None

Cognitive ability for self care activites
Knows how and when to feed, toilet or groom self

Feeding
- ❑ 0.0 Complete
- ❑ 0.5
- ❑ 1.0 Partial
- ❑ 1.5
- ❑ 2.0 Minimal
- ❑ 2.5
- ❑ 3.0 None

Toileting
- ❑ 0.0 Complete
- ❑ 0.5
- ❑ 1.0 Partial
- ❑ 1.5
- ❑ 2.0 Minimal
- ❑ 2.5
- ❑ 3.0 None

Grooming
- ❑ 0.0 Complete
- ❑ 0.5
- ❑ 1.0 Partial
- ❑ 1.5
- ❑ 2.0 Minimal
- ❑ 2.5
- ❑ 3.0 None

Dependence on others
Level of functioning
Physical & cognitive disability
- ❑ 0.0 Completely independent
- ❑ 0.5
- ❑ 1.0 Independent in special environment
- ❑ 1.5
- ❑ 2.0 Mildly dependent-limited assistance
  Non-resident helper
- ❑ 2.5
- ❑ 3.0 Moderately dependent-moderate assist
  Person in home
- ❑ 3.5
- ❑ 4.0 Markedly dependent
  Assistance with all major activities, all times
- ❑ 4.5
- ❑ 5.0 Totally dependent
  24 hour nursing care

Psychosocial adaptability
Employability
As full time worker, homemaker, student
- ❑ 0.0 Not restricted
- ❑ 0.5
- ❑ 1.0 Selected jobs, competitive
- ❑ 1.5
- ❑ 2.0 Sheltered workshop, noncompet.
- ❑ 2.5
- ❑ 3.0 Not employable

Total score (sum all scores) ____________

Figure 12.2 Disability Rating Scale (DRS). (From Rappaport M, Hall KM, Hopkins HK, et al. Disability rating scale for severe head trauma: Coma to community. Arch Phys Med Rehabil 1982; 63:118–123).

attention, concentration, memory, comprehension, reasoning, self-monitoring and impulse control, self- and other-awareness and executive function. Executive functions involve the ability to formulate context-appropriate goals and to initiate, plan and organize, sequence, and adapt behavior based on anticipated or actual consequences of actions (51).

Maladaptive behaviors occur as a result of cognitive deficits interacting with neuroanatomic and neurochemical dysfunction. These deficits are typically seen whether the TBI is mild, moderate, or severe (51) and include impulsivity, perseveration, irritability and poor control of temper, and social disinhibition. Limited self-awareness or a lack of insight may slow rehabilitation progress, as well as the ability to participate successfully in academic, vocational, or social roles. Despite a common lack of awareness, TBI survivors are at greater risk for suicide; suicide rates vary between 2.7 and 4.1 times that of the general population when matched for age and sex (52,53).

Medical/Surgical Management

The focus of medical management in the acute phase is preservation of life and the prevention of secondary damage. Maintaining an effective airway and circulatory function are critical life-preservation steps immediately after injury. An endotracheal tube may be placed to support breathing. After arrival at the hospital, diagnostic tests are begun to identify the location and severity of all injuries. The patient typically receives a computerized axial tomography scan (CAT). If this reveals an intracranial hematoma, immediate surgical decompression is performed. Constant monitoring of consciousness occurs, as the duration and depth of coma are significant indicators of both mortality and morbidity (54).

Physicians from neurology, neurosurgery, internal medicine, or orthopedics may direct overall medical management in the acute phase. More than 50% of persons with severe head injury have associated injuries. Hydrocephalus, or the abnormal accumulation of cerebrospinal fluid in the brain, is a serious complication for up to 75% of individuals with TBI. Fractures are common as well, as 82% of those with TBI have one or more extracranial fractures, with 10% of these cervical spinal cord injuries. In the latter case, medical management is therefore needed for both a brain injury and a high-level spinal cord injury (55,56). As a result of rigid abnormal posturing and other motor disturbances, up to 84% of those with TBI develop contractures of the neck, trunk, and extremities. The longer the duration of coma, the greater is the potential for the development of contractures. About one third of those hospitalized with TBI aspirate food into their lungs, resulting in aspiration pneumonia. These persons usually have a delayed or absent swallowing reflex (55,56).

Intensive care medical management is constant. An indwelling urinary catheter is placed and closely monitored. A nasogastric tube is positioned and used for high caloric feeding. Close attention to skin integrity is essential, and the person's total body position is changed frequently. Daily passive range of motion helps prevent contractures. Suctioning of the endotracheal tube and vigorous respiratory therapy helps prevent additional pulmonary problems. Monitoring of the level of consciousness occurs frequently (54). Rehabilitation in the intensive care unit may begin as soon as neurological stability is achieved. The focus of early rehabilitation is graded and specific sensory stimulation, with the assumption that selective sensory input may speed or improve neurological recovery.

Medications used with the person with TBI must be carefully selected and monitored because of potential adverse side effects. Categories of frequently prescribed medications include anticonvulsants and antispasticity medications. Phenytoin and phenobarbital are traditional drugs used as anticonvulsants, but may cause adverse cognitive side effects. Phenytoin has now been shown to be successful in preventing early but not late posttraumatic seizures, and is typically withdrawn within a few weeks of injury under most circumstances (57). Newer anticonvulsant drugs are now available, including levetiracetam, tiagabine, oxcarbamazepine, zonisamide, and lamotrigine, but these can all be sedating (58–60).

In addition levetiracetam has been found to cause irritability and hostility (60).

Antispasticity medications have traditionally included diazepam and phenytoin, again with sedating side effects. Newer medications include the use of phenol blocks, botulinum toxin, and baclofen, all of which act peripherally and not centrally. Phenol results in permanent chemical denervation of the sensory roots. Botulinum toxin was introduced in the 1980s, and acts by temporarily blocking the release of acetylcholine at the neuromuscular junction. The duration of effect is typically 2 to 4 months, and there are few side effects (59). Intrathecal baclofen pumps have been used to treat spasticity of central origin since the 1990s (59). Baclofen also has few side effects. A surgical procedure is required to place the pump, and the pump must be reliably refilled to avoid a life-threatening syndrome. As a result, use of the baclofen pump is often not considered until at least 1 year after injury (61).

Animal and still-limited human studies suggest that recovery following focal brain injury may be modulated by the use of medications affecting specific neurotransmitters, and thereby improving the outcome for persons with TBI. One such drug is amphetamine. In a study of five placebo-treated and five amphetamine-treated persons following stroke, it was found that those treated with amphetamine coupled with a session of focused physical therapy showed significant improvements in motor scores as compared to persons treated with a placebo (62). Levodopa, which mediates central norepinephrine levels, has also been shown to improve motor function (63). Both amphetamine and levodopa have been shown to be effective in small groups of patients with severe TBI (63). However, additional research needs to be completed before clinical effectiveness can be established.

Medical stability, cognitive level, and the ability to benefit from intensive rehabilitation are used to identify the appropriate time for transfer to the rehabilitation phase (54). Intensive rehabilitation is usually directed by a **physiatrist**, a physician specializing in rehabilitation medicine. Goals of the rehabilitation program are to restore the person to an optimal level of functioning in all areas, and to minimize additional physical or psychosocial disability (54). Along with the primary physician, core rehabilitation members include specialists in occupational therapy, physical therapy, speech and language pathology, nursing, neuropsychology, and social work. The long-term rehabilitation goals in occupational therapy are to reestablish occupational performance skill, sensorimotor integration and control, and the integration of perceptual, cognitive, and communication skills with daily tasks. Where remediation is not possible or when maximal neurological recovery can be assumed to occurred, the use of compensation strategies may be appropriate. As basic goals are accomplished, discharge from the hospital may occur, with more advanced skills learned on an outpatient basis. Outpatient occupational therapy goals include instrumental activities of daily living, community reintegration and work re-entry.

Impact of Conditions on Client Factors

All areas identified in the Occupational Therapy Practice Framework are affected with TBI. The deeply comatose person, with cognitive levels I through III, shows depressed function in all occupations. With further recovery improvement in performance skills and patterns, as well as in client factors, may occur and enable the performance of preferred or required occupations. In a study of 1,170 records from the Traumatic Brain Injury Model Systems database, Bushnik et al. (21) found that individuals with TBI as a result of a vehicular accident were initially admitted with significantly lower functional independence measure motor scores than those who were admitted because of violence, falls, or other causes. However, at discharge from rehabilitation, no significant differences were found among patients in the four etiology groups for most psychosocial and functional outcome measures. In fact, 85% to 96% of all patients demonstrated sufficient basic ADL skills to live in a private residence upon discharge.

Employment is a significant and strong contributor to improved quality of life for individuals with TBI (64,65). However, most persons have major difficulties returning to work after injury whether the injury is mild or severe. Ruffolo et al. (66) reported that while 42% of people with mild brain injury returned to work, only 12% returned to their premorbid level of employment. Cognitive and behavioral issues were cited for this decreased function. For those with moderate to severe injuries, the ability to return to work has been correlated with a lesser severity of injury, prior work experience, younger age, greater education, higher socioeconomic status, and handicap, defined as physical, cognitive, or emotional dependence on others (2,67). Additionally, psychosocial skills that affect social integration show a stronger correlation with successful return to work than either cognitive or sensorimotor skills, or any combination of the three factors (68). Bushnik et al. (21) found the unemployment rate for persons with TBI because of violence to be 70%, significantly greater than the rate of approximately 50% for those with TBI from all other causes. The DRS has been found to predict employment. In a study of 145 persons with TBI, Cope et al. (69) found that 62% of those with scores of 1 to 3 on rehabilitation admission were employed or in school at 1 year after discharge, while 39% of those with scores of 4 to 6 and only 11% of those with a DRS score of 7 to 20 were similarly employed. For those returning to work, supported part-time employment has been shown to be a viable and cost-effective option (2). However, limited employment opportunities with typically lower wages and decreased work hours often result in the need for public assistance (2,29).

Brain damage also can compromise the ability to drive. Physical disabilities, as well as cognitive and visual or perceptual deficits, can significantly impair driving function. Additionally, limited awareness of these deficits can make driving a potentially hazardous occupation. Despite these problems, 40% to 60% of TBI survivors resume driving after hospitalization (70,71), with the likelihood of driving inversely correlated with the severity of the injury. Driving is frequently more limited in frequency and distance compared to pre-injury (70). Persons more likely to return to driving include those discharged from rehabilitation with independence or modified independence in most ADL.

CASE STUDY

Case Illustrations

■ CASE 1

J.D., age 20, survived an automobile accident with a moderate TBI. After 2 weeks each in intensive care and an acute medical unit, he is to begin intensive rehabilitation. His occupational therapist cannot get reliable information from him, so she relies on a medical record review for his medical history and a discussion with his mother to identify his previous occupations.

His mother does not seem to be very aware of his activities. She states that he has had three jobs as a garage mechanic in the last 2 years. She says he seemed to get tired of routine and did not get along well with his bosses. He moved into her two-bedroom apartment about 6 months ago so he could start saving money for a new car. He does not participate in any home-care tasks but does help with the rent. Leisure activities included fixing up his old car and "hot-rodding" around. J.D.'s mother does not care for many of his friends, but becomes tearful when asked about his relationship with Kathy. She says they were planning to be married in the fall.

The medical record review reveals that J.D. sustained a right tibia-fibula fracture with the TBI. After 3 days of general unresponsiveness, he began to obey simple commands (LCFS level III). In a few days, he became agitated and confused. A few words could be understood, including swear words. He persistently pulled out both his urinary catheter and his nasogastric tube.

The agitation has lessened somewhat, but he continues to be intermittently disoriented, as when he calls his occupational therapist "Kathy." There is a 1- to 2-second delay before any requested movement. His gaze appears divergent, and he performs best when closing one eye. When fatigued or perhaps frustrated, he is irritable and the therapist has used protective measures she was taught to both protect herself and J.D. from injury as he jabs his fist out toward her.

Motor deficits include poor sitting balance and right hemiplegia, with moderate to severe spasticity. The left upper extremity is within functional limits in range of motion and strength. Transfers require moderate assistance.

J.D. is independent in eating but requires assistance for all other tasks. He requires moderate assistance and verbal cuing for showering using a shower chair, donning and removing a T-shirt, and transferring to and from the bed and wheelchair. Wheelchair mobility is slow but he can wheel himself from one area to another with verbal cuing for the route. J.D. is unable to read, and perseveration is apparent when writing his name. J.D. has come a long way, but there is still a longer way to go to achieve maximal possible independence.

■ CASE 2

Carol's family had the misfortune of being in the wrong place at the wrong time. Returning late one night, tanned and happy from 2 weeks at the lake, her husband could not avoid the oncoming car that went through a red light and sideswiped them. While her husband and two small children received mild injuries, Carol was hurt most of all as she had been sitting where the greatest damage to the car occurred.

At the hospital, she was initially able to respond to simple motor requests, then became unresponsive during the third hour after injury. After surgical intervention for increased intracranial pressure, she regained awareness and progressed to RLA level IV within 2 weeks, at which time intensive rehabilitation began.

Surprisingly, Carol had no broken bones and her sensorimotor status improved rapidly. By the time of discharge from the hospital, she was walking independently in a slow but stable manner. Her primary physical problems were decreased right upper extremity coordination and limited endurance. Cognitively, she had difficulty with organization, sequencing, and task initiation. She did not anticipate any problems in resuming her roles as wife, mother, and homemaker. She did not think she could return to being a secretary just yet.

At the time of admission to an outpatient rehabilitation program, Carol had deficits in a number of occupations. Keyboard use was slow, at 20 words per minute, with many spelling errors, and limited to approximately 10 minutes before she complained of eyestrain. Carol was not bothered by these problems, as she stated she did not plan to return to work.

She is neat and clean in appearance at all times. However, her clothes are all tight-fitting, as she gained 25 pounds during her rehabilitation stay despite being put on a strict diet. She has always been proud of her clean home but now does not clean it thoroughly. When pressed, she admitted that she has trouble organizing her day to accomplish all the tasks she did previously. Many tasks have been assumed by other family members. She is able to prepare simple meals, but the family has learned that she is often unable to read her recipe cards correctly, instead substituting whatever she finds in the cupboard. Her memory problems have made stove use hazardous.

Carol was outgoing, assertive, and pleasant before her injury. At present she seems content to stay at home. She expresses no interest in going out with the family or resuming any of her previous activities. When she is not asked to participate in a task, she frequently watches television, although she often can't say what the program is about. Conversation is limited. She seldom initiates conversation other than basic social remarks. When she speaks, it is usually about herself, and she seldom asks about others. Occasionally, the noise created by two healthy children and their friends bothers her, and she becomes unexpectedly angry. Her children now spend more time at their friends' homes than previously. Carol recognizes that she is different and blames her change on her memory and vision problems. Although she cannot identify just how she is different, she does recognize those differences when they are pointed out. She would like to "get better."

Case Study Comments

J.D. and Carol represent one person at one point in the continuum of recovery, with individual backgrounds, unique mechanisms of injury, and specific factors affecting recovery. The occupational therapist working with persons with brain injury must first identify and evaluate the many occupations and performance skills, and patterns affected by the injury. Goals must be established either to remediate or maintain occupations or performance areas, or to compensate for lost skills.

References

1. Brain Injury Association of America. Facts about brain injury. August 2005. Available at: http://www.biausa.org/aboutbi.htm. Accessed July 4, 2006.
2. Wehman P, Kregel J, Keyser-Marcus L, et al. Supported employment for persons with traumatic brain injury: a preliminary investigation of long-term follow-up costs and program efficiency. Arch Phys Med Rehabil 2003;84:192–196.
3. Jennett B, Bond M. Assessment of outcome after severe brain damage. Lancet 1975;1:480–484.
4. Bazarian JJ, McClung J, Shah MN, et al. Mild traumatic brain injury in the United States, 1998–2000. Brain Injury 2005;19:85–91.
5. Dawodu ST. Traumatic Brain Injury: Definition, Epidemiology, Pathophysiology. eMedicine: eMedicine.com, Inc., 2005. Available at: http://www.emedicine.com/pmr/topic212.htm. Accessed July 4, 2006.
6. Meythaler JM, Peduzzi JD, Eleftheriou E, et al. Current concepts: Diffuse axonal injury—associated traumatic brain injury. Arch Phys Med Rehabil 2001;82:1461–1471.
7. Adams JH, Graham DI, Murray LS, et al. Diffuse axonal injury due to non-missile head injury in humans. An analysis of 45 cases. Ann Neurol 1982;12: (6):557–563.
8. Strich SJ. Lesions in the cerebral hemispheres after blunt head injury. J Clin Pathol 1970;23:154.
9. Jennett B. Scale and scope of the problem. In: Rosenthal M, Griffith, ER, Bond, MR, et al, ed. Rehabilitation of the adult and child with traumatic brain injury. 2nd Ed. Philadelphia: F.A. Davis, 1990:59–74.
10. Jennett B. Posttraumatic epilepsy. In: Rosenthal M, Griffith ER, eds. Rehabilitation of the head-injured adult. Philadelphia: F.A. Davis, 1983.
11. Beyerl B, Black PM. Posttraumatic hydrocephalus. Neurosurgery 1984;15:257–261.
12. Rimel RM, Jane JA. Characteristics of the head injured patient. In: Rosenthal M, Griffith ER, eds.

Rehabilitation of the head injured adult. Philadelphia: F.A. Davis, 1983.
13. Bontke CF. Medical complications related to traumatic brain injury. In: Horn LJ, Cope DN, eds. Physical Medicine and Rehabilitation: State of the Art Reviews. Traumatic Brain Injury. Philadelphia: Hanley & Belfus, 1989:43–58.
14. National Center for Injury Prevention and Control. Centers for Disease Control and Prevention (CDC). The injury fact book 2001–2002. July 2002. Available at http://www.cdc.gov/ncipc/fact_book/01_Preface.htm Accessed July 4, 2006.
15. Centers for Disease Control and Prevention. Traumatic Brain Injury in the United States—A Report to Congress. Atlanta, GA, 1999. Available at http://www.cdc.gov/ncipc/tbi/tbi_congress/index.htm Accessed July 4, 2006.
16. Bruns JJ. The epidemiology of traumatic brain injury: a review. Epilepsia 2003;44:2–10.
17. Centers for Disease Control and Prevention (CDC). Traumatic brain injury in the United States: A report to congress. 2001. Available at http://www.cdc.gov/ncipc/tbi/tbi_congress/index.htm Accessed July 4, 2006.
18. Whitman S, Coonley-Hoganson RT. Comparative head trauma experiences in two socioeconomically different area communities: Chicago—a population study. Am J Epidemiol 1984;119:570–580.
19. Department of Transportation. National Highway Traffic Safety Administration (NHTSA). Traffic safety facts 2006. Available at http://www.nhtsa.gov/portal/site/Accessed July 4, 2006.
20. Bogner JA, Corrigan JD, Mysiw J, et al. A comparison of substance abuse and violence in the prediction of long-term rehabilitation outcomes after traumatic brain injury. Arch Phys Med Rehabil 2001;82:571–577.
21. Bushnik T, Hanks RA, Kreutzer J, et al. Etiology of traumatic brain injury: Characterization of differential outcomes up to 1 year postinjury. Arch Phys Med Rehabil 2003;84:255–262.
22. Corrigan JD. Substance abuse as a mediating factor in outcome from traumatic brain injury. Arch Phys Med Rehabil 1995;76:302–309.
23. Gordon WA, Mann N, Willer B. Demographic and social characteristics of the traumatic brain injury model system database. J Head Trauma Rehabil 1993;8:26–33.
24. Sosin DM, Sniezek JE, Thurman DJ. Incidence of mild and moderate brain injury in the United States, 1991. Brain Injury 1996;10:47–54.
25. Thurman D. The epidemiology and economics of head trauma. In: Miller L, Hayes R, eds. Head trauma: Basic, Preclinical, and Clinical Directions. New York, NY: Wiley & Sons, 2001.
26. Consensus Conference. Rehabilitation of persons with traumatic brain injury. NIH consensus development panel of rehabilitation of persons with traumatic brain injury. JAMA 1999;282:974–983.
27. Lehmkuhl LD, Hall KM, Mann N, et al. Factors that influence costs and length of stay of persons with traumatic brain injury in acute care and inpatient rehabilitation. J Head Trauma Rehabil 1993;8:88–100.
28. National Institutes of Health. Rehabilitation of persons with traumatic brain injury. NIH consensus statement. 1998;16:1–41.
29. Johnstone B, Mount D, Schopp LH. Financial and vocational outcomes 1 year after traumatic brain injury. Arch Phys Med Rehabil 2003;84:238–241.
30. Kandel ER, Schwartz JH, Jessell TM. Principles of neural science. In: Kelly DD, ed. Disorders of sleep and consciousness. Norwalk, CT: Appleton & Lange, 1991:805–819.
31. Gouvier WD, Blanton PD, LaPorte KK, et al. Reliability and validity of the disability rating scale and the levels of cognitive functioning scale in monitoring recovery from severe head injury. Arch Phys Med Rehabil 1987;68:94–97.
32. Sohlberg MM, Mateer CA. Introduction to Cognitive Rehabilitation. Theory and Practice. New York: Guilford Press, 1989.
33. Bushnik T. The Level of Cognitive Functioning Scale. The Center for Outcome Measurement in Brain Injury 2004. Available online at http://www.tbims.org/combi/lcfs Accessed July 4, 2006.
34. Weintraub AH, Opat CA. Motor and sensory dysfunction in the brain-injured adult. In: Horn LJ, Cope DN, eds. Physical Medicine and Rehabilitation: State of the Art Reviews. Traumatic Brain Injury. Philadelphia: Hanley & Belfus, Inc., 1989, 59–84.
35. Pansky B, Allen DJ, Budd GC. Review of Neuroscience. New York: Macmillan Publishing Company, 1988.
36. Freed S, Hellerstein LF. Visual electrodiagnostic findings in mild traumatic brain injury. Brain Injury 1997;11:25–36.
37. Costanzo RM, Becker DP. Smell and taste disorders in head injury and neurosurgery patients. In: Meiselman HL, Rivlin RS, eds. Clinical Measurement of Taste and Smell. New York: Macmillan, 1990:565–578.
38. Padula WV, Argyrio SJR. Visual-evoked potentials (vep) evaluating treatment for post-trauma vision syndrome (PTVS) in patients with traumatic brain injury. Brain Injury 1994;8:125–133.
39. Sakai CS, Mateer CA. Otological and audiological sequelae of closed head trauma. Semin Hear 1984;5:157–173.
40. Lazarus C, Logemann J. Swallowing disorders in closed head trauma patients. Arch Phys Med Rehabil 1987;68:79–84.
41. Logemann JA, Pepe J, Mackay LE. Disorders of nutrition and swallowing: Intervention strategies in the trauma center. J Head Trauma Rehabil 1994;9:43–56.
42. Mackay LE, Morgan AS, Bernstein BA. Swallowing disorders in severe brain injury: Risk factors affecting return to oral intake. Arch Phys Med Rehabil 1999;80:365–371.
43. Ponsford J, Willmott C, Rothwell A, et al. Factors influencing outcome following mild traumatic brain injury in adults. J Int Neuropsychol Soc 2000;6:568–579.

44. Horn LJ, Cope DN. Physical Medicine and Rehabilitation: State of the Art Reviews. Philadelphia: Hanley & Belfus, Inc., 1989.
45. Rosenthal M, Bond MR. Behavioral and psychiatric sequelae. In: Rosenthal M, Griffith ER, Bond MR, eds. Rehabilitation of the adult and child with traumatic brain injury. Philadelphia: F.A. Davis, 1990: 179–192.
46. Rappaport M, Hall KM, Hopkins HK, et al. Disability rating scale for severe head trauma: Coma to community. Arch Phys Med Rehabil 1982;63:118–123.
47. Novack TA, Bergquist TF, Bennett G, et al. Primary caregiver distress following severe head injury. J Head Trauma Rehabil 1992;6:69–77.
48. Hall KM, Cope DN, Rappaport M. Glasgow outcome scale and disability rating scale: Comparative usefulness in following recovery in traumatic head injury. Arch Phys Med Rehabil 1985;66:35–37.
49. Hall KM, Hamilton B, Gordon WA, et al. Characteristics and comparisons of functional assessment indices: Disability rating scale, functional independence measure, and functional assessment measure. J Head Trauma Rehabil 1993;8:60–74.
50. Cicerone KD, Dahlberg C, Kalmar K, et al. Evidence-based cognitive rehabilitation: Recommendations for clinical practice. Arch Phys Med Rehabil 2000;81: 1596–1615.
51. Hawley CA. Behaviour and school performance after head injury. Brain Injury 2004;18:645–659.
52. Engberg AW, Teasdale TW. Psychosocial outcome following traumatic injury in adults: A long-term population-based follow-up. Brain Injury 2004;18: 533–545.
53. Teasdale TW, Engberg AW. Suicide after traumatic brain injury: A population study. J Neurol Neurosurg Psychiatry 2001;71:436–440.
54. Mack A, Horn LJ. Functional prognosis in traumatic brain injury. In: Horn LJ, Cope DN, eds. Physical Medicine and Rehabilitation: State of the Art Reviews. Traumatic Brain Injury. Philadelphia: Hanley & Belfus, Inc., 1989:13–26.
55. Eames P, Haffey WJ, Cope DN. Treatment of behavioral disorders. In: Rosenthal M, Griffith ER, Bond M, et al., eds. Rehabilitation of the adult and child with traumatic brain injury. Philadelphia: F.A. Davis, 1990:410–432.
56. Hanscom DA. Acute management of the multiply injured head trauma patient. J Head Trauma Rehabil 1987;2:1–12.
57. Temkin NR, Dikmen SS, Wilensky AJ, et al. A randomized, double-blind study of phenytoin for the prevention of posttraumic seizures. N Engl J Med 1990;323:497–502.
58. Bergin AM, Connolly M. New antiepileptic drug therapies. Neurol Clin North Am 2002;20:1163–1182.
59. Glenn MB, Wroblewski B. Twenty years of pharmacology. J Head Trauma Rehabil 2005;20:51–61.
60. Hoch DB, Daly L. Anticonvulsants. J Head Trauma Rehabil 2003;18:383–386.
61. Meythaler JM. Intrathecal baclofen for spastic hypertonia in brain injury. J Head Trauma Rehabil 1997;12:87–90.
62. Walker-Batson D, Smith P, Curtis S, et al. Amphetamine paired with physical therapy accelerates motor recovery after stroke-further evidence. Stroke 1995;26:2254–2259.
63. Goldstein LB. Neuropharamacology of tbi-induced plasticity. Brain Injury 2003;17:685–694.
64. O'Neill J, Hibbard MR, Brown M, et al. The effect of employability on quality of life and community integration after traumatic brain injury. J Head Trauma Rehabil 1998;13:68–79.
65. Webb CR, Wrigley M, Yoels W, et al. Explaining quality of life for persons with traumatic brain injuries 2 years after injury. Arch Phys Med Rehabil 1995;76:1113–1119.
66. Ruffolo CF, Friedland JF, Dawson DR, et al. Mild traumatic brain injury from motor vehicle accidents: Factors associated with return to work. Arch Phys Med Rehabil 1999;80:392–398.
67. Wagner AK, Hammond FM, Sasser HC, et al. Return to productive activity after traumatic brain injury: Relationship with measures of disability, handicap and community integration. Arch Phys Med Rehabil 2002;83:107–114.
68. Conti GE. Factors Affecting Return to Work for Persons with Traumatic Brain Injury. Eastern Michigan University, Unpublished thesis. 1992.
69. Cope DN, Cole JR, Hall KM, et al. Brain injury: Analysis of outcome in a post-acute rehabilitation system. Part I: General analysis. Brain Injury 1991;5: 111–125.
70. Fisk GD, Schneider JJ, Novack TA. Driving following traumatic brain injury: Prevalence, exposure, advice and evaluations. Brain Injury 1998;12:683–695.
71. Coleman RD, Rapport LJ, Ergh TC, et al. Predictors of driving outcome after traumatic brain injury. Arch Phys Med Rehabil 2002;83:1415–1422.

Recommended Learning Resources

Consumer and Professional Resources

Brain Injury Association of America Inc.
8201 Greensboro Drive
Suite 611
McLean, VA 22102

FamilyHelpline@biausa.org
Tel: 800–444–6443
Fax: 703–761–0755
www.biausa.org

Brain Trauma Foundation
523 East 72nd Street)8th Floor
New York, NY 10021
www.braintrauma.org
Tel: 212–772–0608
Fax: 212–772–0357

Centers for Disease Control and Prevention
1600 Clifton Rd.
Atlanta, GA 30333
Public Inquiries
Tel: (800) 311–3435
www.cdc.gov

Family Caregiver Alliance
690 Market Street
Suite 600
San Francisco, CA 94104
info@caregiver.org
www.caregiver.org
Tel: 800–445–8106
Fax: 415–434–3508

National Institutes of Health (NIH)
9000 Rockville Pike
Bethesda, Maryland 20892
www.nih.gov

National Rehabilitation Information Center (NARIC)
4200 Forbes Boulevard
Suite 202
Lanham, MD 20706
naricinfo@heitechservices.com
www.naric.com
Tel: 301–459–5900
Fax: 301–562–2401
www.tbims.org
www-nrd.nhtsa.dot.gov

Suggested Readings

Umphred DA. Neurological Rehabilitation. 4th Ed. St. Louis: Mosby, Inc., 2001.

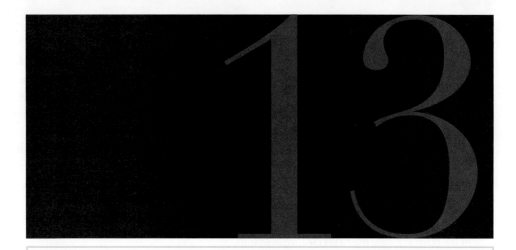

Burns

Elizabeth L. Phillips

Key Terms

Allograft	Compression garment	Full-thickness burn
Autograft	Debridement	Hypertrophic scar
Burn scar contracture	Eschar	Superficial burn
Collagen	Fluid Resuscitation	Partial-thickness burn

Sam, age 15, is scheduled for a burn dressing change at the outpatient burn clinic. Sam suffered 46% mixed partial and **full-thickness burns** to his face, neck, chest, and bilateral arms 4 months ago when he added gasoline to a brush fire. The resulting explosion set Sam's clothes on fire. Sam panicked and started running. A neighbor who heard the explosion from inside his house tackled Sam and smothered the flames with a blanket. Sam spent 2 months as an in-patient on the burn unit where he received extensive grafting to his face, neck, arms, and chest. He was discharged 2 months ago but continues to have scattered small open areas. Sam arrives at the clinic, accompanied by his mother, and immediately requests assistance to remove his coat. When he is asked to try to remove his coat himself, he is able to complete the task but is noted to have extremely limited range of motion (ROM) and severe bilateral axillary contractures. It is noted that both his clothing and temporary **compression garment** have been cut apart at the arms and shoulder and duct-taped together. When asked why this was done he replies that it is easier to remove his clothes this way. His mother states, "I told him he shouldn't do that."

Incidence/Etiology

The third leading cause of accidental death in the United States is burn trauma (1). Each year approximately 2 million Americans seek treatment for burn injuries, over 100,000 are hospitalized and more than 5,000 die (2). Advancements in the treatment of burn injuries, such as early excision and skin grafting, improved antibiotic treatment and the use of cultured epithelium, have decreased morbidity and mortality rates. Factors that increase the risk of death following a burn injury include increasing burn size, age of patient, and the presence of an inhalation (pulmonary) injury (3).

Burn injuries can result from a variety of mechanisms. Types of burns that have been identified include scald (hot liquid), flame or flash (from explosion), contact (with hot or cold surface), radiation, chemical, and electrical (2). Awareness of potential mechanisms for burn injury can focus prevention education to assist individuals and families in decreasing their risk. Actions such as having a smoke detector, placing covers on electrical outlets, turning pot handles toward the back of the stove, and turning the temperature down on hot water heaters to 130°F degrees can greatly decrease the risk for burn injuries in children and adults (1).

Anatomy and Physiology of the Skin

The skin is the largest organ of the body (4). The thin nonvascular outer layer, called the epidermis, consists of layers of epithelial cells. Beneath the epidermis is the thicker dermis, which makes up the bulk of the skin. Housed within the dermis are hair follicles, blood vessels, sweat glands, nerve ending, and sebaceous glands, which play an integral part in the functions

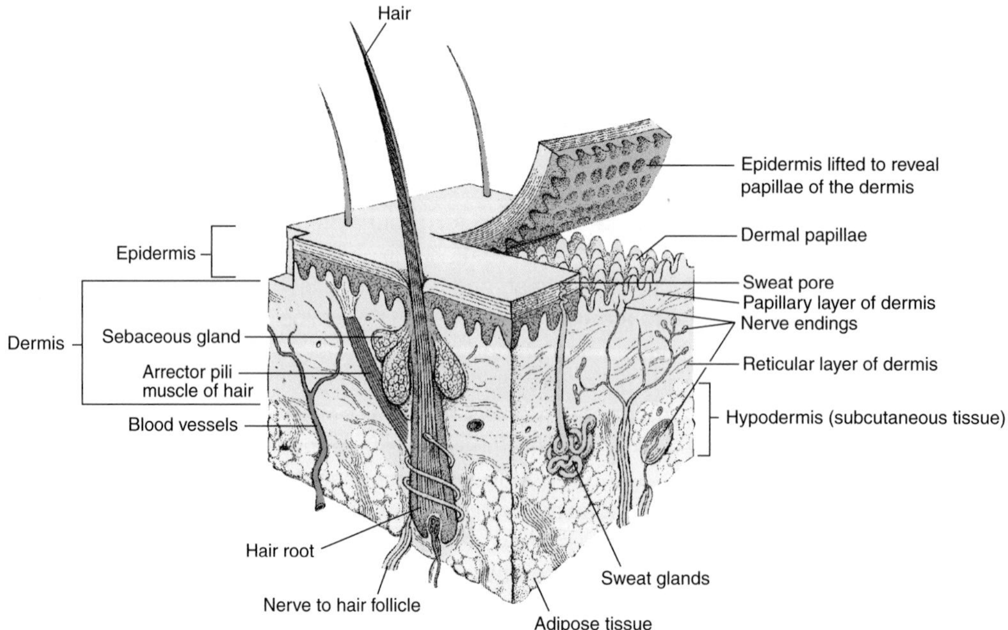

Figure 13.1 Structure and components of the skin. (Adapted from Stedman's Medical Dictionary. 27th Ed. Baltimore: Lippincott Williams & Wilkins 2000.)

of the skin (Fig. 13.1). The functions of the skin include (5):

- Protection against infection
- Prevention loss of body fluid
- Control of body temperature
- Functioning as an excretory organ
- Production of Vitamin D
- Helping to determine personal identity

Pathophysiology of Burns

The two primary factors that influence the amount of tissue destruction that occurs following a burn injury are temperature and duration of exposure (5). The tissue damage that occurs following a burn injury can be divided into three zones. The zone of coagulation is the area of irreversible tissue destruction. Surrounding this is the zone of stasis, where damage results in decreased perfusion. The outer zone is referred to as the zone of hyperemia (6). The tissues in these outer zones are damaged and considered at risk but with proper care should recover and heal. Without proper care of these at risk tissues, further damage will result and increased tissue loss can occur (5). The aim of care after a burn injury is to reduce or prevent dermal ischemia, therefore avoiding further tissue death. The residual necrotic layers of skin destroyed by direct heat damage or the injury occurring secondary to heat damage is referred to as **eschar** (7).

Depth of Burn

The depth of a burn injury reflects how deep into the skin layers a burn extends and influences survival rates, healing time, treatment, and scar formation. The depth of the burn wound is not always clear on admission and burn depth is often underestimated at initial examination (8). The old terminology used to categorize burn depth; first degree, second degree, and third degree have been replaced by the terms, superficial, superficial partial thickness versus deep partial thickness, and full thickness.

Superficial Burn Injury

A **superficial burn** injury involves only the epidermal layers of the skin (5). This burn is characterized by redness and pain. The wound is dry and does not form blisters. The wound blanches readily and is exquisitely sensitive to air and/or light touch. A superficial burn injury can result from a variety of causes such as a sunburn or flash from an explosion. This wound will generally heal within 3 to 6 days and does not produce any residual scarring (1).

Partial Thickness Burn Injury (Superficial versus Deep)

A partial-thickness injury destroys the epidermal layer and extends down into the dermal layer of the skin. Some portion of the dermis remains in a partial-thickness injury, which allows this wound to eventually regenerate skin cells (5). The differentiation between superficial partial-thickness and deep partial-thickness is dependent upon how deep the burn extends into the dermal layer. A **partial-thickness burn** is characterized by large thick-walled blisters, which will increase in size, and is a deep red to waxy white in color. This wound leaks body fluid, is moist to the touch and blanches readily. The wound is soft and elastic in texture and is sensitive to pressure. This wound will generally heal in 7 to 20 days if it is properly managed (1). This wound does leave a residual scar, which ranges from pigment changes in superficial partial thickness to hypertrophy and the potential for contracture formation in deep partial thickness (5).

Full-Thickness Burn Injury

A full-thickness burn injury destroys the entire epidermal and dermal layers of the skin and extends down into subcutaneous fat. Because both layers of the skin are destroyed this wound will not heal spontaneously. Some very small full-thickness injuries can regenerate from the margins of the wound but this delays healing time and is associated with significant scarring (6). A full-thickness injury may be a variety of colors. The wound can be charred black, cherry red, tan, or pearly white in color. This wound may present with small fragile, thin-walled blisters that break easily and do not increase in size. Overall, the wound is dry and leathery hard in texture (5). Since nerve endings are destroyed, the wound is initially anesthetic but remains sensitive to deep pressure. Because burn wounds often have a mixture of differing depths, pain is never a good indicator of depth of wound. Healing time is dependent upon the availability of donor sites. This wound will leave a residual scar and is at severe risk for contracture formation (1).

Extent of Burn

It is important to accurately estimate the total body surface area (TBSA) involved in the burn injury, as this will guide management. There are two common methods utilized to estimate extent of burn. The Rule of Nine (Fig. 13.2) is a convenient and rapid method that may be effectively used at the scene of accident to estimate extent of burn (5). It divides the body surface into areas, representing 9% or multiples of 9%. This method has limited accuracy when used with children. The Lund and Browder scale (Fig. 13.3) should be used when calculating the extent of burns in children. This scale modifies the percentages of areas according to age thus reflecting the fact that the head and neck of the child make up a greater percentage of the body surface area than does that of an adult (1). In the presence of scattered, spotty burns, one helpful rule of thumb is that the surface of the patient's palm is roughly 1% of their TBSA (5).

Medical Management

Burn injuries require specialized care not available at all hospitals. The American Burn Association has identified criteria (Table 13.1) for burn injuries that should be transferred to a hospital with a designated burn/trauma unit, capable of providing the specialized care required by significant burn injuries (2). A burn injury has the potential to affect all body systems. The two major systems affected are the cardiac and pulmonary systems. Immediately following a burn injury, during the emergency phase of treatment, pulmonary and/or cardiac complications are the most common cause of death.

The most common pulmonary complications that can occur are carbon monoxide poisoning, upper-airway obstruction and restrictive defects. Almost all products release carbon monoxide during combustion. It is an odorless, colorless gas that has a greater affinity for binding hemoglobin than oxygen, thus displacing oxygen and leading to asphyxia (5). Upper airway-obstruction occurs because toxic byproducts of combustion, such as various gases, are released during the burning process and are inhaled. These gases are highly irritating to the respiratory mucosa causing upper-airway edema (9). Restrictive defects can lead to respiratory distress when the presence of a tight, circumferential, restrictive eschar on the chest, neck, or abdomen causes difficulty with inspiration and expiration (8).

It is essential to assess for the presence of respiratory difficulty, as this may indicate pulmonary complications. Signs and symptoms that may indicate the potential for respiratory complications include: the presence of facial

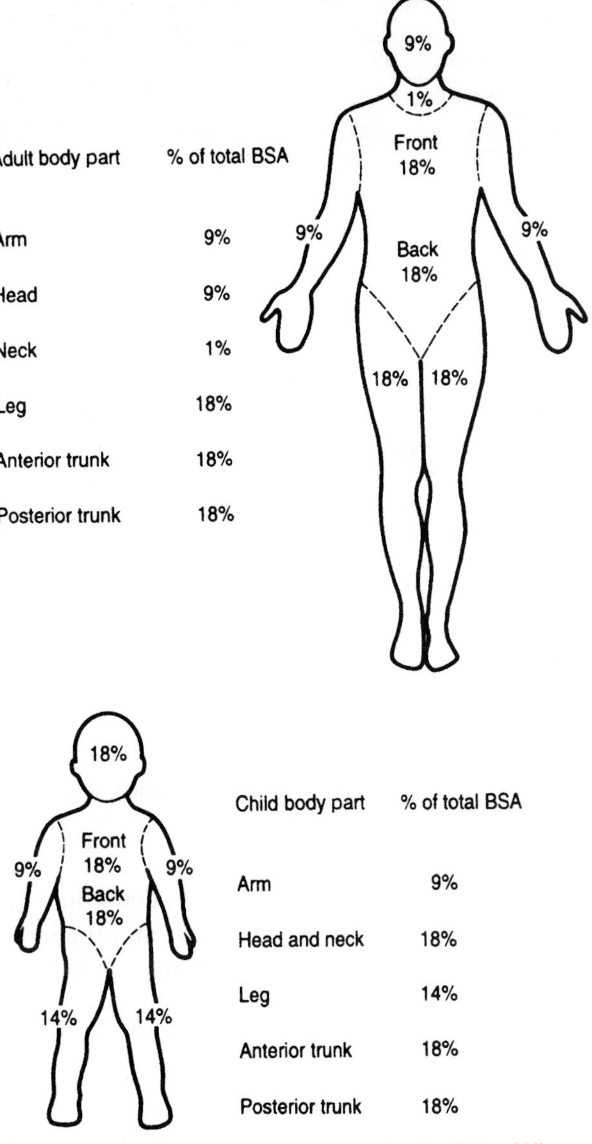

Adult body part	% of total BSA
Arm	9%
Head	9%
Neck	1%
Leg	18%
Anterior trunk	18%
Posterior trunk	18%

Child body part	% of total BSA
Arm	9%
Head and neck	18%
Leg	14%
Anterior trunk	18%
Posterior trunk	18%

Figure 13.2 Estimation of burn size using the Rule of Nines.

burns, singed nasal hair and/or darkened oral mucosa, hoarse voice, cough, drooling, stridor, tachypnea, and hypoxia (9). Those patients whose injuries occurred in an enclosed space, such as a house fire, are at a much greater risk for developing pulmonary complications. Treatment is aimed at maintaining adequate oxygenation through the administration of humidified 100% oxygen by mask. Intubation and ventilator support may be indicated in the presence of severe respiratory obstruction or restrictive defects. In the presence of restrictive eschar on the chest or abdomen, the patient may require escharotomies. Escharotomies are incisions through the eschar down to viable tissue to release the restriction and allow for expansion of the chest wall during inspiration and expiration (8).

The primary cardiac complication that occurs after a burn injury is referred to as

Age	0–1	1–4	5–9	10–14	15
A – ½ of head	9½%	8½%	6½%	5½%	4½%
B – ½ of one thigh	2¾%	3¼%	4%	4¼%	4½%
C – ½ of one leg	2½%	2½%	2¾%	3%	3¼%

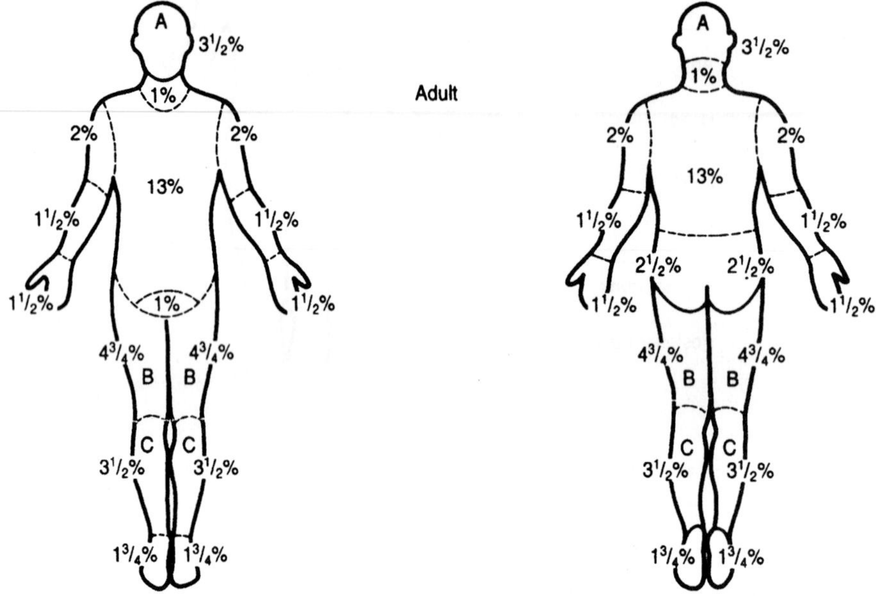

Figure 13.3 Estimation of burn size using the Lund and Browder method. (Reprinted with permission from Hernden D. Total Burn Care. London, WB Saunder; 1996:36)

"burn shock" (9). Unlike other causes of shock the problem is not a loss of blood but rather the fluid or plasma portion of the circulating blood volume. Immediately following a burn injury an increase in capillary permeability allows fluid in the intravascular space to shift into the interstitial space producing burn wound edema. The effect on the cardiovascular system is a marked increase in peripheral vascular resistance accompanied

Table 13.1 AMERICAN BURN ASSOCIATION CRITERIA FOR BURN CENTER REFERRAL

Partial-thickness burns >10% TBSA.
Burns involving face, hands, feet, genitalia, perineum, and major joints.
Full-thickness burns in any age group.
Electrical burns, including lightning.
Chemical burns.
Inhalation injury.
Burn injuries in patients with complicating pre-existing medical conditions.
Burns with concomitant additional trauma in which burn injury poses the greatest risk of morbidity or mortality.
Burned children in hospitals without qualified personnel or equipment.
Burn injury in patients requiring special social, emotional, or long-term intervention.

by a decrease in cardiac output. This shift is greatest in the first eight hours post injury but continues for 24 hours postinjury (8). After the first 24 hours, capillary wall function returns and gradually burn-wound edema will shift back into the intravascular volume and be excreted by the kidneys. In the presence of a burn wound greater than 25%, this fluid shift occurs throughout the body and edema develops in areas that have not been burned (9). In burns less than 25% the fluid shift is usually confined to the burn area.

When hypovolemia from this fluid shift is untreated, shock, organ failure (most commonly renal) and tissue hypoxia occur (2). The treatment for burn shock is **fluid resuscitation**, which is the administration of intravenous fluid. The fluid replacement of choice is crystalloid, or lactated Ringer's solution (9). The goal of fluid resuscitation is to maintain the intravascular volume in sufficient amounts to ensure adequate perfusion and oxygenation to all tissues and organs. Once fluid resuscitation is initiated, burn-wound edema increases. If circumferential burn wounds are present on the extremities; distal areas should be checked frequently for compromised blood supply. If compromised perfusion is detected escharotomies will need to be performed to improve circulation (8).

The Baxter (also called Parkland) formula is commonly utilized to calculate the amount of fluid required (10). This formula calculates fluid requirements based on the patient's weight and TBSA burned. According to the Baxter (Parkland) formula, the patient should receive 4 mL/kilogram body weight/% burn, as a volume of fluid needed for the initial 24-hour fluid resuscitation. One half of this amount is given in the first 8 hours postinjury. The remaining half is given over the next 16 hours. Adequate assessment of the effectiveness of fluid resuscitation is important, as excessive fluids can cause increased burn-wound edema and compromised local blood supply. Inadequate fluid resuscitation can lead to hypovolemia and renal failure. Monitoring hourly urine output is a reliable guide to evaluate the effectiveness of fluid resuscitation. The use of the Baxter (Parkland) formula as a guide to predict fluid requirements has been proven effective but continuous monitoring of the patient is needed to insure adequate treatment of burn shock (10–12).

A large burn injury triggers a significant and prolonged stress response in the body and initiates the release of stress hormones such as catecholamines, prostaglandins, glucagon, and cortisol (13). The release of these hormones initiates and mediates a hypermetabolic response in the body. This hypermetabolic state will result in increased energy catabolism, skeletal muscle catabolism, immune deficiencies, peripheral lipolysis, and reduced bone mineralization and growth. Nutritional support is needed to meet the resulting increase in basal energy expenditure. Most patients cannot consume enough calories through eating and require nutritional support via the enteral route (nasogastric feedings). Early initiation of nutritional support via enteral feedings will help reduce the risk of bacterial translocation from the gut and the development of sepsis (5).

Burn Wound Management

Eschar facilitates bacterial access and acts as the common denominator for burn sepsis. After the emergency phase of burn treatment the patient enters the acute phase. In the acute phase of treatment the most common cause of death is sepsis. Until the burn wound is healed the patient remains vulnerable to invasive infection. **Debridement** is the cleansing and removal of nonadherent and nonviable tissue (14). Daily cleansing and debridement of the burn wound is necessary to decrease the potential for burn-wound sepsis, to facilitate healing and to prepare the wound for grafting if this procedure is needed to achieve wound closure.

Debridement is a painful procedure and it is important to make sure the patient has been premedicated with analgesics and sedative medication prior to starting the dressing change. Commonly used analgesics include morphine, fentanyl, or codeine. A common drug given to sedate the patient is ketamine. Anxiolytics, such as diazepam or midazolam, are drugs given to control anxiety. Anxiety influences pain perception. The use of anxiolytics is beneficial in reducing anticipatory anxiety regarding future dressing changes (13). The use of alternative therapies such as guided imagery, relaxation techniques, and music along with pharmaceuticals may further decrease the pain response during burn-wound dressing changes.

Hydrotherapy (tub bath) is the optimal place for burn-wound cleansing as the jets help loosen nonviable tissue and facilitates ROM exercises. If a patient's condition is unstable, burn-wound dressing changes are done in bed. A mild soap, soft washcloth, tweezers, and scissors are utilized to aid in debridement. To decrease the potential for hypothermia, time in the bath is limited and the temperature of the room should be kept at 82.4°F to 87.8°F (28°C to 31°C) (2). Once the wound has been cleansed, an antimicrobial agent and outer bandages are applied. The burn dressings act as a barrier to the environment, decrease temperature loss through the wound and promote comfort (7). Dressing changes are usually only done once a day. If outer bandages become saturated with drainage, however, it is necessary to replace them with dry outer bandages to prevent the wicking of bacteria down to the surface of the wound.

Topical antimicrobial agents are used to delay and/or minimize burn-wound colonization (13). The topical antimicrobial agent of choice is silver sulfadiazine 1% (Silvadene). Silvadene is a broad-spectrum antimicrobial agent effective against gram-positive and gram-negative bacteria with some antifungal activity. Silvadene does not penetrate burn eschar. It controls bacterial growth only on the surface of the wound, has few side effects and is usually well tolerated by the patient. When there is a need to penetrate the eschar, such as on the ears to prevent chondritis, 10% mafenide (Sulfamylon) is used (14). Sulfamylon is effective against a broad range of microorganisms but does not treat yeasts. This drug may produce metabolic acidosis and application is painful, so the use of Sulfamylon is limited to small areas (13). The use of intravenous antibiotic therapy is reserved for documented wound infections and is not given prophylactically (14).

In full-thickness injuries, the risk of bacterial entrance and fluid/heat loss through the wound continues until the wound is closed either temporarily or permanently through the application of synthetic dressings (Biobrane; Integra) or biological coverage (7). Grafting priorities are influenced by location and size of the burn. If the patient requires long-term intravenous fluid administration, skin grafting may be needed on the chest to allow for insertion of a central line. Hands, because of their functional importance, are given grafting priority. Faces and ears have a dense cross-section of dermal appendages and are given additional time to ascertain if healing will occur without surgical intervention (5).

If the patient does not have available donor sites the burn wound can be excised down to viable tissue and temporarily closed through the application of a synthetic dressing such as Biobrane or a biological coverage such as an **allograft**. An allograft (also referred to as a homograft or cadaver skin) is donor skin taken from another person. The body, through cell-mediated immunity, will reject an allograft usually within 10 to 14 days after application (5). These temporary means of wound closure provide the time needed to achieve a permanent method for closing the wound.

The only way to achieve permanent wound closure in large full-thickness burn injuries is through surgical intervention and the application of either an **autograft** or cultured epithelium. An autograft is the surgical transplantation of the patient's own skin from one area to another. A split-thickness skin autograft is the standard method of achieving wound closure (6). Donor skin is taken from areas of unburned skin. The harvested skin is 0.008 to 0.012 inches in thickness. This leaves a wound, referred to as a donor site, that takes about 7 to 10 days to heal. Once healed, donor sites can be reharvested but will take longer to heal. Burn eschar is excised down to viable tissue, and bleeding is controlled prior to placement of the skin graft. A split-thickness skin autograft can be applied as a mesh graft or a sheet graft. A mesh graft is a graft that has had small holes placed evenly throughout the graft, which allows it to be expanded (2:1, 3:1). Use of a mesh graft allows more area to be covered then the actual size of the donor skin taken. Unfortunately this results in an unsightly "cobblestone" appearance in the scar (5). Because of this, mesh grafts are avoided in areas where there are concerns about the appearance of the scar, such as on the face or hands. Split thickness grafts can be applied as a sheet graft in areas with aesthetic concerns. A sheet graft is a graft in which the donor skin has been laid intact over the area to be grafted. While sheet grafts are preferred because of cosmetic reasons, limited availability of donor sites in large burn injuries limits their use.

In large burns with limited availability of donor sites, cultured epithelium can be used to achieve wound closure. A biopsy of unburned skin is taken and sent to a laboratory that can grow cultured epithelium. It takes 3 to 4 weeks for cultured epithelium to be available for grafting. The resulting grafts are extremely fragile and sensitive to infection. Because of the expense of this form of treatment and the fragile nature of the graft, the use of cultured epithelium is controversial and is reserved for patients with massive burn injury (5).

Immediately after grafting, with either an autograft or cultured epithelium, the graft is fragile and susceptible to loss. Factors that can cause graft failure include shearing/motion, hematoma formation, and infection (5). To prevent loss of graft, the grafted area is immobilized in a functional position and remains in that position until the first dressing change. If grafts are placed on the chest or back the bandages are sutured to the body to decrease the risk of shearing when repositioning the patient. Extremities are elevated to prevent/minimize edema formation. The timing of the first dressing change is controversial and each physician will have his or her own preference. ROM to the grafted area is avoided until the graft is stable which is usually about 4 to 5 days after surgery.

Rehabilitation

Healing begins immediately after the burn injury so it is important to consider and initiate rehabilitation activities upon admission. While the scope of this book is not focused on specific rehabilitation approaches and methods, an overview is provided here with the expectation that the reader will be studying specific procedures in a course designed for that purpose. Rehabilitation needs are influenced by the phase of treatment the patient is experiencing. During the emergency phase and fluid resuscitation, edema formation is to be expected and may be profound. The emphasis should be placed on preservation of joint function and maintaining appropriate positioning of the affected area (15). ROM exercises help to reduce edema and maintain joint mobility. ROM exercises should be preformed during the dressing change and throughout the day when the patient is awake. Timing ROM exercises to occur when the patient has been medicated for pain will help patients tolerate the discomfort associated with this activity (8).

Splints are constructed to prevent the formation of contracture deformities and should be worn when the patient is asleep or resting (15). In the acute phase of treatment reconditioning exercises are started and ROM exercises and splinting are continued. Once the patient's condition is stable, ambulation is initiated and patients are encouraged to participate in activities of daily living (ADL). Assistive devises may be needed to help patients participate in (ADL).

When burn wounds have been grafted/healed the patient enters the rehabilitation phase of treatment. The focus of rehabilitation includes reconditioning, ROM, scar revision, contracture release, and reconstruction (4). Healed burn scars are initially fragile, dry, itchy and susceptible to sunburns (16). Destruction of sebaceous glands in partial- and full-thickness injuries cause dry skin and itching. It is important that patients receive proper education regarding how to care for their burn scars. Use of an unscented soap and application of a moisturizing lotion several times a day will help lubricate the skin and reduce itching. Antihistamines (such as Benadryl) can be taken orally to control itching and promote comfort. Application of a sunscreen is important if burn scars are exposed to the sun.

Burn scars are prone to **hypertrophic scar** formation. Hypertrophic scars are scars in which the tissues are enlarged above the surrounding skin and typically present as red, raised, and rigid (17). Hypertrophic scars are differentiated from keloid scar formation by the fact that they remain within the boundary of the original wound and will eventually fade in color, flatten, and become more pliable as they mature. Hypertrophic scar formation is more common in children, people of color, and over areas involved in stretch or motion (5). Hypertrophic scar formation is frequently seen in deep dermal wounds that heal spontaneously but take a longer time to heal (8). The exact mechanism of hypertrophic scar formation is unclear. Excessive deposition of tissue **collagen** appears to play a significant role, leading to a thickening of the scar (18). Collagen is a basic structural fibrous protein found in all tissue. There is no single effective method to prevent hypertrophic scar formation.

Methods that may help control hypertrophic scar formation include the use of compression garments, scar massage, topical silicone, steroid injection, and surgery (8). Compression garments are the preferred conservative method to treat hypertrophic scars and have been in use since the early 1970s. Compression garments are thought to reduce oxygen flow to the scar thereby decreasing collagen production (17). Shortly after the burn wound is healed, measurements are taken and compression garments are custom-made for each patient. Compression garments are fit for all areas of partial- and full-thickness injuries and apply a pressure of 25 mm Hg to the scar. The garments need to be worn 23 hours a day; they should be removed only for bathing and the application of a moisturizing lotion.

It is important to verify that compression garments fit properly as excessive pressure may contribute to skin breakdown. Children who are growing and adults who have a significant weight gain after discharge from the hospital may need to be refitted for new compression garments. Compression garments will need to be worn until burn scars are mature which can take from one to two years depending upon the individual. Mature burn scars are softer, more pliable and are no longer hyperemic in color, their color is similar to surrounding unburned skin. Once burn scars are mature nothing can be gained by the continued use of compression garments.

Wound healing involves three processes: epithelialization, connective tissue deposition and contraction. Wound contraction is an active process generated by fibroblasts and myofibroblasts and is one of the most powerful mechanical forces in the body (18). **Burn scar contracture** is the shortening and tightening of the burn scar. Burn scar contracture deformities are most problematic over large joints. They can severely limit ROM and interfere with the ability to perform ADLs (19). Mature burn scars do not have the capacity to stretch that is found in normal skin. A child with large full-thickness injuries may develop burn scar contractures years after their initial burn injury as they literally grow out of their scar.

Immature burn scars have a greater capacity to stretch but are prone to the development of contracture deformities. Prevention of burn scar contracture through exercise, positioning, and splinting is important until the burn scar is mature. It is essential for practitioners, patients, and family members to realize that position of comfort often results in contracture formation. A prime example of this is the use of a pillow during sleep, while more comfortable, this action may facilitate the development of neck contractures. Simple acts such as having the bed flat when sleeping or avoiding the use of straws when drinking cause the patient to have to assume a position that provides a stress tension on the scar and helps to prevent contracture deformities. ROM exercises help reduce the risk of contracture formation. An individualized exercise plan should be developed that meets the needs of the patient. It is important to involve both the patient and their family members in the development and execution of this plan to increase the likelihood that it will be followed. Incorporating exercises into activities that a patient likes to do may increase the likelihood that patients will adhere to an exercise regimen. Engaging a child in play that involves large and/or fine motor groups is a great way for a child to perform ROM exercises. The use of splints at night will aid in maintaining the stretch achieved during the day through ROM exercises. Even with a patient's best efforts contracture deformities may develop that will require surgical intervention to release.

Impact on Occupational Performance

A burn injury is a devastating injury that has far-reaching consequences that continue even after the wound is healed. The impact of a burn injury on an individual's occupational performance is influenced by the size, location, and depth of the burn injury. A burn injury may impact an individual's ability to perform basic ADLs, work activities, or play/leisure activities. Burn injuries that have the greatest potential to impact occupational performance include deep partial-thickness or full-thickness burns, burns involving major joints and larger burn injuries. It is critical to follow up with the patient on a routine basis after discharge to identify and initiate early intervention if significant hypertrophic scar formation and contracture deformities are detected that are impacting a patient's occupational performance.

It is important to recognize and assist patients and families in dealing with the psychological and psychosocial impact of a major burn injury. Burn support groups can be helpful in assisting patients and families in dealing with the lifelong disfigurement and dysfunction that may result from a major burn injury. Having patients meet with a burn survivor can help them realize what challenges they may face and ways to overcome these challenges. Family members may experience many emotions such as fear, guilt, or sadness. If these emotions are not addressed family members may feel the need to "take care of their loved one" and to do things for the patient that they need to do for themselves. Having family members meet with another burn survivor and their families will help prepare them for the challenges ahead and assist them to deal with their emotions. This preparation will enable the family to provide the patient both the support and independence they will need to achieve the best outcome.

Additionally, children can benefit from school re-entry and summer burn camp programs. School re-entry programs prepare classmates on what to expect and help in the transition back to school. Summer camp for burn children can also help to improve self-esteem and allow children to realize that they can overcome the difficulties they face.

CASE STUDY

Case Illustration

■ CASE 1

L.S., a 5 year old, is playing outside when her father arrives home. He is having difficulty with his car, which is overheating. Unaware that L.S. has come over to watch him work on the car he removes the radiator cap. Hot radiator fluid and steam strikes L.S. and she sustains a 32% mixed partial- and full-thickness burn injury to her face, neck, chest, and scattered area on bilateral arms.

During the emergency phase she required fluid resuscitation and intubation to maintain her airway during the initial fluid shift and resulting swelling. She was extubated on postburn day 3 and has had no further problems with her airway. Three weeks have passed and L.S. has been to surgery twice. During the first surgery mesh grafts were placed on her chest and arms. During the last surgical procedure, a sheet graft was placed on her neck. Her grafts are intact and healing well, but scattered open areas remain at the margins of the grafts. L.S. has donor sites on her bilateral thighs and buttock, which are healing without difficulty.

Neuromuscular components of ROM, strength and soft tissue integrity have all been affected by the burn injury L.S. sustained. She has participated in ROM exercises since she was extubated. ROM exercises were halted for a few days, after the grafting procedures, to facilitate adherence of the graft. Currently, L.S. has some restriction of ROM to bilateral axillary areas and has been fitted with an airplane splint to be worn when sleeping. This splint will maintain a 90-degree abduction to the axillary area. While she currently does not demonstrate any restriction of neck ROM, she is at great risk for developing contractures in this area. Her parents have been instructed to not allow L.S. to sleep with a pillow and to avoid the use of straws when drinking to promote adequate stretch on the neck. L.S. has been fitted for her compression garments, which should arrive in the next 2 weeks.

ADLs and play or leisure activities are the occupational performance areas that have been affected. Currently, L.S. has few limitations on ROM to most joints, but because of the discomfort experienced during ROM she is hesitant to move. Her parents have been instructed to apply lotion twice daily to facilitate stretching of the scar during ROM activities. Both parents express a great deal of difficulty with the discomfort that L.S. has experienced during her treatment and are hesitant to make her do things that may cause discomfort. L.S.'s father expresses a lot of guilt surrounding the circumstances that caused the burn injury. Arrangements are made for parents to meet with another burn survivor and the survivor's family prior to discharge.

References

1. Morgan ED, Bledsoe SC, Barker J. Ambulatory management of burns. Am Fam Physician 2000;62:2015–2026.
2. Herndon DN, Spies M. Modern burn care. Sem Pediatr Surg 2001;10:28–31.
3. Muller MJ, Pegg SP, Rule MR. Determinants of death following burn injury. Br J Surg 2001;88: 583–587.
4. Latenser BA, Kowal-Vern A. Pediatric burn rehabilitation. Pediatr Rehabil 2002;5:3–10.
5. Kao CC, Garner WL. Acute burns. Plastic Reconstr Surg 2000;101:2482–2492.
6. Shakespeare P. Burn wound healing and skin substitutes. Burns 2001;27:517–522.
7. Konigova R, Matouskova E, Broz L. Burn wound coverage and burn wound closure. Acta Chir Plast 2000;42:64–68.
8. Sheridan RL. Burns. Crit Care Med 2002;30: S500–S514.
9. Yowler CJ, Fratianne RB. Current status of burn resuscitation. Clin Plast Surg 2000;27:1–10.
10. Engrav LH, Colescott PL, Kemalyan N, et al. A biopsy of the use of the Baxter formula to resuscitate burns or do we do it like Charlie did it? J Burn Care Rehabil 2000;21:91–95.
11. Cartotto RC, Innes M, Musgrave, MA, et al. How well does the Parkland formula estimate actual fluid resuscitation volumes? J Burn Care Rehabil 2002;23:258–265.
12. Inoue T, Okabayashi K, Ohtani M, et al. Circulating blood volume in burn resuscitation. Hiroshima J Med Sci 2002;51:7–13.
13. Murphy KD, Lee JO, Herndon, DN. Current pharmacotherapy for the treatment of severe burns. Expert Opin Pharmacother 2003;4:369–384.
14. Palmieri TL, Greenhalgh DG. Topical treatment of pediatric patients with burns. Am J Clin Dermatol 2002;3:529–534.
15. Jordan RB, Daher J, Wasil K. Splints and scar management for acute and reconstructive burn care. Clin Plast Surg 2000;27:71–85.
16. Ho WS, Chan HH, Ying SY, et al. Skin care in burn patients: a team approach. Burns 2001;27:489–491.
17. Puzey G. The use of pressure garments on hypertrophic scars. J Tissue Viability 2001;12:11–15.
18. Atiyeh BS, Ioannovich J, Al-Amm CA, et al. Improving scar quality: A prospective clinical study. Aesthetic Plast Surg 2002;26:470–476.
19. Celis MM, Suman OE, Huang TT, et al. Effect of a supervised exercise and physiotherapy program on surgical interventions in children with thermal injury. J Burn Care Rehabil 2003;24:57–61.

Recommended Learning Resources

Herndon DN, ed. Total Burn Care. 2nd Ed. London: WB Saunders, 2002.
Associated online support at: www.totalburncare.com

American Burn Association
625 North Michigan Ave, Suite 2550
Chicago, IL 60611
Tel: 312–642–9260
Toll free: 800–548–2876
Fax: 312–642–9130
www.ameriburn.org

Shriners Burn Institutes
2900 Rocky Point Dr
Tampa, FL 33607–1460
Tel: 813–281–0300
www.shrinershq.org/Hospitals/BurnInst/

The Phoenix Society for Burn Survivors, Inc
1835 R W Berends Dr SW
Grand Rapids, MI 49519–4955
Tel: 800–888–2876
Fax: 616–458–2831
www.phoenix-society.org

Burn Summer Camps for Kids
(Information available at Kids Camps)
2500 N. Military Trail Suite 450
Boca Raton, FL 33431
Tel: 877–242–9330
Fax: 866–665–2904
www.kidscamps.com/special_needs/burn.html

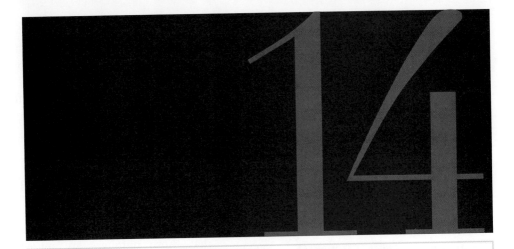

Progressive Neurological Disorders

Diane K. Dirette

Key Terms

Agnosia
Cogwheel rigidity
Demyelination
Dysesthesia
Dysarthria
Electroencephalogram
Myelin
Nystagmus
Optic neuritis

Shortly after the birth of her second child, Joan started getting the sensation of pins and needles in her hands and feet. Within a couple of months, she noticed some numbness and weakness in her arms and legs. She was having difficulty walking for long distances and began to worry that she might drop her 2-year-old son or even her newborn. When the children napped in the afternoon, she found herself slumped on the couch for a much-needed rest. Convinced that this was just part of her postpartum recovery, Joan did not inform her doctor of this difficulty. However, when she found herself struggling one day to focus on the words of her son's bedtime story, she decided to seek medical advice.

Over time, Joan found out she had a progressive neurological disorder called multiple sclerosis (MS). Progressive neurological disorders are a group of diseases that affect various areas of the central nervous system (CNS), are chronic in nature, and cause a deterioration of function over time. This chapter discusses three of the most common progressive neurological disorders: MS, Parkinson's disease (PD), and amyotrophic lateral sclerosis (ALS).

There is little known about the underlying etiology and there is no known cause of any of these three progressive neurological disorders, but research indicates that the etiology is a combination of interrelated factors (1–3). These include genetic predisposition, viruses, and environmental influences. A genetic predisposition is suspected because these diseases are more prevalent among families and certain racial groups. Viruses and their resulting autoimmune response also may be involved as an external cause of these progressive neurological disorders. Specific viruses have not been isolated, but particular interest has focused on a viral subgroup called retroviruses. What causes them is unknown and they can remain silent for years before the onset of a disease. Environmental factors, including exposure to such toxins as lead or pesticides, have also been associated with a higher incidence of progressive neurological disorder (2,4,5). None of these factors, however, have been isolated as the single cause of any of the progressive neurological disorders.

Multiple Sclerosis

Etiology

MS is a debilitating immunological and neurodegenerative disease characterized by the person's own body attacking the **myelin** sheath that surrounds the brain and spinal cord neurons (3,6–9). The latest evidence regarding MS suggests that a viral infection triggers the immune system to wage an attack on the nerve cells of people who are genetically susceptible (10). **Demyelination** of the neurons in the CNS results in scar tissue formation that reduces the axons' ability to conduct impulses (3). The location of demyelination varies from person to person. The visual, motor, sensory, cognitive, psychological, and bowel and bladder systems can be affected.

Incidence and Prevalence

MS affects approximately 1% of the population of the United States and there is evidence that those numbers are increasing (3,6). Currently, an estimated 300,000 to 400,000 people in the United States have MS (3), and the distribution of these individuals varies geographically. The closer a person lives to the equator, the less likely he or she is to have MS (8). For example, in the southern United States, the rate of incidence is 20 to 39 for every 100,000 persons. In the northern United States and Canada, the rate is more than 40 out of every 100,000 persons. (8). If a person migrates from a location near the equator prior to age 15, the incidence of MS is reduced, which contributes to the theory of a possible childhood infection having a role in the onset (10). The incidence of MS also varies according to gender. Multiple sclerosis affects females more often than males at a ratio of between 2 and 3 females for every 1 male with the disease (10).

Population prevalence studies and family aggregation studies provide evidence of a genetic contribution to the disease (3). MS occurs more frequently among people of European ancestry than other white racial groups. People of Scandinavian and Scottish descent are most susceptible to MS. It is twice as common among Caucasians than other races and it is rare among people of Mongolian, Japanese, Chinese, Native American, Eskimo, African, and Aborigine descent (8,10). Studies of offspring, twins, siblings, and adopted children demonstrate that the closer a relation genetically, the more likely a person is to have MS. The incidence of MS decreases as biological relationship decreases. If a person has MS, the identical twin, full siblings, half-siblings, and offspring have increased risk of also having MS in that order (3). In adoption studies, increased risk was only noted in biological relatives. Immediate relatives of a person who has MS are 12 to 20 times more likely than an unrelated person of the same ethnicity living in the same climate to develop the disease (8).

Signs and Symptoms

Some of the more common symptoms of MS include visual deficits such as diplopia or unilateral **optic neuritis**, sensory disturbances such as **dysesthesia** or paresthesia, urinary incontinence or retention, muscle weakness, gross and fine motor incoordination, fatigue, ataxia, dysphagia, **dysarthria**, and cognitive or emotional disturbances. Each person with MS has symptoms that result from lesions in specific areas of the CNS. The types of symptoms, their intensity, and their effects on the person's functional status are highly individualized (11). Table 14.1 includes a summary of common signs and symptoms.

Visual disturbances often are among the earliest signs of MS. They usually appear as a partial loss of vision (scotoma), double or blurred vision, or ocular pain. Sudden loss of vision with pain in or behind the eye is caused by optic neuritis. These early symptoms may subside after 3 to 6 weeks without any residual deficit. For others, visual loss may be insidious and painless. Nonetheless, nearly 80% of all persons who have MS have some loss of visual acuity. Oculomotor control may also be affected because of lesions of the supranuclear connection to the oculomotor nuclei in the brainstem. As a result, the person loses horizontal eye movement either unilaterally or bilaterally.

The individual with MS can experience a variety of other sensory disturbances such as numbness; impairment of vibratory, proprioceptive, pain, touch, and temperature sensation; and distortion of superficial sensation. Because of these sensory losses, the person also may lose various perceptual skills such as stereognosis, kinesthesia, and body scheme (12).

Fatigue is the most common complaint and is often identified as the most debilitating symptom (7,11). Increased energy is required for nerves to conduct their impulses in a demyelinated nervous system, making it difficult for the individual to initiate movement and perform sustained activities. The individual also may experience muscle weakness. As the disease progresses, the person requires more frequent rest periods between activities, and decreased levels of activity lead to further debilitation.

Table 14.1 COMMON SIGNS AND SYMPTOMS OF MULTIPLE SCLEROSIS

Tactile Awareness	Motor	Visual	Cognitive	Psychological
Numbness Disturbance in pain sensation Hypersensitivity	Spasticity Limitations in tolerance/low energy Weakness Ataxic-like symptoms Intention tremor	Double vision Pain behind the eyes Blurred vision Partial blindness/ scotoma **Nystagmus**	Memory loss or disturbance Difficulty with complex ideas Decreased attention span	Depression or euphoria Impulsivity Lability

Adapted from Umphred DA, ed. CV Mosby, Rehabilitation, 1st ed. St. Louis;1985:401.

Approximately 50% of individuals with MS experience some change in their cognitive ability. Short-term memory, attention, processing speed, visuospatial abilities, and executive functions have all been identified as deficit areas in people with MS (13). For some it is difficulty with verbal or spatial-motor memory (11). Others have disorders of judgment, decreased attention and concentration, various types of **agnosia**, or diminished ability to think conceptually (14). As with all aspects of MS, there is considerable variability among individuals with the disease depending on the area of the brain affected (13). An emotional component to this disease results in some individuals having bouts of depression, euphoria, or lability (14) caused by lesions in the frontal lobes of the brain.

Course and Prognosis

MS is the most common progressive neurological disorder found in young adults. Multiple sclerosis is usually diagnosed between the ages of 20 and 40 years (8). It is rarely seen in children or diagnosed in adults older than age 50. No two people with MS follow the same course, and each person experiences variation in symptoms over time (6). The clinical course of this disease can be roughly organized into four types or patterns: benign, relapsing–remitting-nonprogressive, relapsing-remitting-progressive, and progressive. The first is benign, in which the person experiences one or two episodes of neurological deficits with no residual impairments. This person's chance of remaining symptom free increases with each nonsymptomatic year. The next pattern of progression is relapsing-remitting-nonprogressive. In this pattern the person returns to the previous level of function after each exacerbation. With the third type, relapsing-remitting-progressive, however, the person has some residual impairment with each remission. Finally, there is the progressive pattern, which involves a steady decline in function without remissions and exacerbations. Individuals with MS may shift from one pattern to another, with no reliable predictors of these shifts (7,15,16). Eighty percent of people have one of the relapsing-remitting forms of MS in which they experience neurological symptoms followed by complete or partial recovery (10).

Overall, about 60% of individuals with MS remain fully functional up to 10 years after their first exacerbation, and about 30% remain functional 30 years after their first attack (17). In a longitudinal study concluded in 1971, more than two thirds of subjects were ambulatory 25 years after onset (18). In spite of the seriousness of this disease, it does not significantly decrease the person's life expectancy. A few people, however, do become severely disabled and die prematurely because of recurring infections or complications resulting from inactivity (12,17).

Diagnosis

The diagnosis of MS involves excluding other conditions that share the symptomatology of MS such as B12 deficiency, AIDS, rheumatoid arthritis, lupus, Sjogren's syndrome, and Lyme disease (3). To make a definitive diagnosis of MS, the physician examines the person's medical history, symptoms reported by the person, and signs detected by various tests (6). These tests include magnetic resonance imaging (MRI) to detect plaques or lesions in two distinct areas of the central CNS, neurological examination, evoked potentials (visual, brainstem auditory, and somatosensory), and spinal tap to assess cerebrospinal fluid (CSF) proteins.

The results of these diagnostic procedures help contribute to a diagnosis of MS, but they do not determine the diagnosis independently. Many other conditions can elicit positive results. The physician and the individual must work together to rule out other causes before a diagnosis can be made. A definitive diagnosis of MS is made when the person has episodes of exacerbation and remission and slow or step-by-step progression over 6 months. There also must be evidence of lesions in more than one site in the white matter (as determined by MRI) and no other neurological explanation for the clinical picture (12).

Medical/Surgical Management

For each of the progressive neurological disorders discussed in this chapter, surgical intervention is not part of the routine care given. Several medications are used to alleviate the myriad of symptoms caused by each of these diseases. The medications most often prescribed to treat the symptoms of MS include antispasmodics, muscle relaxants, and anticonvulsants. Some current medications include methylprednisolone for functional skills, Prokaryon for fatigue, interferon B-1a for cognition-attention, information processing, and memory/learning (13). Interferon B-1b shows some potential to provide a reduction in lesions for relapsing-remitting MS (19). Possible future treatments include antiviral medications, vaccinations, transplantation of Schwann cells, cell lines, or stem cells, and/or gene therapy (19). Cognitive rehabilitation has shown some promise for amelioration of the effects of cognitive deficits (13).

Parkinson's Disease

Etiology

PD is a progressive neurological disorder identified by depigmentation of the substantia nigra and the presence of Lewy bodies (1). The substantia nigra, which is located in the basil ganglia, produces dopamine, a neurotransmitter, and transports it to the striatum. This leads to deficits in the speed and quality of motor movements, postural stability, cognitive skills, and affective expression (4,20,21). There are variations in the clinical and pathological presentation of PD and there is overlap with other parkinsonian disorders (22). The differentiation of PD from other parkinsonian disorders does not have definitive, validated tests. The underlying cause of PD is unknown although there is some evidence that implicates both genetic and environmental factors. As many as 50% of persons with PD have an affected relative. This lends some evidence to the hypothesis of a genetic factor in PD.

Incidence and Prevalence

Worldwide, the prevalence of PD is estimated at 1% of the population, with an estimated 500,000 cases in the United States (20). These cases appear to be evenly distributed throughout the world, based on available diagnoses. Diagnostic data, however, vary from one medical care system to another.

PD has been reported to affect males slightly more than females, but recent studies report an equal distribution among the genders (20). PD occurs in all races worldwide (20). However, in the United States, there is a lower incidence among African Americans compared to Caucasians (4).

Signs and Symptoms

The major symptoms of PD are resting tremor, muscle rigidity, bradykinesia, and postural instability (4,20,22) (Table 14.2). The most obvious and familiar of these symptoms is tremor, which is usually noted initially in the hand on one side and sometimes in the foot. In the hand, the movement is frequently described as "pill-rolling." The tremors are usually variable. They disappear when the person is asleep or calmly resting and they increase under stress or intense mental activity (20). Infrequent eye blinking is often an early sign of PD followed by progressive loss of facial expression.

Table 14.2 PRIMARY AND SECONDARY SIGNS AND SYMPTOMS OF PARKINSON'S DISEASE

Primary Signs and Symptoms	Tremor (resting, pill-rolling) **Rigidity (cogwheel)** Bradykinesia (slowness of movement) Postural changes (stooped, unsteady)
Secondary Signs and Symptoms	Gait disturbances (shuffle, reduced reflexes, falling) Impaired dexterity and coordination Involuntary immobilization (freezing) Speech difficulties (soft, monotone, rapid) Swallowing difficulties (drooling) Poor balance Oculomotor impairments (deficits in fixation, scanning, tracking) Reduced facial expression Sleep disturbances Reduced bowel and bladder function Painful cramping of muscles Sexual dysfunction Low blood pressure Sensory disturbances (numbness, tingling, burning sensations) Seborrhea (oily skin, dandruff) Fatigue

Secondary symptoms of PD include gait disturbances referred to as a "festinating gait" (short-stepped or shuffling with reduced arm swing), dexterity and coordination difficulties, involuntary immobilization, micrographia (small handwriting), cognitive impairments (visuospatial, memory, and frontal lobe functions), sensory loss, muffled speech, frequent swallowing, poor balance, oculomotor impairments, reduced facial expression, sleep disturbances, reduced bowel and bladder function, painful cramping, sexual dysfunction, low blood pressure, seborrhea, depression or anxiety, and fatigue (1,4,20,23,24). This array of symptoms varies among people with PD. It is highly unlikely that any person with PD would develop all of the symptoms listed above. Some people may not experience a specific symptom, whereas for another person, that symptom might be a major complaint. For example, some people may experience cognitive deficits, such as executive functions impairment, as the initial symptoms, while others may never demonstrate any cognitive decline.

Course and Prognosis

PD is usually first diagnosed when a person is older than 50 years (4). The average onset age is about 60 years. It rarely affects people younger than age 40 (20). As with MS, the progression of PD differs with each person. Generally, PD is a slow, progressive disorder (1). The three phases of the disease include the preclinical period when neurons have begun to degenerate, but no symptoms are yet evident (22). The second phase of PD is the prodromal period that can last months or even years. During this phase generalized symptoms such as depression, anxiety, fibromyalgia, or shoulder pain may appear. The third phase is the symptomatic period when the PD symptoms are evident (22). According to a clinical scale by Hoehn and Yahr, the third phase can be divided into five stages, as follows:

Stage I: Signs of PD are strictly one-sided, affecting one side of the body only.
Stage II: Signs of PD are bilateral and balance is not impaired.
Stage III: Signs of PD are bilateral and balance is impaired.
Stage IV: PD is functionally disabling.
Stage V: Person is confined to bed or a wheelchair.

Progression through these stages is variable for each person. Usually, a person will have PD for 15 to 20 years before entering the most severe stages. Some people may be in the first asymptomatic, preclinical phase and remain there until death (22). There are also fluctuations within each stage. The loss of function is not a linear progression. Each person experiences some periods of improvement scattered throughout the progressive loss of function. Because of advances in medical treatment, life expectancy is not significantly affected by a diagnosis of PD.

Diagnosis

A definitive diagnosis of PD can only be made by autopsy (22). Therefore, a person is given a diagnosis of probable PD. To determine this diagnosis, the physician observes the current symptoms, eliminates other diseases as the cause of those symptoms, and evaluates the person's response to medications used to treat PD (4). At least one of the primary symptoms (resting tremor, rigidity, bradykinesia, or postural instability) must be present. Several tests, such as computerized axial tomography scan, MRI, or **electroencephalogram** (EEG), are used to eliminate the possibility of other neurological disorders. The physician may also use positron emission tomography (PET) to detect a loss of dopamine, which is indicative of PD.

Medical/Surgical Management

The medications usually prescribed to treat the symptoms of PD include dopamine replacement medications, acetylcholine inhibitors, and antiviral compounds. Some of the dopamine replacement medications include carbidopa/levodopa, pergolide, bromocriptine, ropinirole, and pramipexole. Some possible side effects of these medications include nausea, loss of appetite, dyskinesias, dry mouth, sleepiness, confusion, and hallucinations.

Many surgical procedures have also been developed to treat the symptoms of PD. These procedures include thalamotomy, pallidotomy, and deep brain stimulation (neurostimulation) (25). Thalamotomy is a surgical procedure in which heat via an electrode or γ-knife radiosurgery is used to destroy part of the thalamus. The thalamus is an area of the brain involved in movement. A thalamotomy can reduce tremors associated with PD and may sustain the improvement for over ten years. A pallidotomy is a surgical procedure in which heat via an electrode or γ-knife radiosurgery is used to destroy part of the globus pallidus. The globus pallidus is also an area of the brain involved in movement. A pallidotomy can reduce tremors, shuffling gait, flat affect, rigidity, and slowness of movement. These symptoms may be dramatically reduced following this procedure and the effects may last for at least 5 years. Deep brain stimulation (neurostimulation) is the implantation of a type of "brain pacemaker" that delivers electrical impulses to the subthalamic nucleus, the internal globus pallidus or the thalamus to reduce tremors associated with PD. The potential side effects of this procedure include depression, slurred speech, tingling in the head and hands, and problems with balance. The generator usually needs to be replaced every 3 to 5 years.

A more controversial surgery that treats the symptoms of PD is also being studied (25). Tissue implantation using fetal brain tissue or fetal pig tissue has shown some promise for alleviating the symptoms of PD. In this surgical procedure the dopamine-producing tissue is implanted into the parts of the brain responsible for the symptoms of PD. More research is needed to determine the potential and long-term effects of such procedures.

Amyotrophic Lateral Sclerosis

Etiology

ALS is a fatal, progressive, degenerative motor neuron disease in which scars form on the neurons in the corticospinal pathways, the motor nuclei of the brainstem, and the anterior horn cells of the spinal cord (26–29). Degeneration of motor neurons leads to progressive atrophy of muscles, usually beginning with the loss of strength in the small muscles of the hands or feet (7,26). When the motor neurons are affected, the reflexes can become hyperactive. Progressive loss of muscle movement, difficulty speaking and swallowing, loss of emotional control, and reduced body temperature regulation (7,26) are common. The actual mechanism of neuro-degeneration remains a mystery. There is speculation that cystoptotic and mitochondrial pathway dysfunction results in the buildup of proteins that lead to motor neuron death (30). There is also evidence of an inflammatory component in the mechanisms of the disease process (29).

There is no known cause of ALS, but it is speculated that several disorders with several causes lead to this motor neuron disease (29). Recent advances have discovered a genetic mutation as one cause for familial ALS (30). There is also evidence of genetic causes using familial patterns of susceptibility. Family history of a first- or second-degree relative with ALS is a significant risk factor for the disease. In most cases, however, ALS occurs sporadically and is presumed to be acquired. There is also some speculation regarding viral, retroviral, and environmental causes, but concrete evidence is lacking (30).

Incidence and Prevalence

The prevalence of people with ALS is estimated to be 4 to 7 out of every 100,000 people uniformly worldwide (28,29). It is the most common motor neuron disease in adults. ALS affects males more often than females with a ratio of 1.7:1 (30). Ongoing investigation indicates the possibility of increasing prevalence of ALS worldwide (28,31).

Signs and Symptoms

The most common initial symptom of ALS is weakness of the small muscles of the hand or an asymmetrical foot drop (26). Night cramps, particularly in the calf muscles, also may be present. The signs and symptoms of ALS are progressive, most commonly in a distal to proximal pattern. The symptoms can be divided into three areas: lower motor neuron, corticospinal tract, and corticobulbar tract dysfunction (Table 14.3).

Table 14.3 SIGNS AND SYMPTOMS OF AMYOTROPHIC LATERAL SCLEROSIS

Lower Motor Neuron	Corticospinal Tract	Corticobulbar Tract
Focal and multifocal weakness Atrophy (progressive distal to proximal Muscle cramping Muscle twitching	Spasticity Hyperreactive reflexes Dysphagia (difficulty swallowing) Dysarthria (impaired quality of speech production)	Dysphagia (difficulty swallowing) Dysarthria (impaired quality of speech production)

The lower motor neuron dysfunction symptoms include focal and multifocal weakness, atrophy, cramps, and muscle twitching. Spasticity and hyperresponsive reflexes are associated with corticospinal tract dysfunction. Dysphagia and dysarthria are associated with corticobulbar dysfunction (26,32).

Course and Prognosis

The age of onset of ALS occurs between 16 and 77 years, but it is usually diagnosed when a person is between the ages of 50 and 70 years (32). The course of ALS is usually progressive and relatively rapid. The duration of survival after diagnosis is usually 1 to 5 years, with a mean survival of three years (26,32). The younger a person is and the more mild the symptoms at the time of diagnosis, the longer the course. There is some evidence of a "resistance in ALS," in which a person may demonstrate improvements and live longer than 10 years. This is seen in approximately 10% to 16% of people with ALS (32). Death is usually from respiratory failure (29).

Diagnosis

As with the other progressive neurological disorders, the physician pieces together clinical symptoms, electromyogram (EMG) results, and tests to exclude other causes of the clinical presentation to make a definite diagnosis of ALS (26,32). The EMG findings will include motor denervation and fasciculation (twitching) with intact sensory responses. A CT scan or MRI of the CNS may be used to rule out other causes of the symptoms. Blood tests are usually normal. CSF is often normal but may show raised protein levels.

Medical/Surgical Management

The medical treatments that are currently available do little to alter the fatal course of ALS (29). The medications prescribed to treat the symptoms of ALS include antispasmodic medications, nonsteroidal anti-inflammatory medications, and antibiotics. There is evidence that riluzole helps people stay in the milder stages for a longer time. Experimental medications that have been in clinical trials include celecoxib (Celebrex) and minocycline, which are anti-inflammatory drugs, and topiramate, gabapentin, riluzole (Rilutek), which are antiglutamatergic drugs (29).

Gastrostomy and noninvasive positive-pressure ventilation have been shown to increase both quality and possibly length of life (28). Low-dose radiation and botulinum toxin injections into the salivary glands are sometimes used to treat drooling.

There is some evidence that attending a clinic staffed by a multidisciplinary team (neurologists, specialist nurses, physical, occupational, and speech therapists, and a pulmonologist, nutritionist, psychologist, and social worker) is effective for improving quality and length of life (33). Palliative care may also be very important for people with ALS and their families. It has been estimated that 62.4% die in a hospice-supported environment (28).

Impact of Conditions on Client Factors and Occupational Performance

Each of these progressive neurological disorders is progressive and can affect all client factors, performance patterns, performance skills, and areas of occupation. The extent of this effect depends on the stage and severity of the disease. In each case, a person may have any combination of the deficits listed.

Activities of Daily Living

Self-care skills are affected by changes in the person's sensorimotor skills. Changes are usually noted in gross and fine motor coordination, postural control, muscle tone, endurance, and sensation (except in ALS). Loss of independence in bathing, dressing, personal device care, and toilet hygiene may occur. Toileting can become problematic for persons with MS or PD because of the loss of bladder and bowel control. The individual may experience any combination of the complications noted earlier in this chapter.

Eating may be difficult, either because the person loses the strength and coordination to self-feed or because of chewing or swallowing difficulties (dysphagia). The latter is caused by weakness or incoordination of the pharyngeal musculature, which also can make it difficult for an individual to ingest oral medications.

Functional mobility is another critical concern. Neuromuscular and motor problems make ambulation difficult or impossible, either independently or with assistive devices, even in an electrically propelled wheelchair. Acquiring alternate methods of mobility requires the ability to adapt. The person must be able to change motor patterns, requiring concurrent new and varied perceptual and cognitive strategies. At the same time, the individual is challenged psychologically to make the necessary adjustments to new and different types of mobility. As the person's function decreases, issues of home and work accessibility must be considered, and the necessary adaptations must be made to maintain performance in activities of daily living.

Instrumental Activities of Daily Living

Deficits in neuromusculoskeletal, movement-related functions and motor skills because of progressive neurological disorders usually lead to reduced ability to perform all instrumental activities of daily living. In addition to neuromusculoskeletal losses, reduced sensory, cognitive, and perceptual functions may also interfere with independence in this area. In the early stages of these diseases adaptations need to be made to afford the person the opportunity to maintain function for as long as possible. Most of these tasks, however, eventually need to be delegated to other members of the household further creating issues of dependence and loss of role function.

A normal activity for many persons, including those with progressive neurological disorder is the care of others, including a spouse or significant other, children, or older, dependent adults. The individual with a progressive neurological disorder may have increasing difficulty fulfilling this role. In fact, he or she may have to rely on these care receivers to provide support and care, creating a major role reversal. These changes in responsibilities can be very stressful for all concerned; they challenge everyone's ability to maintain the integrity of the relationships.

Education

Because of the age of onset for these progressive neurological disorders, many people will not be involved in formal educational activities. Those who are may gradually experience a reduced ability to physically participate due to decline in underlying neuromusculoskeletal and movement-related functions and motor skills. Deficits in cognitive and perceptual functions may further limit learning ability. Adaptations such as computer-based courses for formal and informal education may be a viable option.

Work

All client factors have the potential to affect work activities. Work is a crucial area of occupational performance and, for many adults, is an important part of self-identity. As motor skills decline, the ability to perform specific work tasks also declines. "Invisible symptoms" such as fatigue, weak or blurred vision, and difficulties with bladder control often confound the issue. Co-workers may not understand why someone who does not look ill cannot work. Again, this affects the person psychologically, with changes in societal roles and self-concept. This is particularly true for an individual whose job requires a high degree of physical stamina and skill. For example, assembly workers or truck drivers may lose their jobs fairly early in the course of these diseases. An individual who has been the breadwinner of the family and whose identity is closely tied to physical strength and endurance may have serious adjustment problems. Cognitive deficits also may make it difficult for the person to function and continue to find satisfaction in work.

Play and Leisure

Many leisure activities can be affected by the changes that result from progressive neurological disorders. Alternative leisure activities must be explored as more and more performance deficits occur. A balance between work and play should be maintained as long as possible. However, if the person can no longer engage in usual work and daily living activities, it is even more critical to have meaningful and fulfilling leisure pursuits. These activities will grow in importance as a means of self-actualization and satisfaction.

Social Participation

Communication, mobility, sexual dysfunction, and eating problems may all affect the person's normal socialization with individuals or groups. Dysarthria, or imperfect articulation, is caused by a lack of control of the tongue and other oral muscles essential to speech. This problem can affect the person's ability to communicate thoughts, needs, and desires and can limit social interaction. The individual may lose upper extremity function, making it difficult to compensate for speaking problems with written communication.

Sexual dysfunction may also be present. Because of depression and diminished self-concept, the person may no longer feel attractive, which causes problems in sexual expression. Also, loss of specific motor and sensory function can affect physical performance.

Because of the unpredictable nature of the course of each progressive neurological disorder, potential dependency issues are ongoing problems. This may lead to secondary psychosocial issues caused by these lifestyle changes. Progressive neurological disorders require an initial social-psychological adjustment as well as continual readjustment because of erratic progression of symptoms. A person who was active and outgoing may have a diminished self-concept because of the inability to engage in activities that were once of interest and value. The result is a variety of role changes in the family or society.

Role expectations, which exist in every social situation, are ways of behaving or reacting that fit with one's self-image and the expectations of others. These include attitudes, activities, patterns of decision-making, expressing feelings, and meeting the needs of significant others (34). Some individuals with loss of bladder control may avoid going out in public. Mothers may be unable to care for their children. Some may come to see themselves as no longer useful or attractive to others. Marriages may break up under the strain of living with progressive neurological disorders. Occasionally, individuals with progressive neurological disorders threaten suicide. An individual with a progressive neurological disorder must think seriously about current role expectations and how these might be threatened by the progressive neurological disorder (34).

CASE STUDY

Case Illustrations

■ CASE 1: MULTIPLE SCLEROSIS

M.A. is a 28-year-old woman who was diagnosed with MS 5 years before this hospital admission. She was admitted because she noticed a progressive deterioration of function during the past 6 months. The main problems she identifies are an increase in fatigue, difficulty with bowel and bladder function, and several falls. She complains of feeling moody and forgetting information.

She is married and has two children, an 11-year-old girl and a 5-year-old boy. She is self-employed as a paralegal, which requires her to spend many hours typing on the computer. Her husband works full-time and has been very supportive. At the time of admission, he seemed overwhelmed.

M.A. tries to do her morning self-care but is finding it more difficult and frustrating. Getting dressed is particularly fatiguing, and she admits that at times she goes to bed fully dressed to avoid having to get dressed in the morning. She has been using a manual wheelchair off and on for the past 2 years.

Her daughter is currently helping with the laundry, cooking, and simple cleaning. M.A. states that she has problems doing household tasks because she must hold onto something stable before reaching for, or lifting, an object.

She currently enjoys no leisure activities. At one time, she liked to knit, but it has become too frustrating to be pleasurable.

She complains of bladder urgency but often cannot void. She also has a mild dysarthria, spasticity of the lower extremities, weakness of the upper extremities (able to move against gravity withstanding minimal resistance), poor sitting balance, poor fine and gross motor coordination, blurred vision, and loss of stereognosis and light touch.

When the occupational therapist spoke with her, it became apparent that she did not comprehend the nature and course of MS. She is feeling frustrated and depressed about her recent decline of function.

She is currently taking acetaminophen (Tylenol), senna (Senokot), psyllium (Metamucil), Colace, heparin, and multivitamins and is using Dulcolax suppositories.

■ CASE 2: PARKINSON'S DISEASE

C.R. is a 72-year-old man with stage III PD. He has recently experienced a severe loss of balance and functional mobility. He reports difficulty moving quickly and gracefully. He also complains of poor handwriting, problems sleeping, and numbness in both hands.

C.R. is a single, retired accountant who lives independently in a two-story home. His bedroom and bathroom are on the second floor. There are four steps to enter the home. He has no children. He has one sister who lives within walking distance of his home. She, however, is suffering from arthritis and has difficulty offering much assistance.

C.R. has been caring for himself thus far, but his sister reports she is concerned about his safety, especially with activities such as cooking and bathing. She reports that he has fallen on several occasions recently and spends most of his time sitting in his chair in his living room.

His sister brings him meals as often as possible but is unable to bring meals in the morning or during bad weather. Her children live out of state and are only able to offer assistance to him during occasional visits when they try to do some of the major household chores such as painting, repairs, and cleaning.

C.R. was once interested in music and art. He played the piano and painted with watercolors. He reports that he has not participated in these leisure activities for "a long time." He also played tennis on a regular basis at the local club. He is still a member of the club but has not been there in more than a year.

C.R. is reportedly self-conscious of his illness and, therefore, does not like to go out in public very much. His sister, who has always been very close to her brother, expresses concern about his "depression and lack of motivation." She states that she has tried on several occasions to get him to go to local musical concerts or museums, but she feels he is just too depressed.

He is currently taking levodopa–carbidopa (Sinemet CR) and trihexyphenidyl hydrochloride (Artane). His sister, however, reports that he does not consistently take his medications because they "make him feel sick."

■ CASE 3: AMYOTROPHIC LATERAL SCLEROSIS

T.M. is a 48-year-old man who has recently been diagnosed with ALS. Six months before being referred to occupational therapy services, he began to experience some weakness in his hands and he began dropping objects, such as tools. He reports loss of strength in his arms and legs. The weakness in his legs has become so severe that he now uses a borrowed wheelchair part of the time. He complains of difficulty sleeping due to cramps in his legs. He also reports that he has lost almost 20 lbs in the last 6 or 8 months.

T.M. is married and has two sons, ages 6 and 4. He independently owns and operates a lawnmower shop at which he sells and repairs lawnmowers. He reports significant difficulty performing the repair parts of his job because of weakness in his hands and arms. Most of the repairs have become backed up in the shop and he is considering hiring assistance or sending the work to another shop.

His wife is employed full-time as a legal secretary. She has helped with the business as much as possible by completing some of the bookkeeping after hours. She is very busy caring for their boys and trying to maintain the household. She appears to be very supportive of T.M., but also seems very burdened by her responsibilities.

T.M. has many interests in sports and outdoor activities. He has been racing in "Iron Man" triathlons and marathons for the last several years. He was a high school track and cross-country star. He enjoys biking and camping. Every summer, he and his family take a 2-week trip to a remote location where they hike and camp. He is also supportive of his sons' sports events and enjoys teaching them various sports. Last year, he was a soccer coach for his oldest boy's team.

The course and prognosis of ALS has been explained to T.M. and his wife and they have reportedly been discussing future plans. They are, however, "hoping for a miracle." At this time, he is taking pain relievers to reduce the pain from the cramping in his legs.

References

1. Hutton JT, Dippel RL. Caring for the Parkinson Patient: A Practical Guide. Buffalo, NY: Prometheus Books, 1989.
2. Armon C, Kurland LT, Beard CM, et al. Psychologic and adaptational difficulties anteceding amyotrophic lateral sclerosis: Rochester, Minnesota, 1925–1987. Neuroepidemiology 1991;10(3):132–137.
3. Kenealy SJ, Pericak-Vance MS, Haines JL. The genetic epidemiology of multiple sclerosis. J Neuroimmunol 2003;143:7–12.
4. Lieberman AN, Williams FL, Imke S, et al. Parkinson's Disease: The Complete Guide for Patients and Caregivers. New York: Simon & Schuster, 1993.
5. O'Sullivan SB, Cullen KE, Schmitz TJ. Physical Rehabilitation: Evaluation and Treatment Procedures. Philadelphia: FA Davis, 1981.
6. Kalb RC. Multiple Sclerosis: The Questions You Have, the Answers You Need. New York: Demos Vermande, 1996.
7. Maloney FP, Burks JS, Ringel SP, eds. Interdisciplinary Rehabilitation of Multiple Sclerosis and Neuromuscular Disorders. Philadelphia: JB Lippincott, 1985.
8. Matthews B. Multiple Sclerosis: The Facts. 3rd Ed. Oxford: Oxford University Press, 1993.
9. Pryse-Phillips W. The epidemiology of multiple sclerosis. In: Cook SD, ed. Handbook of Multiple Sclerosis. New York: Marcel Dekker, 1992:1–24.
10. Hanson LJ, Cafruny WA. Current concepts in multiple sclerosis: part 1. S D J Med 2002;55(10):433–436.
11. Delisa JA, Hammond MD, Mikulic MA, et al. Multiple sclerosis: part 1. Common physical disabilities and rehabilitation. Am Fam Physician 1985;32(4): 157–163.
12. Umphred DA. Neurological rehabilitation. 2nd Ed. St Louis: CV Mosby, 1990.
13. Bobholz JA, Rao SM. Cognitive dysfunction in multiple sclerosis: a review of recent developments. Curr Opin Neurol 2003;16:283–288.

14. Chusid JG. Correlative neuroanatomy and functional neurology. 16th Ed. Los Altos, CA: Lange Medical Publications, 1976.
15. Delisa JA, Miller RM, Mikulic MA, et al. Multiple sclerosis: part 2. Common functional problems and rehabilitation. Am Fam Physician 1985;32(5): 127–132.
16. Ferguson JM. Helping an MS patient live a better life. Rehabil Nurs 1987;50(12):22–27.
17. Andreoli TE, Carpenter CC, Plum F, et al. Essentials of Medicine. Philadelphia: WB Saunders, 1986.
18. Percy AK. Multiple sclerosis in Rochester, Minnesota: a 60 year appraisal. Arch Neurology 1971;25:105.
19. Noseworthy JH. Management of multiple sclerosis: current trials and future options. Curr Opin Neurol 2003;16:289–297.
20. Duvoisin RC, Sage J. Parkinson's Disease: A Guide for Patient and Family. Philadelphia: Lippincott-Raven, 1996.
21. Taylor AE, Saint-Cyr JA, Lang AE. Parkinson's disease: cognitive changes in relation to treatment response. Brain 1987;110:35–51.
22. Albanese A. Diagnostic criteria for Parkinson's disease. Neurol Sci 2003;24:S23–S26.
23. Carbon M, Marie R. Functional imaging of cognition in Parkinson's disease. Curr Opin Neurol 2003;16: 475–480.
24. Cooper JA, Sagar HJ, Jordan N, et al. Cognitive impairment in early, untreated Parkinson's disease and its relationship to motor disability. Brain 1991;114:2095–2122.
25. Surgical procedures for Parkinson's Disease, 2003. Available at: http://www.swedish.org/15575.cfm. Accessed March 3, 2005.
26. Beresford S. Motor Neurone Disease (Amyotrophic Lateral Sclerosis). London: Chapman & Hall, 1995.
27. Rusk HA. Rehabilitation Medicine. 3rd Ed. St Louis: Mosby, 1971.
28. Przedborski S, Mitsumoto H, Rowland LP. Recent advances in amyotrophic lateral sclerosis research. Curr Neurol Neurosci Rep 2003;3:70–77.
29. Weydt P, Weiss MD, Moller T, et al. Neuro-inflammation as a therapeutic target in amyotrophic lateral sclerosis. Curr Opin Invest Drugs 2002;3(12): 1720–1724.
30. Shaw CE, Al-Chalabi A, Neigh N. Progress in pathogenesis of amyotrophic lateral sclerosis. Curr Neurol Neurosci Rep 2001;1:69–76.
31. Durrleman S, Alperovitch A. Increasing trend of ALS in France and elsewhere: are the changes real? Neurology 1989;39:768–773.
32. Mitsumoto H, Hanson MR, Chad DA. Amyotrophic lateral sclerosis: Recent advances in pathogenesis and therapeutic trials. Arch Neurol 1988;45:189–202.
33. Traynor BJ, Alexander M, Corr B, et al. Effect of a multidisciplinary amyotrophic lateral sclerosis (ALS) clinic on ALS survival: a population based study, 1999–2000. J Neurol Neurosurg Psychiatry 2003;74:1258–1261.
34. Holland NJ, Kaplan SR. Social adaptations. In: Scheinberg LC, Holland NJ, eds. Multiple Sclerosis: A Guide for Patients and Their Families. New York: Raven Press, 1987:219–239.

Recommended Learning Resources

Multiple Sclerosis

National Multiple Sclerosis Society
www.nmss.org

The Multiple Sclerosis Foundation
www.msfacts.org

The Multiple Sclerosis Association of America
www.msaa.com

Parkinson's Disease

National Parkinson Foundation
www.parkinson.org

Parkinson's Disease Foundation, Inc.
www.pdf.org

The American Parkinson Disease Association, Inc.
www.apdaparkinson.com
Amyotrophic Lateral Sclerosis

The ALS Association
www.alsa.org

World Federation of Neurology Amyotrophic Lateral Sclerosis
www.wfnals.org

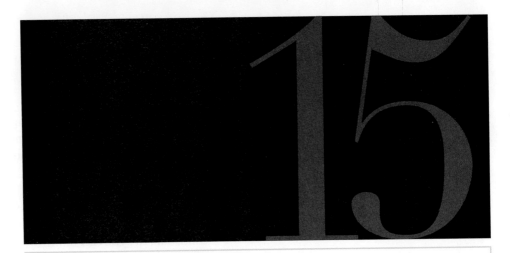

Rheumatoid Arthritis

David P. Orchanian

Key Terms

- Anemia
- Ankylosis
- Antibodies
- Apophyseal
- Arthritis
- Boutonniere deformity
- Bursitis
- Carpal Tunnel Syndrome
- De Quervain's tenosynovitis
- Diarthroses
- Epstein-Barr virus
- Inflammation
- Juvenile rheumatoid arthritis
- Osteoarthritis
- Pannus
- Rheumatoid arthritis
- Rheumatoid factor
- Rheumatologist
- Sjögren's syndrome
- Swan-neck deformities
- Synovial
- Tenosynovitis

Augustin-Jacob Landre-Beauvais is given credit for the earliest description of **rheumatoid arthritis** (RA) in his thesis of 1800. It was not until 1858 that A.B. Garrod coined the actual phrase rheumatoid arthritis, and it was in 1941 that the American Rheumatism Association (ARA) adopted the terminology. The appearance and distribution of lesions in ancient skeletons suggests that rheumatoid arthritis may have existed in North America 3,000 years ago (1).

More than 100 different forms of **arthritis** are documented. Arthritis is divided into eight major categories, with RA included under the synovitis category. Though less common than other forms of the disease, such as **osteoarthritis**, it is considered to be more serious.

The total cost of arthritis and other rheumatic conditions (AORC) in the United States in 1997 was $86.2 billion (including $51.1 billion in direct costs and $35.1 billion in indirect costs), approximately 1% of the U.S. gross domestic product (2). Total costs attributable to AORC by state ranged from $121 million in Wyoming to $8.4 billion in California. Costs for arthritis remain high and underscore the need for better interventions to reduce the economic burden of arthritis of all types (3).

Data indicate that the economic costs linked with RA are on a level with those of coronary heart disease. Annually, per person medical costs have been estimated at upwards of $5,400 (1994 figures) (4).

Anatomy

It is essential to have an accurate awareness of the joint anatomy and its related structures (Fig. 15.1) before discussing the etiology, signs and symptoms, and course of RA. The word "arthritis" derives from the Greek words "athron" (meaning joint) and "itis" (meaning **inflammation** or infection). Therefore the word is defined as "inflammation or infection of the joint" (5). The base word "rheum" in rheumatoid refers to the stiffness, general aching, weakness, and fatigue that is experienced throughout the body.

The basic anatomy of a healthy joint as shown in Figure 15.1 should be referred to when, later in the chapter, the disease process and its effects on the joint are discussed.

Etiology

RA results from interplay among immunogenetic risk factors, environmental insults, and random modulations of the musculoskeletal and immune systems (6). RA develops when the synovium changes into disorganized lymphoid granulation tissue. Multiple factors involving both resident and infiltrating cells contribute to **synovial** lining hyperplasia and cartilage or bone erosion. Deposition of infectious agents and immune complexes into the synovial layer triggers complement activation and inflammation in joint tissue (7).

Some recent studies report increased lymphoma risks linked to RA disease activity. The hypothesis that disease-modifying drugs, and in particular methotrexate, increase the lymphoma risk receives little support. Observation times for the tumor necrosis factor (TNF)-blocking therapies are still short, but so far no clear increased risk for lymphoma has been observed. Presence of **Epstein-Barr virus** (EBV), as analyzed with Epstein-Barr virus-encoded ribonucleic acid (EBER) in situ hybridization, appears to be uncommon in RA-related lymphomas. Hypothetically, an increased proliferative drive caused by self or non-self antigens may play a role in lymphoma development in RA patients, but this has to be further studied.

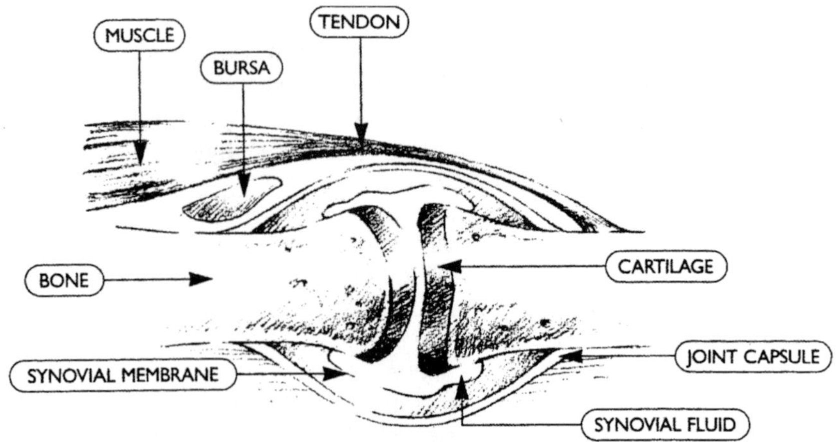

Figure 15.1 Anatomy of a joint. Arthritis can affect different parts of a joint.

Rheumatologists need to be aware of the increased lymphoma risk in their RA patients. The reason for the increased lymphoma risk in RA patients is still unclear, but available studies support the hypothesis of a link between RA disease severity and the risk of lymphoma rather than increased risks associated with specific treatment regimens (7).

RA is a chronic, inflammatory, systemic disease that produces most prominent manifestations in the diarthrodial joints (Fig. 15.2). **Diarthroses** are the most mobile joints and are by far the most common articular pattern (8). Because these joints possess a synovial membrane and contain synovial fluid, diarthrodial joints are more commonly referred to as synovial joints.

Synovial joints are subclassified according to shape: ball and socket (hip), hinge (interphalangeal), saddle (first carpometacarpal [CMC]), and plane (patellofemoral) joints. These widely varying configurations demonstrate the fact that form parallels function in the design of diarthrodial joints (8). In all cases noted, a well-lubricated bearing develops from essentially congruent cartilaginous surfaces that slide freely against each other. The shape and the size of the opposing surfaces define the direction and extent of the available motion. Within the limits of each joint, a wide variety of designs permit motion in flexion (bending), extension (straightening), abduction (movement away from the midline of the body), adduction (moving toward the midline of the body), and rotation. It is seen that individual joints can act in one (humeroulnar joint), two (wrist), or up to three (shoulder) axes of movement (8).

Persistent and progressive synovitis develops in peripheral joints. The initial event inciting the inflammatory response is unknown. An infectious etiology of RA has been vigorously pursued without yielding convincing evidence (9). Genetic and environmental factors control the progression, extent, and pattern of the inflammatory response and are, as such, responsible for the heterogenous clinical features. Genetic factors have been identified as potentially influential in the disease. RA is not inherited; it is not passed directly from parents to children. A susceptibility or tendency to develop RA can be inherited, but not everyone who inherits this susceptibility will have the disease develop (10).

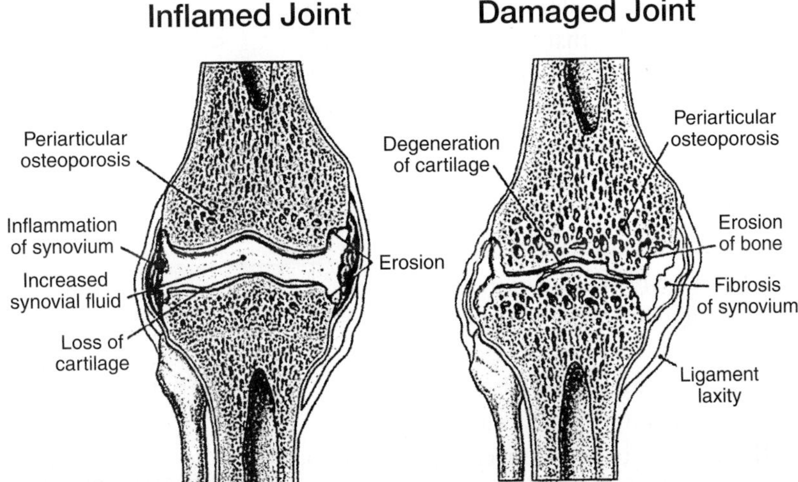

Figure 15.2 The postinflammatory response to joint inflammation is fibrosis, not unlike the scarring (fibrosis) that results from a surgical incision. The function of the postinflammatory joint depends on the degree of fibrosis and the destruction that occurred during the inflammatory stage. The damage influences the alignment, angle of tendon pull (joint integrity), range of motion, and stability. (Reprinted with permission from the Arthritis Foundation. The AHPA Arthritis Teaching Slide Collection. 2nd Ed. 1988.)

Epidemiology

RA has a worldwide distribution and involves all ethnic groups. Though the disease can occur at any age, the prevalence increases with age and the peak incidence is between the fourth and sixth decade. Data from population-based prevalence and incidence studies have to be interpreted cautiously because there is no unique feature to establish the diagnosis of RA. Studies of incidence and prevalence have not had a major impact on the understanding of the disease pathogenesis. Insignificant differences in prevalence rates among ethnic groups are likely explained by variations in disease assessment and age distribution of the study populations (11, 12).

It is speculated that a high proportion of individuals with RA demonstrate circulating **antibodies** to an antigen present in the EBV. The inflammatory problem involves a triggering of a chronic inflammation that begins in the synovial membrane of the joints and progresses to erosion of the joint capsule, tendons, ligaments, and eventually cartilage and bone. The inflammation usually spreads to other joints, resulting in further joint damage (13).

Leukocytes (white blood cells) have been studied for hereditary factors that predispose a person to RA. One type of leukocyte, the T cell, matures under the influence of the thymus and mediates cellular immunity. This cell-mediated immunity provides the body's main defense against intracellular organisms and involves the identification and removal of foreign substances (antigens) from the body. The entire process depends on the interaction of the antigen with receptors on the surface of the T cell; therefore, T cells are further classified into genetic classes containing human leukocyte antigen (HLA) receptors. A large accumulation of data links specific HLA antigens with particular disease states in the human (10).

The T cell has a binding cleft (receptor site) with specific sensitivity to certain antigens and is complimentary to the structures found in antibodies. One particular class, the HLA-DR4 type, does not distinguish between antigens and healthy tissue and is associated with a susceptibility to RA. As a result, substances that facilitate inflammation of the synovial lining are released.

The following description helps to provide an understanding of the molecular process. Initially, an antigen such as EBV comes in contact with the T-cell receptor; the T-cell membrane becomes activated and is transformed into a large blast cell that then proliferates. The sensitized T cells indirectly stimulate macrophage-like cells of the synovial lining of the joints. During this inflammatory phase the affected joint demonstrates increased heat, swelling, pain, redness, and decreased range of motion (ROM) (13).

Later there is a proliferation of connective tissue and a heavy infiltration by more lymphocytes, as well as plasma cells. The activated synovial cells grow out as a malignant **pannus** (cover) (see Fig. 15.3) over the cartilage, leading to cartilage breakdown. This granulation

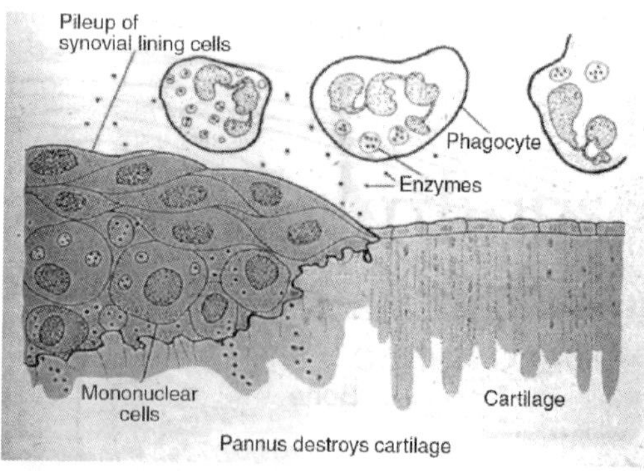

Figure 15.3 Synovial lining cells multiply, creating a mass called pannus. Substances in this mass further damage the underlying cartilage, which softens, weakens, and ultimately is destroyed. The waste products of cartilage cell destruction further stimulate the inflammatory process. New phagocytes rush to the area to clean up the debris. Some lymphocytes and other mononuclear cells are mistakenly rendered capable of attacking cartilage. Lysosomal enzymes and collagenase are released, thus perpetuating the abnormal process. (Reprinted with permission from the Arthritis Foundation. The AHPA Arthritis Teaching Slide Collection. 2nd Ed. 1988.)

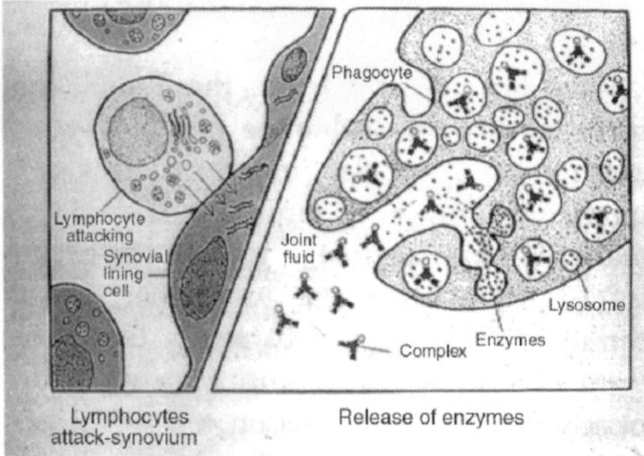

Figure 15.4 In the development of inflammatory rheumatic diseases, the normal protective process of inflammation goes awry. Lymphocytes can no longer distinguish between antigens and healthy tissue, and they secrete substances that cause the synovial lining to become inflamed. Phagocytes become overloaded with immune complexes and release lysosomal enzymes into the joint fluid. The enzymes then attach to the cells of the joint lining eventually destroying them. (Reprinted with permission from the Arthritis Foundation. The AHPA Arthritis Teaching Slide Collection. 2nd Ed. 1988.)

tissue continues to spread, the joint space is slowly effaced by fibrous adhesions, and eventually fibrous **ankylosis** appears. The byproduct of the synovial lining destruction further stimulates the inflammation process, leading to more tissue damage than tissue repair (10) as shown in Figure 15.4. Additional research has demonstrated that individuals who have inherited a specific gene sequence from both parents have a higher risk of developing much more severe RA that could involve internal organs as well as joints. Continued research on genetic factors may facilitate genetic counseling to identify people at higher risk of developing severe forms of RA or of needing more intensive treatment (13,14).

Juvenile Rheumatoid Arthritis

Juvenile rheumatoid arthritis is the most common rheumatic disease in childhood. The diagnostic criteria for JRA are onset at age younger than 16 years, persistent arthritis in 1 or more joints for at least 6 weeks, and exclusion of other types of childhood arthritis (Table 15.1) (15). The three classifications for JRA are summarized in Table 15.2. Estimates of prevalence vary from 30 to 150 per 100,000 per year in Europe and the United States (16). There has been ongoing dialogue among pediatric rheumatologists from different parts of the world about classification of the juvenile arthritides for several decades (17,18).

Childhood arthritis overlaps with many other conditions, and the clinical features lack definitive laboratory test findings. The known genetic and serologic markers are not yet universally applicable or biologically meaningful. Despite these difficulties, an effort has been made to include clinical and laboratory findings, autoantibodies, systemic organ involvement, and genetic risk factors (19).

The international community of pediatric rheumatologists continues to be divided by the classification criteria controversy. Readers of the rheumatology literature need to be cognizant of the origin of the study and the classification system employed. There will likely be more refinement of the classification system. A final system is contingent on homogeneity of subgroups defined by immunogenetics and pathogenesis of the diseases. Systemic JRA (S-JRA) affects 10% of children with JRA. Intermittent fever spikes of more than 101 degrees characterize it. Children with SJRA often experience a rash with the high fever; the rash may be present only when temperature is elevated and is most commonly seen on the trunk. SJRA usually affects multiple joints and may facilitate other problems, such as pericarditis, pleuritis, stomach pain, **anemia**, and an increase in white blood cells. General feelings of fatigue, weakness, and weight loss may be experienced as well. The prognosis is decided by the severity of the arthritis that usually develops with the fever and rash. Onset of JRA may begin at any age; however, the peak of onset is 1 to 6 years old. Boys and girls are equally affected (20).

Table 15.1 CRITERIA FOR THE DIAGNOSIS OF JUVENILE RHEUMATOID ARTHRITIS

I. General
The JRA Criteria subcommittee in 1982 reviewed the1977 Criteria (86) and recommended that JRA be the name for the principal form of chronic arthritic disease in children and that this general class should be classified into three onset subtypes: systemic, polyarticular, and pauciarticular. The onset subtypes may be further subclassified iinto subsets as indicated below. The following classification enumerates the requirements for the diagnosis of JRA and the three clinical onset subtypes and lists subsets of each subtype that may be useful in further classification.

II. General criteria for the diagnosis of juvenile rheumatoid arthritis:
  A. Persistent arthritis of at least 6 weeks duration in one or more joints
  B. Exclusion of other causes of arthritis (see list of exclusions)

III. JRA onset subtypes
The onset subtype is determined by manifestations during the first 6 months of disease and remains the principal classification, although manifestations more closely resembling another subtype may appear later.
  A. Systemic onset JRA: This subtype is defined as JRA with persistent intermittent fever (daily intermittent temperatures to 103°F or higher) with or without rheumatoid rash or other organ involvement. Typical fever and rash will be considered probable systemic onset JRA if not associated with arthritis. Before a definite diagnosis can be made, arthritis, as defined, must be present.
  B. Pauciarticular onset JRA: This subtype is defined as JRA with arthritis in four or fewer joints during the first six months of disease. Patients with systemic onset JRA are excluded from this onset subtype.
  C. Polyarticular JRA: This subtype is defined as JRA with arthritis in five or more joints during the first 6 months of disease. Patients with systemic JRA onset are excluded from this subtype.
  D. The onset subtypes may include the following subsets:
    1. Systemic onset
      a. Polyarthritis
      b. Oligoarthritis
    2. Oligoarthritis (pauciarticular onset)
      a. Antinuclear antibody (ANA) positive-chronic uveitis
      b. RF positive
      c. Seronegative, B27 positive
      d. Not otherwise classified
    3. Polyarthritis
      a. RF positively
      b. Not otherwise classified

IV. Exclusions
  A. Other rheumatic diseases
    1. Rheumatic fever
    2. Systemic lupus erythematosus
    3. Ankylosing spondylitis
    4. Polymyositis or dermatomyositis
    5. Vasculitic syndromes
    6. Scleroderma
    7. Psoriatic arthritis
    8. Reiter's syndrome
    9. Sjögren's syndrome
    10. Mixed connective tissue disease
    11. Behçet's syndrome
  B. Infectious arthritis
  C. Inflammatory bowel disease
  D. Neoplastic disease including leukemia
  E. Nonrheumatic conditions of bones and joints
  F. Hematologic diseases
  G. Psychogenic arthralgia
  H. Miscellaneous
    1. Sarcoidosis
    2. Hypertrophic osteoarthropathy
    3. Villonodular synovitis
    4. Chronic active hepatitis
    5. Familial Mediterranean fever

V. Other proposed terminology for juvenile chronic arthritis,
JCA and JA are new diagnostic terms currently in use in some places for the arthritides of childhood. The diagnoses of JCA and JA are not equivalent to each other, nor to the other diagnosis of juvenile rheumatoid

(Continued)

Table 15.1 CRITERIA FOR THE DIAGNOSIS OF JUVENILE RHEUMATOID ARTHRITIS (*CONT.*)

arthritis or Still's disease. Hence reports of studies of JCA or JA cannot be directly compared with one another nor to reports of JRA or Still's disease. JCA is described in more detail in a report of the European Conference on the Rheumatic Disease of Children (87) and juvenile arthritis in the report of the Ross Conference (88).

Polyarticular JRA affects approximately 40% of children with JRA and is initiated in several joints at once (five or more). The course usually involves the small joints of the hands and fingers but can also affect the weight-bearing joints. The joints are typically affected symmetrically and fevers may be present. JRA is subdivided into two groups and identified most readily by the absence and presence of **rheumatoid factor** (RF). The prognosis for those with an RF-positive factor is that they are at higher risk for erosions, nodules, growth retardation, lack of adequate bone mineralization, anemia, and poor functional status.

Pauciarticular arthritis, or oligoarthritis, accounts for 50% of those with JRA. This type

Table 15.2 JUVENILE RHEUMATOID ARTHRITIS SUBTYPE CHARACTERISTICS

	Systemic	Polyarticular	Pauciarticular
Frequency of cases	10%	40%	50%
Number of joints with arthritis at onset	Variable	≥5	≤4
Sex ratio (F:M)	1:1	3:1	5:1
Frequency of uveitis	1%	5%	20%
Frequency of rheumatoid factor positivity	<20%	5%–10%	<2%
Frequency of ≥5 joints involved any time during course of JRA	50%–60%	100%	40%
Frequency of active disease >10 years follow-up	42%	45%	41%
Frequency of erosions or joint space narrowing on radiographs	45%	54%	28%
Median time to develop erosions or joint space narrowing on radiographs (years after disease onset)	2.2	2.4	5.4
Frequency of adult height <5th percentile	50%	16%	11%

of JRA characteristically affects the large joints such as the knees, ankles, or elbows and engages only a few joints (four or fewer) at a time. Pauciarticular JRA is divided into two groups: late onset and early onset. Those with late onset JRA are usually girls (outnumbering boys 4 to 1) who are very young (1 to 5 years old), have a 30% to 50% chance of developing chronic eye inflammation with complications, and have the best articular outcome. Late onset JRA affects boys who are HLA-B27 positive, have tendonitis, with the large joints (hip and low back) of the body being the most affected (20).

Incidence and Prevalence

Forty-three million Americans in 2004 reported that a doctor told them they have arthritis or other rheumatic conditions. Another 23 million people have chronic joint symptoms but have not been diagnosed with arthritis. Arthritis is the leading cause of disability in the United States, limiting the activities of more than 16 million adults (21). Approximately one in seven people in the general population are affected, and women are affected three times more than men (21). The prevalence of JRA is approximately 1:1000 of the childhood population, with girls being affected seven times more often than boys (22). The prevalence increases with age until about the seventh decade. Eighty percent of all patients who develop RA are between 35 and 50 years of age. Sex differences diminish in the older age group (13).

Racial factors also appear relevant in RA. African American have a lower occurrence of RA than Caucasians. North American Indians have a higher prevalence of RA, whereas native Japanese and Chinese may have a lower prevalence than whites (23). Reasons for these variations are unknown and may be attributed to both genetic and environmental factors. Epidemiologic studies in Africa indicate that climate and urbanization have a major impact on incidence and severity of RA in groups with similar genetic backgrounds (23).

Signs and Symptoms

Onset of symptoms may be sudden and may vary in degree. RA is frequently characterized by exacerbations (flare-ups) and remissions, in which the disease appears to be quiet and non-existent. Though RA is destructive, the course of the disease is variable from person to person. Some individuals experience only a mild, brief monoarticular involvement and minimal joint damage, whereas others will have an ongoing progressive arthritis with significant joint deformity. Most often, RA affects more than one joint at once. In two thirds of patients, an exacerbation is initiated by feelings of fatigue, generalized weakness, weight loss, malaise, and vague musculoskeletal symptoms until synovitis becomes more obvious. Although joint involvement is generally symmetrical, some patients may experience an asymmetrical pattern (23). An exploration of joint involvement can be divided into two sections: stages of inflammatory joint disease as experienced overall and specific manifestations to particular joints.

Articular and Periarticular Involvement

Table 15.3 presents the stages of the inflammatory process: (a) acute, (b) subacute, (c) chronic-active, and (d) chronic-inactive. As previously mentioned, onset may be sudden, with inflammation occurring in many joints at once. In the acute and subacute phases, fatigue may be extensive enough to cause disability from disuse of joint motion and loss of strength before joint changes actually occur.

Table 15.3 STAGES OF INFLAMMATORY JOINT DISEASE

Stages	Objective Signs	Subjective Symptoms
Acute	Limited range of motion Fever Decreased muscle strength Possible cold, sweaty hands Overall stiffness Gel phenomenon most prominent Weight loss Decreased appetite	Pain at rest and movement most severe Inflammation most severe Hot, red joints Decreased function Tingling and numbness in hands and feet
Subacute	Decreased range of motion Poor endurance Mild fever Decreased muscle strength Morning stiffness Gel phenomenon Weight loss Decreased appetite	Pain and tenderness at rest and movement decreases Joints warm and pink Inflammation subsiding Decreased function Tingling and numbness in hands and feet
Chronic-active	Decreased range of motion Fever has subsided Muscle strength decreased Endurance low	Pain and tenderness at rest minimal Pain on motion decreases Inflammation low-grade Increased activity noted, owing to adjustment to pain
Chronic-inactive	Limited range of motion Muscle atrophy Decreased endurance from limited activity in previous stages Residuals seen from above stages Potential contracture	Pain at motion caused by stiffness from disuse during previous stages and instability of joint No inflammation Residuals seen from above stages Functioning may be decreased due to pain

Various degrees of general soreness and aching are experienced. These are usually followed by progressive, localized symptoms of pain, inflammation, warmth, and tenderness in a joint or multiple joints. Symmetrical involvement of small hand joints, feet, wrists, elbows, and ankles is typical, though initial manifestations may occur in any joint. Pain originates primarily from the joint capsule, which is heavily supplied with pain fibers and is highly sensitive to stretching and distension. Joint swelling results from accumulation of synovial fluid, hypertrophy of the synovium, and thickening of the joint capsule. Synovial thickening, the most specific physical finding, eventually occurs in most active joints. Various degrees of generalized stiffness occur, including the gel phenomenon, which is the inability to move joints after prolonged rest. Morning stiffness that lasts longer than 1 hour is an almost universal feature of inflammatory arthritis, one that distinguishes it from noninflammatory disorders. The length and intensity of the stiffness can be used as a gross assessment of disease activity (23).

In JRA, morning stiffness, gelling after inactivity, and night pain are encountered as frequently as in adult disease. Frequently, children may not discuss these symptoms with anyone, so their presence is detected only by caregiver observation. Initial presentation of disease may be detected by the child's increased irritability, joint guarding, or his outright refusal to walk (15).

Also, adults and children with RA have decreased joint motion, decreased muscle strength and endurance, and a loss of appetite and body weight. Patients frequently experience chills in their hands and feet, as well as numbness and tingling. With pain limiting motion, the inflamed joint is usually held in flexion to maximize joint volume and minimize distension of the capsule.

Once the acute and subacute stages have subsided, limited joint range of motion (ROM) causes contractures to form. Contractures are the result of adhesions that form when the patient avoids movement during the acute, painful phase. Limitations in ROM result from ankylosis, subluxation, or dislocation. Muscle atrophy in chronic stages results from disuse in the earlier, more acute stages (24).

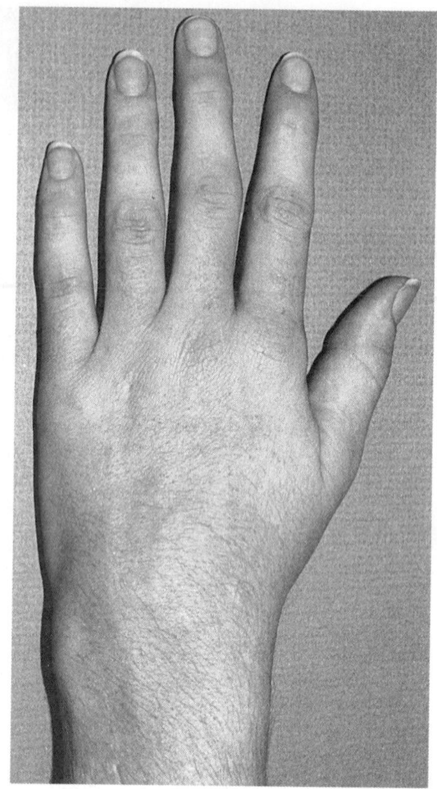

Figure 15.5 Fusiform swelling and erythema about the PIP joints, most significant in the long finger. Swelling at the MCP joints has caused loss of definition of joint margins. The extensor carpi ulnaris tendon sheath (sixth dorsal compartment of the wrist) has synovial thickening and swelling.

Specific Joint Manifestations

Hand

When considering the extremities, the hands are by far the most severely affected by RA (25). Joints with the highest synovium-to-cartilage ratio are those most frequently affected by the disease (23,24). Fusiform or spindle-shaped fingers, a typical sign of RA, result from swelling in the proximal interphalangeal (PIP) joints (Fig. 15.5). This is usually related to bilateral and symmetrical swelling of the metacarpophalangeal (MCP) joints. Pressure on these joints causes tenderness. Distal interphalangeal (DIP) joints are rarely involved which discriminates RA from osteoarthritis and psoriatic arthritis (5,26).

Boutonniere and **swan-neck deformities** are two other common hand deformities that result from RA. A **boutonniere deformity** is a combination of PIP joint flexion and DIP joint hyperextension (Fig. 15.6) More specifically, it is flexion of the PIP joint through the detached central slip of the extensor tendon, which serves as a "button-hole" through which the joint can pop. The DIP joint is then forced into hyperextension. Swan-neck deformities result from contractures of the interosseus and flexor muscles and tendons, which in turn produce a flexure contracture of the MCP joint, compensatory hyperextension of the PIP joint, and flexion of the DIP joint

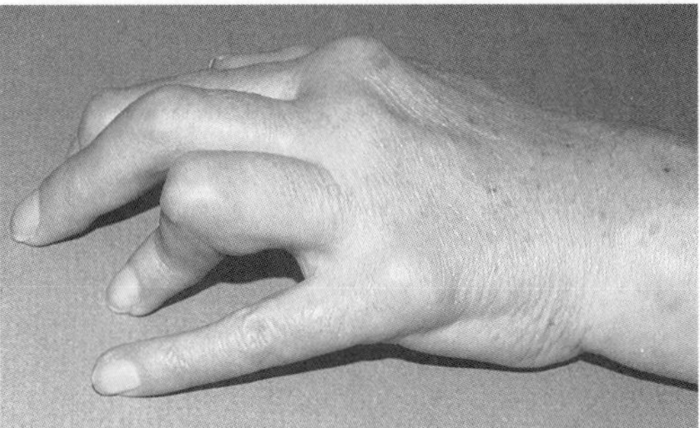

Figure 15.6 A boutonniere deformity of the ring finger, flexion deformity of the long finger PIP joint, and mild swan-neck deformity of the index finger. Extensive synovitis at the MCP joints obscures the usual definition of joint margins.

(Fig. 15.7). Thumb deformities associated with RA have been classified into three categories. In type I, MCP inflammation leads to stretching of the joint capsule and boutonniere-like deformity. In type II, edema of the carpometacarpal (CMC) joint leads to volar subluxation during ankylosis of the adductor pollicis. In type III, after sustained disease of both MCP joints, exaggerated adduction of the first metacarpus, flexion of the MCP joint, and hyperextension of the DIP joint result from the patient's need to establish a compensatory method to pinch (27). Stiffness and crepitary inflammation along the tendon sheath with limitations of flexion and extension may be exhibited (Fig. 15.8). Finger "triggering" occurs when thickening or nodule formation of the tendon interplays with the tenosynovial inflammation, trapping the tendon in a flexed position. Tendon rupture most frequently occurs in the abductors of the thumb and extensor carpi ulnaris of the fourth and fifth fingers. Rupture of the latter is usually caused by a combination of synovitis in the tendon sheaths and mechanical irritation from an eroded and subluxed distal ulna (28).

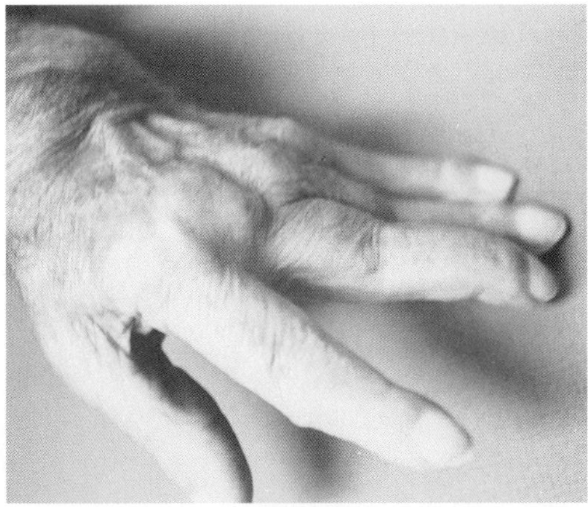

Figure 15.7 Swan-neck deformities of long, ring, and little fingers, with concomitant subluxation of the MCP joints.

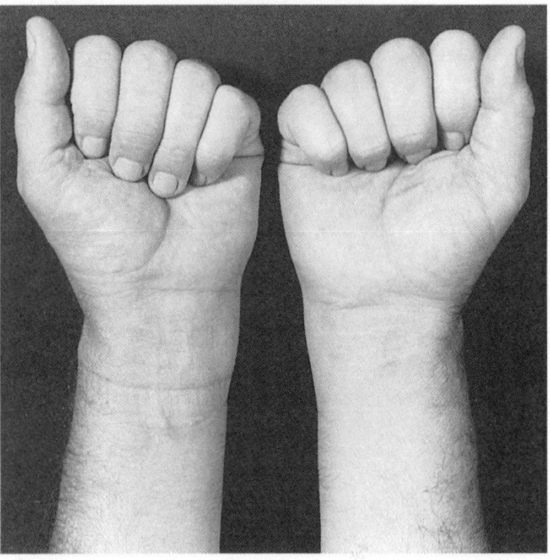

Figure 15.8 Flexor tendinitis at the wrist and in the palm leading to decreased flexion of the fingers of the left hand.

De Quervain's tenosynovitis, (Fig. 15.9) which involves extensors at the thumb, causes severe pain and discomfort, resulting in a decrease in hand function and the ability to grip. Mutilans deformity (opera glass hand) causes transverse folds of the skin of the thumb and fingers, resembling a folded telescope. Pulling on the fingers during examination may lengthen the digit much like opening opera glasses, or the joint may bend in unusual directions just by the pull of gravity. Radiographs of the fingers and thumb identify severe bone resorption, erosions, shortening of the MCP, PIP, radiocarpal, and radioulnar joints (Fig. 15.10) (28). The gross instability of

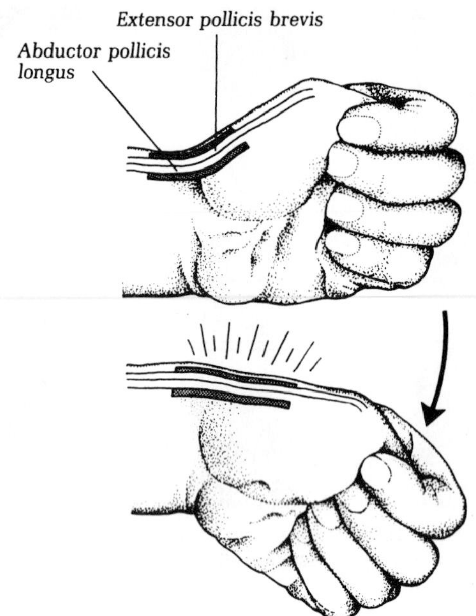

Figure 15.9 Finkelstein's test for de Quervain's disease.

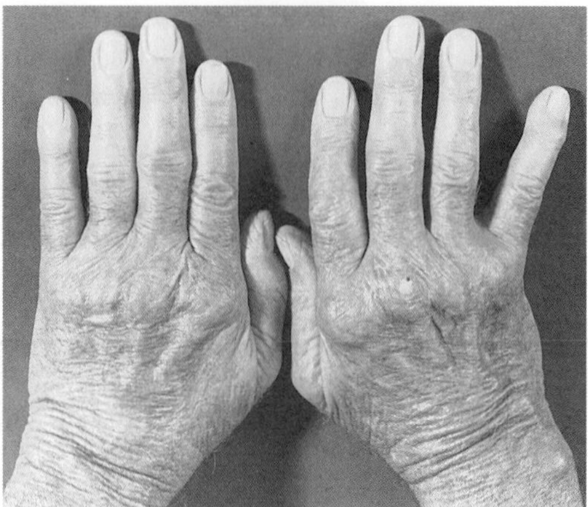

Figure 15.11 Subcutaneous tissue atrophy, MCP joint proliferation synovitis with loss of joint definition, and mild PIP joint enlargement. There is slight volar subluxation of the MCP joints and mild ulnar deviation at the MCP joints of the right hand. Involvement of the dominant (right) hand is more pronounced.

the thumbs and severely deformed phalanges negatively affect hand function and participation in a wide variety of daily living activities.

Wrist

Ulnar deviations and volar subluxation at the MCP joints or radiocarpal deviation are characteristic signs of RA at the wrist as seen in Figure 15.11. These problems develop and result from severe **tenosynovitis** and inflammation where the ligaments surround the joint and eventually lead to edema, joint laxity, erosion of the tendons and ligaments, and muscle imbalance. When ulnar deviation of the MCP is present with radial deviation at the radiocarpal joint, a "zig-zag" presentation of the hand is seen (Figs. 15.12 and 15.13). Dorsiflexion of the wrist often is one of the first movements to be limited. **Carpal tunnel syndrome** is commonly diagnosed, resulting

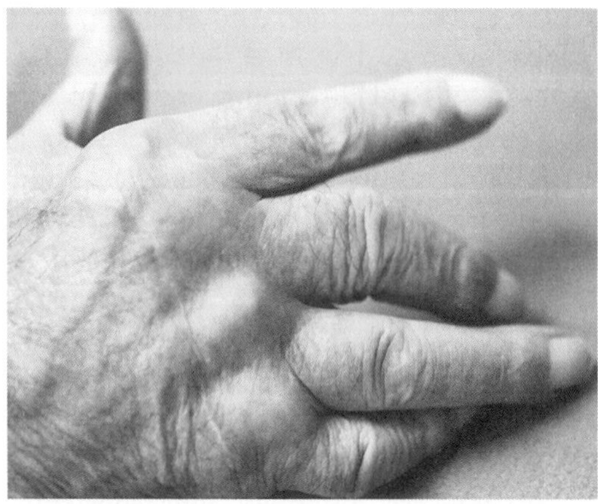

Figure 15.10 Arthritis mutilans. The long PIP joint has been destroyed by RA. Deflection of the distal portion of the phalanx is caused by the pull of gravity.

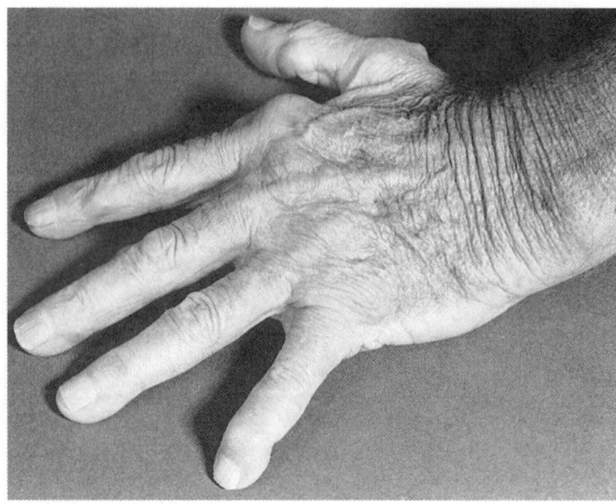

Figure 15.12 "Zig-zag" deformity with ulnar deviation of the fingers at the MCP joints and clockwise rotation of carpus on the distal radius.

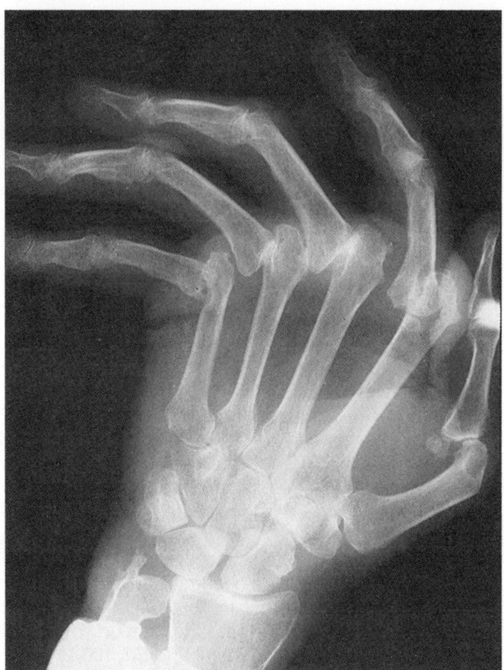

Figure 15.13 Severe MCP joint subluxations in the volar and ulnar directions. There is a concomitant clockwise rotation of the carpus on the distal radius ("zig-zag deformity"). Erosions of the ulnar styloid and metacarpal heads are evident.

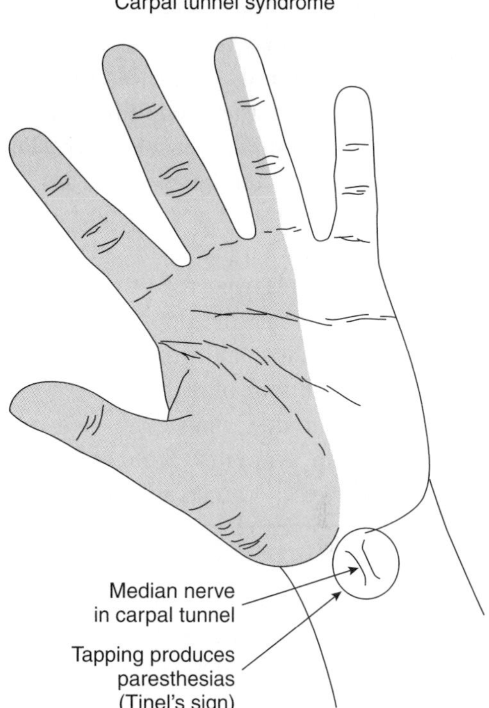

Figure 15.14 Distribution of pain or paresthesias (shaded area) when the median nerve is compressed by swelling in the wrist (carpal tunnel).

from synovial proliferations on the volar aspect of the wrist, which then impinge upon the median nerve (29). This causes paresthesia of the palmar aspect of the thumb, the second and third digits, and the radial aspect of the fourth digit (Fig. 15.14).

Elbow

Loss of motion because of flexion contractures in addition to inflammation are the most prevalent problems with elbow involvement. Synovial swelling and thickening may be observed in the lateral area between the radial head and the olecranon. A bulge will be seen. Synovitis in the radiohumeral joint can result in decreased motion during pronation and supination of the forearm. Lateral epicondylitis, more often referred to as tennis elbow, is reported as sharply painful when firm pressure is placed on this specific area. Other symptoms include paresthesia over the fourth and fifth fingers and weakness in the flexor muscle of the fifth digit.

Shoulder

Shoulder involvement is common and can complicate significantly as RA progresses. The glenohumeral, acromioclavicular, and thoracoscapular joints are the most susceptible. Because the shoulder capsule lies beneath the muscular rotator cuff, inflammation is difficult to detect during physical assessment. Difficulty with shoulder movement and with participation in daily living activities is usually the chief complaint, followed by pain and tenderness (30). Because the shoulder relies on extensive coordinated movement, when any one of these joints becomes affected, dysfunction in activities of daily living (ADL) is seen.

Impairment in ability to manage and carry out self-care tasks may be significant.

Localized pain and tenderness, resulting from tendonitis in the glenohumeral area where the supraspinatus muscle or the long head of the biceps tendon inserts, are frequently seen. Rotator cuff tears are likely where the rotator cuff tendon inserts into the greater tuberosity. Erosion is triggered by the proliferative synovitis that develops there (31). Tendinitis, capsulitis, and **bursitis** (grouped under local conditions of arthritis categories) are causes of shoulder pain diagnosed more frequently than synovitis. Synovitis of the glenohumeral area is seen occasionally in those with RA and is observed as a bulge in the anterior or lateral superior area of the shoulder. Loss of motion is a complication of shoulder synovitis, which is seen in progressed cases and is known as frozen shoulder.

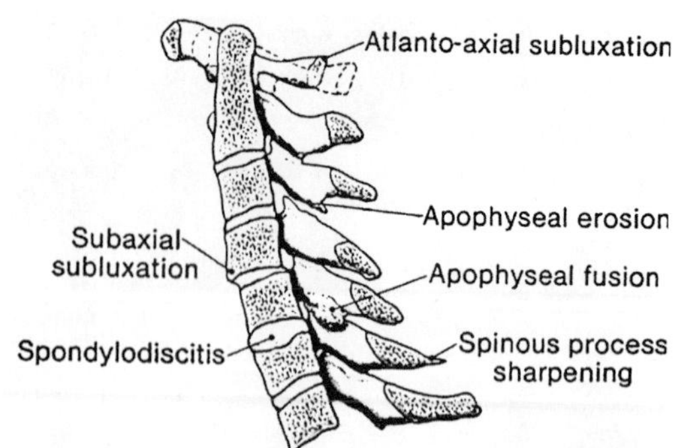

Figure 15.15 Neck abnormalities in RA. The neck is usually involved in adult and juvenile RA. The most common disorder is subluxation of the atlantoaxial joint, which occurs particularly on flexion of the neck. C1 moves forward on C2, and the odontoid process can actually cause pressure on the spinal cord posteriorly. Other findings include erosions at the apophyseal joints, fusion of the apophysial joint, which occurs particularly in JRA, and subluxation at other levels. Disc involvement also may occur, and erosive changes and resorption can cause sharpening of the spinous process. (Reprinted with permission from the Arthritis Foundation. The AHPA Arthritis Teaching Slide Collection. 2nd Ed. 1988.)

Head, Neck, and Cervical Spine

The cervical spine is often involved in RA (32). Involvement of C1 and C2 may produce life-threatening conditions. Neck pain on motion and occipital headaches are common symptoms of cervical spine involvement and occur in those individuals who have had RA longer than 10 years (33). Patients with severe deformities in their hands, as in mutilans deformity, are very likely to have had significant amounts of corticosteroids for RA management (34).

During radiologic examination of this area in advanced cases of RA, the lower cervical and odontoid processes often appear eroded, as do the cervical **apophyseal** and intervertebral joints. The first to the fourth cervical joints are those most commonly affected by inflammation and pain (Figs. 15.15 and 15.16). Involvement of the upper cervical spine in advanced cases leads to subluxation, whereas lower cervical spine involvement produces symptoms of cord-root compression. For example, with a C5 root compression, problems

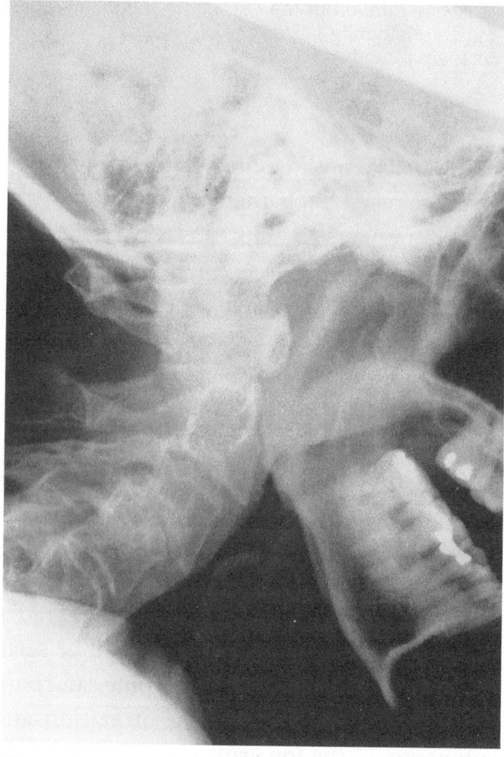

Figure 15.16 A lateral radiograph of a patient with RA who is experiencing severe upper extremity neurological decline caused by C2–C3 and C3 and C4 anterior subluxations. The odontoid is not visible because of severe erosion.

are (a) sensation on the radial aspect of the forearm, (b) muscle weakness and abduction of the shoulder and flexion of the elbow, and (c) decreased biceps jerk reflex. Subluxation also can cause twisting and compression of the vertebral arteries, which can lead to vertebrobasilar artery insufficiency. This may be facilitated by syncope on downward gaze. Flexion and extension of the cervical spine are usually less affected. The temporomandibular joints (TMJ) have varied involvement in RA, ranging from 1% to 60% by some estimates. Women are affected three times more often than men. Both TMJ are usually involved (35). Involvement of this synovial joint results in the inability to open the mouth fully because of side-to-side gliding and protrusion. After persistent inflammation, normal approximation of the upper and lower teeth may be affected.

Hoarseness occurs in up to 30% of patients presenting with RA. This stems from inflamed cricoarytenoid joints, which rotate with the vocal cords as they abduct and adduct to vary pitch and tone of the voice (36).

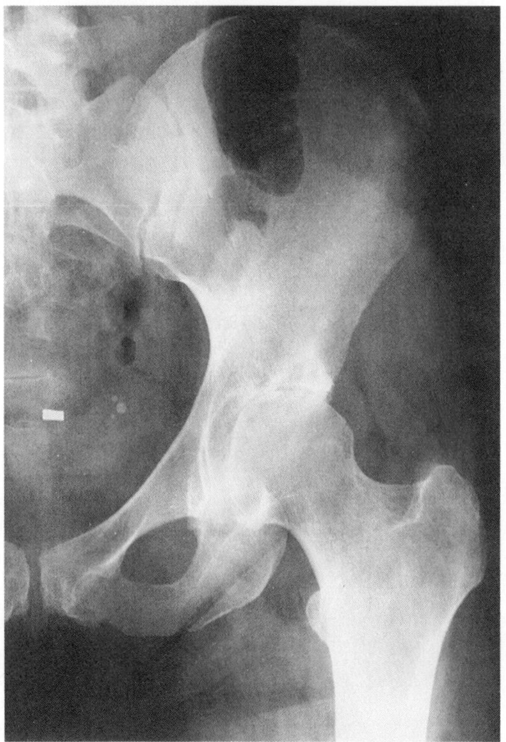

Figure 15.17 Hip radiograph of a patient with RA. There is diffuse joint space narrowing, small cysts in the femoral head and acetabulum, and little reparative bony change.

Hip

Approximately half of the patients diagnosed with RA have radiographic evidence of hip disease as seen in Figure 15.17. Although hip involvement is common, early manifestations of the hip disease are typically not apparent because the location of the joint is deep within the pelvis. With progressive hip involvement, an abnormal gait pattern, possibly in the form of a limp, may be observed. This can result from a variety of factors, including pain, flexion contractures, muscle weakness, or hip instability (37). Fibrous contractures in flexion or external rotation are standard if restriction of motion is prolonged. Because the hip joint capsule is limited in its ability to stretch, severe RA involvement followed by swelling and massive effusion of synovium into the joint capsule may be extremely painful. It is also to be noted that hip involvement will result in discomfort and pain in the groin and the medial aspect of the knee.

As involvement increases (e.g., increased flexion contractures), more functional problems will be experienced in all mobility activities, donning lower extremity garments, sitting in a chair comfortably, ascending stairs, and positioning during sexual activity.

Knee

Hypertrophy and effusion of large amounts of synovium into the joint capsule are common in the knee joint and are more readily demonstrated in the knee than in the hip (Fig. 15.18). Greater than 5 mL of synovial fluid in the knee may be observed as a "bulge" sign; bulges occur behind the patella when fluid is pushed into the suprapatellar

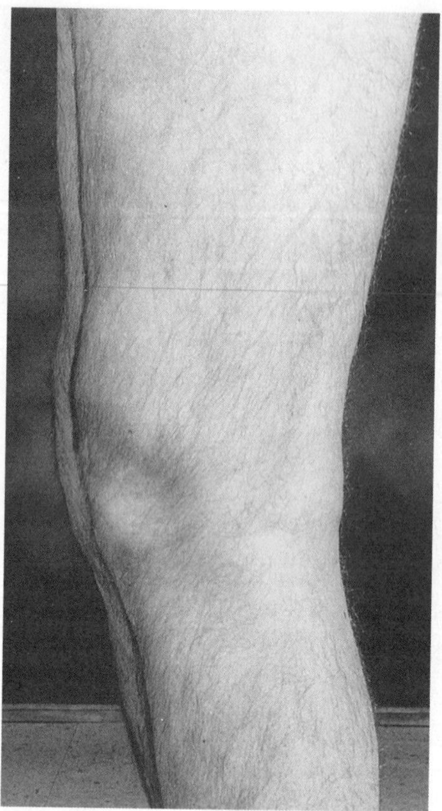

Figure 15.18 Lateral view of a patient with RA affecting the knees. There is quadriceps atrophy, significant synovial proliferation with joint effusion in the suprapatellar pouch, and fullness in the popliteal space because of a small synovial (Baker's) cyst.

pouch and then back into the joint. Swelling, quadriceps muscle atrophy, ligamentous laxity, and joint instability may be more obvious when the patient stands or walks. Pain and swelling on the posterior knee may be caused by significant increases in intra-articular pressure during flexion, which produces an out-pouching, or Baker's cyst. Popliteal cysts such as these may impede superior venous flow in the thigh, producing a dilation of veins and edema (38). When the joint capsule is stretched, a reflex spasm triggers in the hamstring muscles. To relieve joint pain and tension, patients will hold their hips and knees in a flexion position that facilitates contractures. These contractures will cause difficulty in all weight-bearing activities.

Ankle and Foot

True rheumatic disease is less common in the ankle than in other areas of the body and usually is not seen without concurrent midfoot or metatarsophalangeal (MTP) involvement. Tibiotalar swelling and loss of subtalar motion can develop. Ankle synovitis can be palpated in front of, behind, and below the malleoli. The ankle is often very tender and sensitive.

Symptomatic involvement of the feet is reported by 30% to 90% of those who have RA (39). RA of the toes involving the MTP joints results in changes similar to those in the hands. When the MTP joints are affected, normal gait is disrupted. Problems will be exhibited during the push-off phase of ambulation, causing compensatory action with other weight-bearing joints.

Characteristic manifestations of the feet include claw toes, hammer toes, cock-up toes, and hallux valgus (40). Claw toes result from the hyperextension of the MTP and the flexion of the PIP and DIP joints. Hammer toes differ from claw toes in that the DIP joint is hyperextended as seen in Figure 15.19. Cocking up the

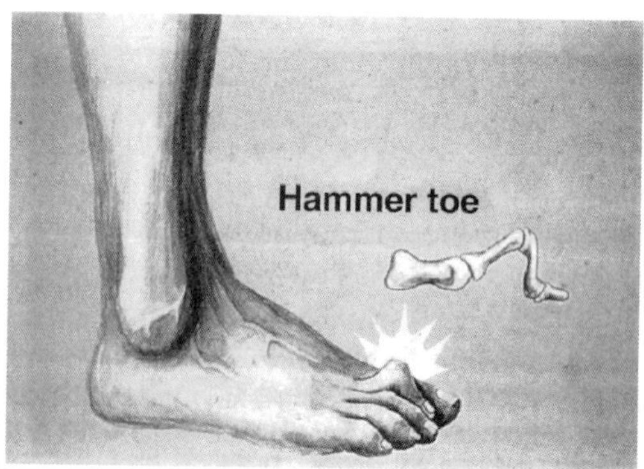

Figure 15.19 In this diagram, the second tow has a cock-up deformity, which is similar to the boutonniere abnormality of the hand. Often this deformity is associated with subluxation of the corresponding MTP joints. This deformity may be hastened in a patient who wears shoes that are too small. Rubbing of the PIP joints on other joints causes pain, callus formation, and possibly ulceration. This abnormality is not restricted to patients with RA. (Reprinted with permission from the Arthritis Foundation. The AHPA Arthritis Teaching Slide Collection. 2nd Ed. 1988.)

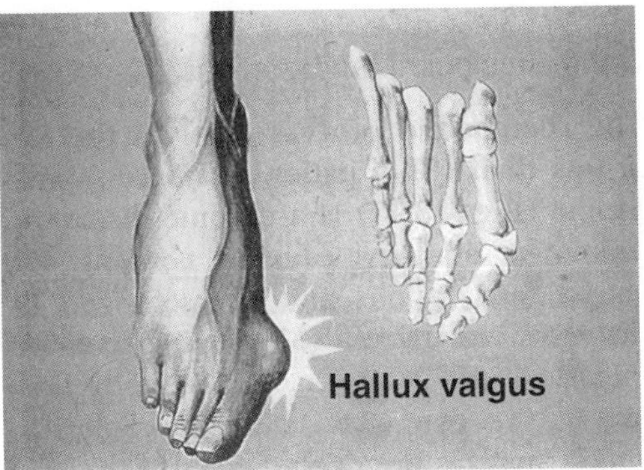

Figure 15.20 An anatomical and clinical diagram of hallux vagus. Pes planus and ligamentous laxity lead to lateral deviation of the great toe with a resultant hallux vagus. This deformity can be hastened by the wearing of narrow-toed shoes. Rubbing of the bunion on the shoe surface produced pain, and the lateral deviation of the great toe may impinge on other digits of the foot. This abnormality is not restricted to patients with RA. (Reprinted with permission from the Arthritis Foundation. The AHPA Arthritis Teaching Slide Collection. 2nd Ed. 1988.)

toes may be associated with subluxation of the metatarsal heads and, finally, a claw-like appearance with an elevation of the tip of the toe above the surface on which the foot is resting. Hallux valgus is a common event in which the fibular deviation of the first through fourth toes occurs. This is similar to ulnar deviation of the hands (Figs. 15.20 and 15.21). Rheumatoid nodules develop over bony prominences that bear more

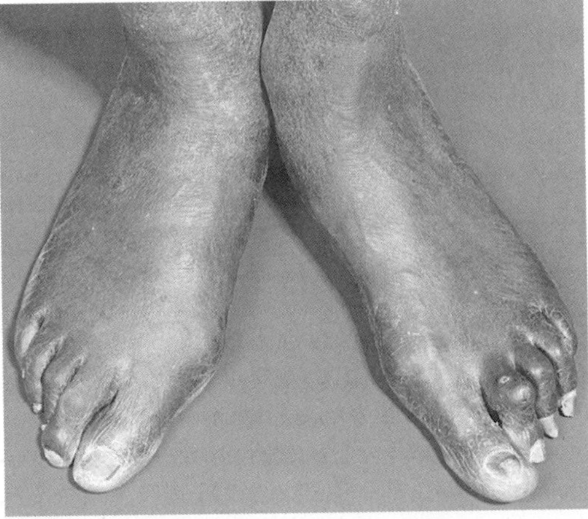

Figure 15.21 Mild hallux valgus, with dorsal subluxation of the MTP joints and resultant "hammer toe" deformities of second through fifth toes. Midfoot instability has lead to eversion, with concomitant flattening of the feet.

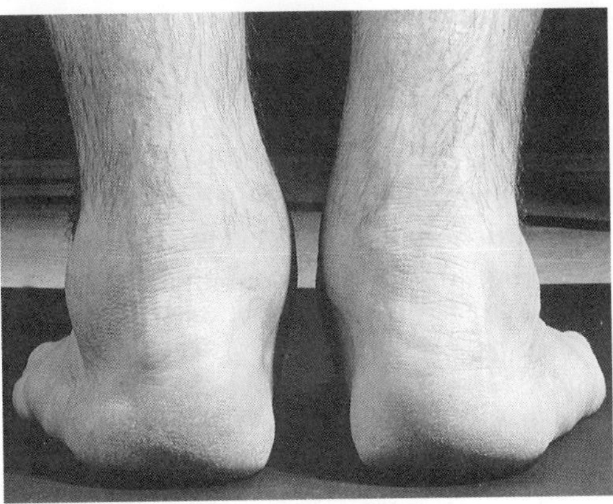

Figure 15.22 Significant ankle and midfoot synovitis. Loss of definition of the arch and eversion at the subtalar joint also are evident.

than normal pressure. For individuals affected by painful forefoot weight bearing, rheumatoid nodules can occur on the heels because of increased weight bearing there (41).Tarsal joint involvement does not occur as often as in the forefoot; however, it can be detrimental to a person's ability to ambulate. As the longitudinal arch in the foot flattens and hind foot valgus occurs, weight-bearing pressure tends to shift medially (Fig. 15.22). This, in turn, facilitates the possible development of callosities and more rheumatoid nodule formation (42).

Muscle Involvement

Most individuals with RA have muscle involvement, including muscle weakness. Researchers have suggested five stages of muscle disease in the RA process:

1. Reduction of muscle bulk associated with muscle atrophy that accompanies the inflammatory process as a result of disuse, bed rest, vascular events, and drug effects. A muscle can lose up to 30% of its bulk in 1 week, with loss of muscle bulk being associated with decline in function.
2. Peripheral neuromyopathy, usually related to mononeuritis multiplex, which is

frequently associated with rheumatoid vasculitis involving localized sensory loss.
3. Steroid myopathy.
4. Active myositis and muscle necrosis (or muscle fiber inflammation resulting in destruction of the muscle fibers).
5. Chronic myopathy resembling a dystrophic process.

Tendon

Tendon damage may result from inflammation of the synovial lining of the tendon sheath (tenosynovitis) and interferes with smooth gliding of the tendon. A lag phenomenon may be seen in patients with tendon damage or muscle weakening, displaying a significant difference between passive and active range of motion.

Extra-Articular Systemic Manifestations

As has been mentioned previously in this chapter, RA affects the joint and is systemic. The number and severity of extra-articular features vary with the duration and extent of the disease and tend to occur in individuals with higher levels of RF in their blood. The following are additional manifestations that may exist in those with RF.

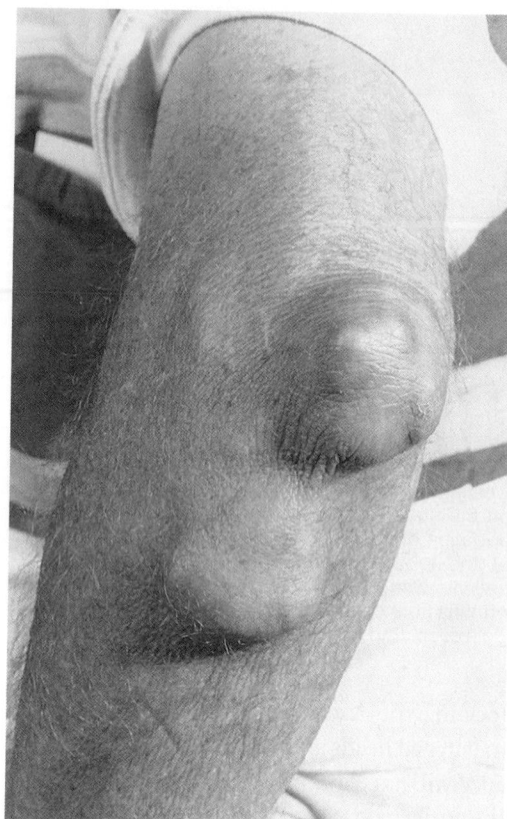

Figure 15.23 Large rheumatoid nodules in the olecranon bursa and along the extensor surface of the proximal ulna. Each mass is a collection of multiple smaller nodules. A small effusion is present in the olecranon bursa.

Rheumatoid or Subcutaneous Nodules

Rheumatoid nodule formation is one of the most common extra-articular manifestations of RA and occurs in up to 50% of individuals at some point during the course of the disease (13,43). Periarticular structures, extensor surfaces, and areas subject to pressure such as the olecranon (Fig. 15.23), the proximal ulna, the Achilles tendon, the occiput, and the sacrum are primary sites for those growths. Most can develop insidiously and regress at any time.

Pulmonary Manifestation

Pleuritis, interstitial fibrosis, pulmonary nodules, pneumonitis, and other forms of pulmonary obstructive disease occur more frequently in those with RA than in the population at large. Evidence of pleuritis is usually found at autopsy, because the disease is generally asymptomatic during life. In a few cases, upper airway obstruction from cricoarytenoid arthritis or laryngeal nodules may develop. Some researchers believe that small-airway dysfunction is related to factors other than RA.

Felty's Syndrome

The condition of leukopenia associated with collagen-vascular disorders, called Felty's syndrome, occurs in less than 1% of patients with RA (44). This syndrome is usually found in those who have progressed and have chronic RA, as well as those who have high levels of RF (13). Splenomegaly, leukopenia, anemia, neutropenia, thrombocytopenia, and granulocytopenia also are features of this syndrome. Although hypersplenism is proposed as one of the causes of leucopenia, splenectomies do not correct the abnormality in many patients.

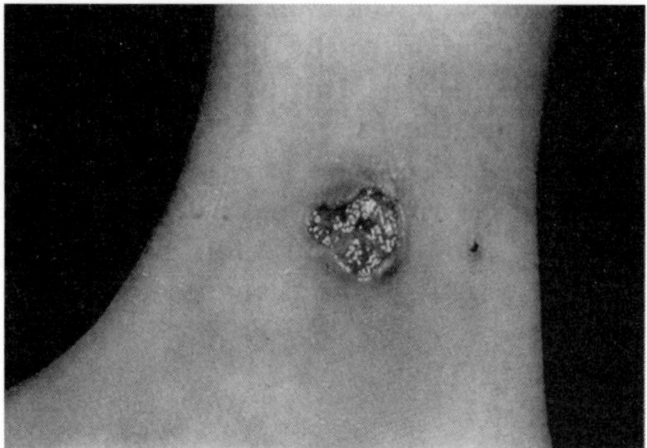

Figure 15.24 Vasculitis, defined as inflammation of the small vessels, is common in RA. The most common vascular abnormality in patients with RA is leg ulceration, which may be indolent and difficult to heal. Ulcers are not usually associated with either arterial or venous insufficiency. Other vasculitis problems among patients with RA include benign digital (fingertip) ulceration and severe systemic vasculitis similar to polyarteritis nodosa. (Reprinted with permission from the Arthritis Foundation. The AHPA Arthritis Teaching Slide Collection. 2nd Ed. 1988.)

Cardiac Manifestations

Asymptomatic pericarditis is found in nearly 50% of autopsied cases (45,46). Most pericardial disease develops with synovitis several years into the course of RA. Manifestations may vary from mild to being the actual cause of death. Other forms of cardiac disease in RA include rheumatoid carditis, endocardial (valve) inflammation, conduction defects, coronary arteritis, and granulomatous aortitis (45,46).

Nervous System

Neurological manifestations may be caused by cervical spine subluxation. As briefly described in the neck, cervical spine, and wrist sections in this chapter, nerve entrapment that is the result of proliferative synovitis or joint deformities may facilitate neuropathies of the median, ulnar, radial, or anterior tibial nerves. In aggressive forms of vasculitis (Fig. 15.24), polyneuropathy and mononeuritis multiplex may result (47). Direct central nervous system involvement does not appear to occur, but vasculitis and rheumatoid nodule-like granulomas can occur irregularly in the meninges (48).

Ophthalmologic Manifestations

The rheumatoid process involves the eye in less than 1% of patients. **Sjögren's syndrome** (Fig.15.25) is a chronic disease of unknown etiology causing corneal and conjunctival lesions and is characterized by dry eyes and mouth (49). Eye discomfort includes the inability to cry and a sandy feeling when blinking. Scleritis, which involves the deeper layers of the eye, may cause pain and visual impairment. Episcleritis is a less serious inflammatory condition and is usually temporary (49).

Eye involvement occurs in 30% to 50% of early onset JRA (Fig. 15.26). In 80% of those children who experience eye involvement, the

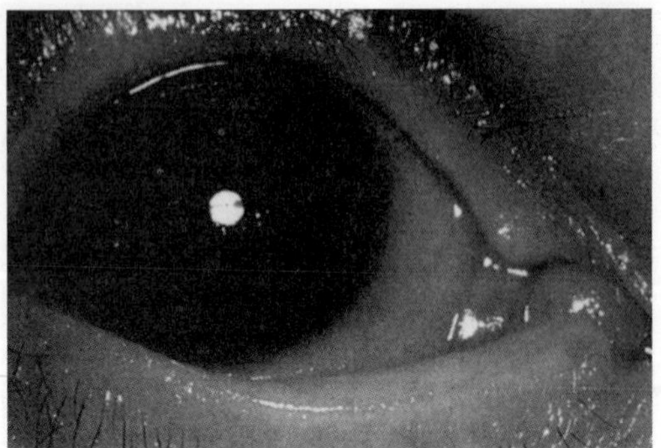

Figure 15.25 Patients with RA may also have Sjögren's syndrome. Sjogren's syndrome is a chronic inflammatory disorder characterized by diminished lacrimal and salivary gland secretions (sicca complex), resulting in keratoconjunctivitis sicca and xerostomia. Patients may complain that the eyes feel "as if they have sand in them." The syndrome also may include decreased vaginal lubrication. Keratoconjunctivitis sicca is demonstrated here by flecks of reddish-purple discoloration in the lower portion of the cornea and conjunctiva, which were stained with rose bengal dye. One-half of all patients with Sjogren's syndrome have RA or some other connective tissue disease, particularly systemic lupus erythematosus or systemic sclerosis. More than 90% of these patients are women, with a mean age of 50 years at the time of diagnosis. Keratoconjunctivitis sicca develops in 10% to 15% of all patients with RA. (Reprinted with permission from the Arthritis Foundation. The AHPA Arthritis Teaching Slide Collection. 2nd Ed. 1988.)

inflammation process primarily involves the anterior chamber of the eye with minimal to no symptoms. Cases have been reported including severe, irreversible eye changes as a result of corneal clouding, cataracts, glaucoma, and partial or total loss of vision. Children with JRA should be screened at regular intervals and treated by eye specialists (50).

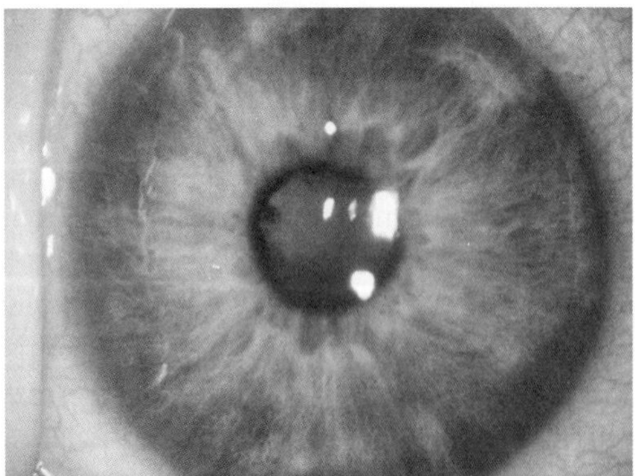

Figure 15.26 Chronic changes in the eye with JRA iritis: posterior synechiae (iris-lens adhesions at pupil margin); iris bombe (shallowing of the anterior chamber caused by blockage of aqueous flow from posterior chamber through pupil); secondary cataract. (Reprinted with permission from Hiles DA. Slide atlas of pediatric physical diagnosis. In: Zitelli BJ, Davis HW, eds. Pediatric Ophthalmology. New York: Gower Medical Publishing, 1987:15.)

Depression

Depression has been identified as a significant problem for those with arthritis. Researchers have determined that the greater the negative impact on an individual's ability to accomplish daily living activities, the greater the likelihood that he or she will develop symptoms of depression (51–57).

Body Composition

Researchers at the United States Department of Agriculture (USDA) Human Nutrition Center on Aging at Tufts University and New England Medical Center found that among persons with RA, changes in their immune system and the substance it produces resulted in higher metabolism, loss of lean body mass, and loss of appetite. This, in turn, suggests that the use of measures for lean mass in those with RA might identify high-risk individuals who could then be identified for interventions, such as nutritional counseling, to improve body composition (58,59).

Course and Prognosis

The course of RA tends to vary from person to person because its effects can differ so dramatically from case to case. Physical and functional outcomes are often difficult for the clinician to predict with accuracy. Onset of the disease is usually gradual or insidious, though too it may be abrupt. As a result of the cyclical nature of the RA process, an individual's ability to function can fluctuate according to the stage and severity of the disease (30). Approximately

Table 15.4 PROPOSED CRITERIA FOR CLINICAL REMISSION IN RHEUMATOID ARTHRITIS

Five or more of the following requirements must be fulfilled for at least 2 consecutive months:

1. Duration of morning stiffness not exceeding 15 minutes
2. No fatigue
3. No joint pain (by history)
4. No joint tenderness or pain on motion
5. No soft tissue swelling in joints of tendon sheaths
6. Erythrocyte sedimentation rate (Westergren method) less than 30 mm/hr for a female or 20 mm/hr for a male

These criteria are intended to describe either spontaneous remission or drug-induced disease suppression, which stimulates spontaneous remission. To be considered for this designation, a patient must have met the American Rheumatism Association criteria for definite or classic rheumatoid arthritis at some time in the past. No alternative explanation may be involved to account for the failure to meet a particular requirement. For instance, in the presence of knee pain that might be related to degenerative arthritis, a point for "no joint pain" may not be awarded. Exclusions: Critical manifestations of active vasculitis pleuritis, or myositis, and unexplained recent weight loss or fever attributed to RA will prohibit a designation of complete clinical remission.

20% of patients will improve spontaneously, and may even achieve remission, especially in the first year of the disease. However, chronic disease progression and functional deterioration occur in the majority of all cases (60). Long-term studies have determined that patients with RA have greater probability of restrictions in daily activities, restrictions in activity days, and 10 times the work disability rate as the general population (5,60–62).

In children with JRA, 70% to 90% make a satisfactory recovery from their disease without serious disability. A small percentage will develop recurrence as adults (15).

Researchers have found that some patients do experience spontaneous remission. Features that appear to have prognostic importance are: (a) number and length of remissions, (b) levels of RF, (c) presence of subcutaneous nodules, (d) extent of bone erosion seen radiographically at the initial evaluation, and (e) sustained disease activity for more than 1 year. Additionally, it has been learned that in patients younger than age 50, women tend to have a worse prognosis with regard to persistence and severity (Table 15.4) (60).

Classification and prognosis of RA also can be assessed by functional analysis as outlined in Table 15.5. The functional capacity of an individual declines as the disease becomes more prevalent. Research has established both an immediate and long-term relationship between

Table 15.5 CLASSIFICATION OF FUNCTIONAL CAPACITY IN RHEUMATOID ARTHRITIS

Class I:	Complete functional capacity with the ability to carry on all usual duties without handicaps
Class II:	Functional capacity adequate to conduct normal activities despite handicap of discomfort or limited mobility of one or more joints
Class III:	Functional capacity adequate to perform only a few or none of the duties of usual occupation or self-care
Class IV:	Largely or wholly incapacitated, with patient bedridden or confined to wheelchair, permitting little or no self-care

arthritis and limitations in function (63). Self-reported functional status and the physical demands of work are the best predictors of disability. Lack of autonomy over the work schedule, the pace of the work, and the nature of the job all increase the likelihood of becoming disabled (64). Early mortality has been linked by researchers to functional disability (65).

Although there is no cure for RA, treatment methods continue to improve. Data suggest that individuals currently admitted to the hospital for RA are likely to have a decreased number of contractures and less fusion of peripheral joints at admission than did a similar cohort of patients 20 years ago (5). Upon completion of a thorough evaluation by a physician, early diagnosis can assist in the development of a treatment approach to reduce joint pain, impede the disease process, and decrease joint deformity. Early classification of the disease facilitates earlier intervention and, ideally a slowing of the disease process and progress.

Emotional and financial supports for treatment contribute to the prognostic outcome and performance of children and adults. Research has demonstrated a high incidence of depression, decreased self-esteem, and social withdrawal. In those individuals with a progressed case of RA, the type of treatment prescribed plays a key part in life expectancy as well as ultimate quality of life.

Diagnosis

Individuals with joint disease delay seeking medical care on average on 2 to 4 years (13). It is much more difficult to establish a diagnosis of RA in the early development of the disease than in the more progressed, later stages. Several visits to a physician for evaluation and testing may be required before a definitive diagnosis can be confirmed. The American

Table 15.6 CLASSIFICATION OF PROGRESSION OF RHEUMATOID ARTHRITIS*

Stage 1—Early
- *1. No destructive changes on roentgenographic examination
- 2. Roentgenological evidence of osteoporosis may be present

Stage II—Moderate
- *1. Roentgenological evidence of osteoporosis with or without slight subchondral bone destruction; slight cartilage destruction may be present
- *2. No joint deformities, although limitation of joint mobility may be present
- 3. Extensive muscle atrophy
- 4. Extra-articular soft tissue lesions, such as nodules and tenosynovitis, may be present

Stage III—Severe
- *1. Roentgenological evidence of cartilage and bone destruction in addition to osteoporosis.
- *2. Joint deformity such as subluxation, ulnar deviation, or hyperextension, without fibrous or bony ankylosis
- 3. Extensive muscle atrophy
- 4. Extra-articular soft tissue lesions, such as nodules and tenosynovitis, may be present

Stage IV—Terminal
- *1. Fibrous or bone ankylosis
- 2. Same criteria of stage III

*An asterisk marks criteria required for classification in the particular stage. See Table 14.5 for clinical remission criteria.

Table 15.7 1987 ARA REVISED CRITERIA FOR THE CLASSIFICATION OF RHEUMATOID ARTHRITIS

1. Morning stiffness	Morning stiffness in and around the joints lasting at least 1 hour before maximal improvement
2. Arthritis of three or more joint areas	At least three joint areas at the same time have had soft tissue swelling or fluid observed by a physician. The 14 possible areas are right or left PIP, MCP, wrist, elbow, knee, ankle, and MTP joints.
3. Arthritis of hand joints	At least one area swollen in a wrist, MCP, or PIP joint
4. Symmetric arthritis	Simultaneous involvement of the same joint areas on both sides of the body (bilateral involvement of PIPs MCPs, or MTPs is acceptable without absolute symmetry)
5. Rheumatoid nodules	Subcutaneous nodules over bony prominences or extensor surfaces or in juxta-articular regions, observed by a physician
6. Serum rheumatoid factor	Demonstration of abnormal amounts of serum RF by any method for which the result has been positive in 5% of normal subjects
7. Radiographic changes	Radiographic changes typical of RA on posteroanterior hand and wrist radiographs, which must include erosions or unequivocal bony decalcification localized in the involved joints.

College of Rheumatology (ACR), formerly the Rheumatism Association (ARA), first developed diagnostic criteria for the classification of RA in 1958, with revisions in 1987 (Tables 15.6 and 15.7). Originally, these criteria were guidelines for classification of disease syndromes to allow correct diagnosis in individuals taking part in clinical research investigations. The criteria have also been used as guidelines for the specific diagnosis of individuals in general (10). The ACR continues to monitor the criteria for accuracy and validity. When diagnosis is still in doubt, further biopsies should be completed, if feasible, on subcutaneous nodules to differentiate them from gouty tophi and amyloid and other types of nodules. Even though RA shares many characteristics of other collagen diseases, particularly systemic lupus erythematosus, the latter can usually be identified by the characteristic skin lesions on the light-exposed areas, temporal frontal hair loss, oral and nasal mucosal lesions, and in joint fluid with a white blood count seen as "overlap syndrome" (13).

Diagnosis of JRA may be a long, emotionally charged process for a family. The diagnosis depends on symptoms experienced in the first 6 months of the illness. The primary steps include many of those taken to diagnose RA in an adult. These include:

- A comprehensive health history to help determine the length of time symptoms have been present.
- A physical examination to look for joint inflammation, rashes, nodules, and eye problems.
- Laboratory tests to rule out other diseases.
- Radiograph examinations of joints to identify other possible conditions.
- Tests of fluids from joints and tissues to evaluate for infections and/or inflammation.

Medical/Surgical Management

The goals of medical management of RA and JRA are: (a) relief of pain and stiffness, (b) reduction of inflammation, (c) preservation of muscle strength and joint function, (d) minimizing medication side effects, (e) maintenance of as much of a normal lifestyle as possible and, for children, and (f) promotion of normal growth and development. Another objective is to attempt to resolve or modify disease progress through, early, aggressive drug therapies advocated because of the diagnosis, prognosis, and reversible damage in the articular cartilage within the first 2 years of the disease (13).

Because the etiology of RA is unknown and the mechanisms of therapeutic interventions uncertain, therapy remains essentially experimental. None of the interventions are curative; therefore, all must be viewed as palliative, aimed at relieving the signs and symptoms of the disease.

A comprehensive therapeutic management program for those with JRA and RA include (a) physical management (including occupational and physical therapy), (b) psychosocial care (includes self-image, pain management work, and school participation, leisure, family functioning, family education, and financial considerations), (c) nutritional aspects, (d) pharmacological management, and (e) other medical aspects including management of comorbidities.

An interdisciplinary approach that focuses on physical, functional, and psychosocial issues is common with RA patients. Physical and occupational therapy interventions, including exercise and rest strategies, physical agent modalities, including ultrasound, heat and gentle ROM, and splinting to allow proper alignment of deformed joints, have all assisted with managing symptoms.

Patient and family education that centers on self-help and self-management of RA have demonstrated positive outcomes. Review of medical and patient education outcomes research shows that medications offer 20% to 50% improvement in arthritis symptoms for most patients and that patient education interventions, such as the various self-help courses available through the Arthritis Foundation, can reduce symptoms an additional 15% to 30% (66–68).

Drug Therapy

A variety of different drugs are used in the medical management of RA. Five different types of drugs are important: analgesic drugs, nonsteroidal anti-inflammatory drugs (NSAIDs), including, salicylates, corticosteroids, disease-modifying antirheumatic drugs (DMARDs), which are considered second-line drugs, and cytotoxics, which are considered third-line drugs.

Treatment is focused on anti-inflammatory and immunosuppressive effects to both prevent destruction of the joint and give pain control. However, as mentioned earlier in this chapter, a wide variety of treatment intervention options are available to the clinician, and should not necessarily be limited to drug therapy alone. During the 1980s, a "pyramid approach" to medical management began with the most conservative methods and then assumed a more aggressive approach as the disease progressed (68). This thought process began to slowly change when methotrexate, a cytotoxic drug, demonstrated that it could control RA with minimal toxicity compared with other second line DMARDs. In the 1990s, the pyramid approach was used less frequently. Instead, more aggressive therapy consisting of immunosuppressives (including cytotoxic drugs) were implemented as the first part of treatment and combined with DMARDs to obtain disease control before severe joint destruction occurred.

Salicylates (e.g., aspirin) or the newer NSAIDs are the primary, and less toxic drugs, available for RA treatment. These provide relief from pain, reduction of inflammation, and though most require a physician's order, are relatively inexpensive (69–70).

Surgery

Surgery plays a role in the management of RA in patients with severely damaged joints. Hip and knee arthroplasties and total joint replacements have offered the most positive outcomes in terms of function and mobility. The goals of surgery are (a) pain reduction, (b) correction of deformity, and (c) functional improvement. As with any major surgery, there are inherent risks that must be thoughtfully weighed. The patient must be prepared for surgery, and demonstrate a willingness to be an active participant in the rehabilitation process (71).

Impact on Occupational Performance

Effects on occupational performance for individuals with RA are usually disruptive but not life threatening. A person with RA will experience varying degrees of improvement, depending on the progression of the disease, anatomical structures involved, systemic problems experienced, comorbidities, financial support available, and overall psychological outlook.

Trombly calls identifying occupational performance problems as the first step in assessment a more "top down" approach (as opposed to the "bottom up" approach of evaluating performance components like range of motion and muscle strength). Taking the top down approach also gives the clinician a better understanding of the context within which the person functions and the priorities he/she believes are paramount (72).

It is important to focus on the context in which the individual must perform daily activities, as this will assist in determining the feasibility and appropriateness of intervention. Christiansen states that hand strength and dexterity limitations have an impact on all ADL and instrumental activities of daily living (IADL), carried out within a variety of contexts (73). Considering that every object in our environment must be grasped, manipulated, moved, smoothed, or pressed, one can understand how RA or JRA can cast a wide shadow over a variety of leisure, work, and self-care activities.

A variety of tools are available to assess performance deficits and assets as well as performance components. For the occupational therapy professional the area of concentrated focus may be on the hand and upper extremity function. A selection of tests of hand and upper limb function for individuals with rheumatic diseases follows:

- Arthritis Hand Function Test (AHFT) (74,75)
- Cochin Rheumatoid Hand Disability Scale (76)
- Disabilities of the Arm, Shoulder, and Hand (DASH) Questionnaire (77)
- Michigan Hand Outcomes Questionnaire (MHQ) (78)
- Sequential Occupational Dexterity Assessment (SODA) (79)

As with all assessments, formal and informal, it is important to focus on the context in which the individual must perform daily activities, as this will determine the feasibility and appropriateness of the occupational therapy intervention.

Impact on Client Factors

Sensory Functions and Pain

The processing of sensory information may be affected in the patient with RA. Tactile, proprioceptive, visual, and auditory abilities specifically, seem to be those most vulnerable. Nerve impingement from the loss of soft tissue integrity can affect both tactile and proprioceptive processing throughout both proximal and peripheral joints. Visual changes occur in approximately 1% of the RA population. Auditory changes can occur in the individual with RA because of the inflammation of the inner ear bony joints.

Neuromusculoskeletal and Movement-Related Functions. By far the most significant deficit in the neuromuscular component is the decrease in both passive and active ROM in the major joints. Subsequent to the loss of ROM, an individual can likely experience loss of muscle mass and strength. Joint deformities are common, especially in the position of flexion. The inflammation of RA causes joint swelling. Joint stiffness, especially in the morning, is a commonly reported complaint. The cumulative effects of immobility, stiffness, and pain result in generalized fatigue that exacerbates the mobility impairment. Patients may present with decreased power during formal functional strength testing. The clinician should be aware that a patient might demonstrate strength in the a "good" range in the pain-free portion of joint range, and a significantly lower score in painful areas of joint range. Strength and function may likewise vary during those times of the day when joint stiffness is decreased.

The most significant motor impairment will be demonstrated as depressed activity tolerance because of decreased neuromuscular status in the individual presenting with RA. Fatigue should be assessed over a 24-hour period or longer in order to gain a full understanding of the client's patterns of behavior and activity participation. Energy-conservation principles involve prioritizing activities; planning and pacing activities over the day, week, or month; and regular physical activity as a mainstay for sustaining endurance for all daily life activities (80). It is beneficial for the clinician to measure heart rate, respiratory rate, and blood pressure during functional activities. Although formal evaluation of passive and active ROM and strength is useful as baseline data, if joint pain and/or poor tolerance to activity is apparent, the clinician must consider incorporating a functional ROM assessment in order to determine availability of motion for performing functional activities that are relevant and necessary for the client. Documenting the time of day during which the assessment takes place can assist in determining if there are cycles or periods when stiffness and diminished functionality are more pronounced. Joint instability can be a significant deterrent to initiation and completion of many daily self-care activities. Researchers have suggested that practice, along with application of joint-protection principles, improves functional ability (81,82). Orthotic devices and splints can help stabilize joints, address underlying biomechanics of motion, reduce pain during activity, and improve hand strength and function (83).

Mental Functions: Affective, Cognitive, and Perceptual. RA does not have a direct effect on cognitive functioning. It has been shown in the literature that difficulty with attention span, short-term memory, sequencing, and problem-solving, as well as other process skills may be caused and/or exacerbated by depression. It is not unusual for an individual with RA to have disease exacerbation as a result of major psychological stressors (84). Breakdown in coping mechanisms may lead to feelings of hopelessness and a sense of helplessness. For some individuals a diminishment of self-concept and the ability to self-manage one's life may occur. Depression and anxiety are other potential conditions that the individual with either RA or JRA may encounter at some time during their life with their condition. It has been shown that nearly 50% of patients with RA report dysfunction in the areas of social interaction, communication with others, and other emotional behaviors (85). The individual with RA or JRA frequently has to implement changes in various aspects of his or her life. Changes in medications, exercise routines, and self-care activities can create anxiety and a sense of loss of control for the individual. Some individuals while seeking to maintain autonomy will disregard the advice and guidance of their caregivers. The caregiver must allow the individual the prerogative to make decisions regarding their own care, and to encourage autonomy and mastery of one's self as well as one's environment. Through mutual respect, the caregiver and the individual dealing with RA or JRA can maximize function while facilitating mastery and self-directedness.

Conclusion

During the past decade and a half, the health care environment has been stressed in regard to reimbursement and funding issues related to assessment and treatment of those with RA, JRA, and all of the other forms of arthritis. Joint problems are now hurting and limiting the functional capacity of 43 million Americans, and according to some estimates they are more costly than cancer or diabetes. The numbers are going up steadily with each passing year. By 2025, the total is expected to top 60 million. As obesity in the United States continues to grow and reach epidemic proportions, more and more individuals will suffer the effects of unrelenting wear and tear on their weight-bearing joints due to arthritis. The active generation of baby boomers now entering their retirement years will likewise be experiencing joint maladies directly attributable to the continuation of active, and sometimes competitive athletics in to their fifth and sixth decades.

Key professionals in the care of this growing population of individuals needing care will continue to be the primary care physician, the family practice physician, physician assistants, and nurse practitioners. Physical and occupational therapists will continue to be essential team members, as will athletic counselors, and educators.

Many people will seek and receive assessment and diagnostic, as well as treatment from medical specialists in the field of rheumatology. Research has shown clearly that positive outcomes have been found with the initiation of early, aggressive intervention.

Patient-centered treatment including self-help, self-management, and education will continue to be advocated by the array of health care providers. The clinician's role in partnering with each client is to assist in the development of realistic goals, to provide encouragement, and to offer a positive environment for the exploration of the various options available now. It will be the continuing responsibility of all health care professionals involved in the assessment and treatment of all types of arthritis to remain informed and aware of advances in the field.

CASE STUDY

Case Illustrations

■ CASE 1

Pete is a 54-year-old landscaper and lawn irrigation system installer living in New Jersey. He is married, has two children in high school, and is active in his company's softball league on weekends. His wife works part-time as a registered nurse. For the past few months Pete has experienced pain and stiffness in the small joints of his hands, and stiffness in both elbows and knees. His wife also has noticed that his fingers look swollen and are warm to the touch.

Pete tends to discount what he considers "minor aches and pains," and attributes his discomfort to "growing pains" and the fact that his hands are in cold water frequently when he is working. Typically, by his first coffee break at 10:15 in the morning, Pete has forgotten his early morning pain and stiffness and is his usual self. After several more months of repeated complaints, Pete's wife arranged for an evaluation with their family practice physician. After a series of tests and some time, he was diagnosed with RA.

■ CASE 2

Marva Witmore is a 34-year-old single mother of two children, a 10-year-old son and an 8-year-old daughter born with spina bifida. Marva was diagnosed with rheumatoid arthritis approximately 4 years ago, and has been managing her home and her self-care, as well as the responsibilities inherent in caring for her young children. Recently, Marva has been experiencing an exacerbation of her symptoms; flare-ups that include increased joint swelling and pain. Marva prides herself on being independent and able to multi-task in order to accomplish many tasks. In her rare free time she enjoys scrap booking and playing poker with her friends in the apartment complex.

Since the onset of her most recent exacerbation, Marva has seen a significant change in her lifestyle and ability to maintain some of the routine activities necessary for balanced family life. Moderate involvement of motor and neuromuscular components affects all occupational performance areas. ROM and muscle strength is affected in all movement of extension in her elbows, wrists and hands. There is a slight, but noticeable ulnar drift at the MP joints bilaterally. Prehension skills are functional for routine activities of daily living, but Marva has noticed that she is having increased difficulty opening containers such as the bottle of shampoo and the dead bolt on the front door. Gross grasp is weakening and Marva has begun purchasing milk for the children in half-gallon jugs rather than the cost-saving larger gallon size.

Marva is experiencing stiffness and pain in the small joints of her fingers. This limits her when she attempts to prepare some dishes for the family dinner. She is also less interested in playing cards when she is feeling this way, she says that it is harder to keep her "poker face" when she is in such discomfort. Recently Marva's sister has been helping out with grocery shopping and clothing shopping for the two children. Her sister is also willing and able to assist by taking Marva's daughter to various clinic visits when necessary. Marva can operate her own car, but her endurance can be drastically affected when the RA is in a flare-up. Marva is hesitant to apply for a handicap-parking permit, but parking and walking distances into and out of stores is getting nearly impossible to do.

Maintaining her self-esteem and morale is becoming more and more difficult as her disease persists. Previously Marva was able to rally herself and work through her pain and the limitations this wrought on her life. Lately she has been staying in bed in the morning after the children leave for school, getting up only to answer the telephone or to make a cup of coffee for breakfast. She can actually feel herself pulling away socially and emotionally from her sphere of friends and at times from her loving family. She feels angry and guilty about no longer being the "super person" she once thought she was.

Marva never was one to look to support groups for answers to her life situation. She vowed to manage the needs of her children, especially her daughter's many physical and medical needs without "leaning on" others. Now she is worried that she is losing ground and many days she feels like she is "sinking into wet concrete." Her sister is planning to attend a local support group for family members of those with RA. The group meets monthly in the basement of a church in the city, and it is a first step toward helping Marva.

■ CASE 3

John Michael is a pleasant, energetic 11-year-old sixth grade student at West Middle School. He enjoys riding his mini-bike in the fields around his neighborhood, playing street hockey, and playing video games with his Playstation 2. He has a variety of friends in school and is never one to be without something to do on most days. There are two other children in his family, a younger brother, Jimmy, age 8, and an older sister Carrie, age 16. His mother is a paraprofessional working in an elementary school with special needs children. His dad is a regional manager for Wal-Mart and he works long hours, sometimes up to 50 to 60 hours per week.

Approximately 4 months ago, John Michael was diagnosed with JRA of the pauciarticular type (four or fewer joints involved). The diagnosis was quite a while in coming from their pediatrician, and was made after a series of laboratory tests, radiographs, and physical examinations. John Michael's mother remembers him complaining of mild, intermittent pain and stiffness in his lower back and hips for almost 3 months prior to the diagnosis.

Performance areas affected include play, self-care, and education. Involved neuromuscular components include; hip and trunk range of motion, lower extremity muscle strength, endurance, and at times postural control. His hip musculature appears stiff at the end of range in the early morning and after sitting for extended periods greater than 1 hour. Muscle strength is measured as 3/3+ on hip extension and flexion and 3+ for trunk extension. On days when he is experiencing significant "stiffness" in his trunk and hips, his postural control is compromised and he cannot react quickly during play. His musculoskeletal endurance diminishes in the afternoon, particularly after a busy day at school. He has adapted his street hockey play to weekends when he tends to have more energy.

John Michael's parents feel it best to share as much information about his condition with his teachers each school year as is practical in an effort to optimize John Michael's learning experience optimal. His teachers appreciate this input and guidance, and have a clear and compassionate perspective on what they may be confronted with on a day-to-day basis in their classrooms. One accommodation that they all have agreed to is to allow John Michael the opportunity to stand and walk around the classroom periodically in order to relieve the stiffness that might be developing from extended static positioning at his desk.

In the self-care arena, John Michael prefers showers to baths. This is actually better for him as there is only a 4-inch step over into the shower stall, and there is also a small bench built into the shower wall in case he needs to sit and rest. The bench seat is positioned approximately 17 inches above the floor and there is a wall safety grab bar positioned on a diagonal to the plane of the seat rest. He uses a squeeze bottle for shampoo and enjoys liquid soap, also administered from a lightweight squeeze bottle. His dad just installed a small shelf in the stall shower to hold these items. Dressing, grooming, feeding, and use of the toilet do not present any problems at this time for John Michael. He tends to avoid wearing tight clothing, and generally wears T-shirts and loose-fitting cargo jeans or shorts on most days. He has just been fitted with braces for his teeth and he is a little concerned about being able to maintain the high level of oral hygiene that his dentist is stressing. John Michael has never been one to floss his teeth, but now he must and his parents will assist him in finding the right tools and technique to accomplish this task.

John Michael is blessed with a very understanding and supportive family. His parents have chosen to not treat him as a "special child." He is required to participate in the routine activities of the family, including some yard work and other household chores. Generally, John Michael has been adjusting well to the limitations imposed by this disease, although there are some occasions when he is severely limited by stiffness and painful movement and these occasions upset and anger him. He is at an age and stage of life where he is trying many news things and experiencing many opportunities in school and leisure. His friends know of his condition, but they have been accepting as a whole and John Michael is fortunate that his positive attitude and warm family atmosphere help him to attract and retain friendships with his peers.

References

1. Rothchild BM, Woods RJ. Symmetrical erosive disease in Archaic Indians: the origin of rheumatoid arthritis in the New World. Semin Arthritis Rheum 1990;19:278–284.
2. Centers for Disease Control and Prevention. Direct and indirect costs of arthritis and other rheumatic conditions. United States, 1997. MMWR Morb Mortal Wkly Rep 2003;52:1124–1127.
3. Michaud K, Messer J, Choi HK, et al. Direct medical costs and their predictors in patients with rheumatoid arthritis: a three-year study of 7,527 patients. Arthritis Rheum 2003;48(10):2750–2762.
4. Schned ES, Reinertsen JL. The social and economic consequences of rheumatic disease. In: Klippel HJ, Weyand CM, Wortman RL, eds. Primer on the Rheumatic Diseases. 11th Ed. Atlanta: Arthritis Foundation, 1997.
5. Arnett F. Rheumatoid arthritis. In: Bennett JC, Plum F, eds. Cecil's Textbook of Medicine, Volume 2. 20th Ed. Philadelphia: WB Saunders Co., 1996.
6. Sen M, Carson DA: RA: learning from its origins and development. JMM 2003;20(11):497–499, 503–506.
7. Baecklund E, Askling J, Rosenquist R, et al. Rheumatoid arthritis and malignant lymphomas. Curr Opin Rheumatol 2004;16(3):254–261.
8. Simkin PA. The Musculoskeletal System: Joints. In: Klippel HJ, Weyand CM, Wortman RL, eds. Primer on the Rheumatic Diseases. 11th Ed. Atlanta: Arthritis Foundation, 1997.
9. Goronzy JJ, Weyand CM. Rheumatoid arthritis: epidemiology, pathology, and pathogenesis. In: Klippel HJ, Weyand CM, Wortman RL, eds. Primer on the Rheumatic Diseases. 11th Ed. Atlanta: Arthritis Foundation, 1997.
10. Goronzy JJ, Weyand CM. Rheumatoid arthritis: epidemiology, pathology, and pathogenesis. In: Klippel HJ, Weyand CM, Wortman RL, eds. Primer on the Rheumatic Diseases. 11th Ed. Atlanta: Arthritis Foundation, 1997.
11. Centers for Disease Control and Prevention. Racial/Ethnic Differences in the Prevalence and Impact of Doctor-Diagnosed Arthritis. United States, 2002. MMWR Morb Mortal Wkly Rep 2005; 54(05);199–123.
12. Escalante A, del Ricon I. Epidemiology and the Impact of Rheumatic Disorders in the United States. Curr Opin Rheumatol 2001;13:104–110.
13. Beers MH, Berkow R, eds. Rheumatoid arthritis. In: The Merck Manual of Diagnosis and Therapy. 17th Ed. New York: John Wiley & Sons, 1999.
14. Nielen MJ, von Schaardenburg D, Reesink HW, et al. Arthritis Rheum 2004;50(8):2427–2430.
15. Cassidy J. Juvenile rheumatoid arthritis. In: Kelley WN, Ruddy S, Harris ED, et al. eds. Textbook of Rheumatology. 5th Ed. Philadelphia: WB Saunders Co., 1997.
16. Gare AB. Juvenile arthritis—who gets it, where and when? A review of current data on incidence and prevalence. Clin Exp Rheum 1999;17:367–374.
17. Petty RE. Classification of childhood arthritis: 1897–1997. Rev Rheum [Eng. Ed] 1997;64(10 Suppl): 161S–162S.
18. Petty RE et al. Revision of the proposed classification criteria for juvenile idiopathic arthritis: Durban, 1997. J Rheum 1998: 10: 1991–1994.
19. Petty RE. Classification of childhood arthritis: a work in progress. Bailliere's Clin Rheum 1998;12(2): 181–190.
20. Lovell DJ. Pediatric rheumatic diseases: juvenile rheumatic diseases and juvenile spondyloarthritis. In: Klippel JH, Weyand CM, Wortman RL, eds. Primer on the Rheumatic Diseases. 11th Ed. Atlanta: Arthritis Foundation, 1997.
21. Arthritis Foundation. Demographic and economic information, 2004. Available at: http://www.arthritis.org. Accessed June 7, 2005.
22. Arthritis Foundation. Status of Pediatric Rheumatology, part I, 1997. Available at: http://www.arthritis.org. Accessed June 7, 2005.
23. Kasper DL, Braunwald E, Fauci A, et al. eds. Harrison's Principles of Internal Medicine. 16th Ed. New York: McGraw-Hill, 2004.
24. Melvin JL, Ferrell KM, eds. Rheumatic Rehabilitation Series: Adult Rheumatic Diseases, Vol. 2. Bethesda: The American Occupational Therapy Association, 2000.

25. Wessel J. The effectiveness of hand exercises for persons with rheumatoid arthritis: a systematic review. J Hand Ther 2004;17(2):174–180.
26. Fowler NK, Nicol AC. Functional and biomechanical assessment of the normal and rheumatoid hand. Clin Biomechanics 2001;16(8):660–666.
27. Neumann DA, Bielefeld T. The carpometacarpal joint of the thumb: stability, deformity, and therapeutic intervention. J Orthop Sports Phys Ther 2003;33(7): 386–399.
28. Ashe MC, McCauley T, Khan KM. Tendinopathies in the upper extremity: a paradigm shift. J Hand Ther 2004;17(3):329–334.
29. Barr AE, Barbe MF, Clark BD. Work-related musculoskeletal disorders of the hand and wrist: epidemiology, pathophysiology, and sensorimotor changes. J Orthop Sports Phys Ther 2004;34(10):610–627.
30. Adams J, Burridge J, Mullee M, et al. Correlation between upper limb functional ability and structural hand impairment in an early rheumatoid population. Clin Rehabil 2004;18(4):405–413.
31. Maloney MD, Ryder S. Multiple overlapping causes and symptoms can complicate the differential: diagnosis and management of shoulder disorders. JMM Journal of Musculoskeletal Medicine. 2003;20(9): 412–418.
32. Mink JH, Gordon RE, Deutsch AL. The cervical spine: radiologist's perspective. Phys Med Rehabil Clin N Am 2003;14(3):493–548.
33. Niere K, Jerak A. Measurement of headache frequency, intensity and duration: comparison of patient report by questionnaire and headache diary. Physiother Res Int 2004;9(4):149–156.
34. Crowther CL. The effects of corticosteroids on the musculoskeletal system. Orthop Nurs 2001;20(6): 33–39.
35. Bayar N, Kara SA, Keles I, et al. Temporomandibular joint involvement in rheumatoid arthritis: a radiological and clinical study. Cranio 2002;20(2):105–110.
36. Blosser S, Wigley FM, Wise RA. Increase in translaryngeal resistance during phonation in rheumatoid arthritis. Chest 1992;102(2):387–390.
37. Stiskal-Galisewski DM. Comparison of the walking performance at two different speeds in adolescents with and without juvenile arthritis using dual-task method. Seton Hall University, College of Education and Human Services. 2003 PhD. (141 pages).
38. Siegel LB, Gall EP. A systematic approach to the physical examination in RA: part 2: the hip, lower extremities, and extra-articular systems. J Musculoskeletal Rehabil Journal of Musculoskeletal Medicine. 1999;16(7):392–394, 397–400.
39. Burra G, Katchis SD. Rheumatoid arthritis of the forefoot. Clin Podiatr Med Surg 1999;16(2):363–371.
40. Costa M, Rizak T, Zimmermann B. Rheumtologic conditions of the foot. J Am Podiatr Med Assoc 2004;94(2):177–186.
41. Jaakkola JI, Mann RA. Managing foot and ankle problems in RA. JMM Journal of Musculoskeletal Medicine 2005;22(1):30–32, 35–36.
42. Burns PR, Scanlan RL, Zgonis T, et al. Pathologic conditions of the heel: tumors and arthritides. Clin Podiatr Med Surg 2005;22(1):115–136.
43. Halverson PB. Extraarticular manifestations of rheumatoid arthritis. Ortho Nurs 1995;14(4): 47–50.
44. Ward MM. Decreases in rates of hospitalizations for manifestations of severe rheumatoid arthritis, 1983–2001. Arthritis Rheum 2004;50(4): 1122–1131.
45. Fye KH. Recognizing the extra-articular manifestations of RA: nonjoint problems may add considerably to morbidity. JMM Journal of Musculoskeletal Medicine 2002;19(8):307–310,312,314–316.
46. Sandhu V, Allen SC. The effects of age, seropositivity and disease duration on autonomic cardiovascular reflexes in patients with rheumatoid arthritis. Int J Clin Pract 2004;58(8):740–745.
47. Bosch PR. Rheumatoid arthritis as an autoimmune disease. Arizona State University 2003 Ph.D. (175 pages).
48. Dessein PH, Shipton EA, Budd K. Nociceptive and non-nociceptive rheumatological pain: recent developments in the understanding of pathophysiology and management in rheumatoid arthritis and fibromyalgia. Pain Rev 2000;7(2): 67–79.
49. Glazer-Hockstein C, Orlin SE. Detecting the ocular manifestations of RA: early recognition can prevent disease progression and loss of vision. JMM 2002;19(12):508–510,512–515.
50. Patel SJ, Lundy DC. Ocular manifestations of autoimmune disease. Am Fam Physician 2002;66(6): 991–998.
51. Jakobsson U, Hallberg IR. Pain and quality of life among older people with rheumatoid arthritis and/or osteoarthritis: a literature review. J Clin Nurs 2002;11(4):430–443.
52. Oliver S. Clinical update. Social and psychological issues in rheumatoid arthritis. Primary Health Care 2004;14(4):25–28.
53. Adam V, St.-Pierre Y, Fautrel B, et al. What is the impact of adolescent arthritis and rheumatism? Evidence from a national sample of Canadians. J Rheum 2005;32(2):354–361.
54. Stevens-Ratchford R, Cebulak BJ. Living well with arthritis: a study of engagement in social occupations and successful aging. Phys Occup Ther Geriatr 2004;(4):31–52.
55. Fifield J, McQuillan J, Armeli S, et al. Chronic strain, daily work stress and pain among workers with rheumatoid arthritis: does job stress make a bad day worse? Work & Stress 2004;18(4):275–291.
56. Burke HM. Depression and cortisol stress responses in adults with rheumatoid arthritis. Arizona State University 2003 PhD. (76 pages).
57. Neugebauer A, Katz PP. Impact of social support on valued activity disability and depressive symptoms in patients with rheumatoid arthritis. Arthritis Rheum 2004;51(4):586–592.

58. Rennie KL, Hughes J, Lang R, et al. Nutritional management of rheumatoid arthritis: a review of the evidence. J Hum Nutr Diet 2003;16(2):97–109.
59. Oku MZ, Yardimci S, Omoglu S. Body fat percent and fat distribution parameters in rheumatic diseases. J Back Musculoskeletal Rehabil 2002;16(2/3):57–61.
60. Goronzy JJ, Matteson EL, Fulbright JW, et al. Prognostic markers of radiographic progression in early rheumatoid arthritis. Arthritis Rheum 2004;50(1): 43–54.
61. Matsunaga S, Sakou T, Onishi T, et al. Prognosis of patients with upper cervical lesions caused by rheumatoid arthritis: comparison of occipitocervical fusion between C1 laminectomy and nonsurgical management. Spine 2003;8(14):1581–1587.
62. Magni-Manzoni S, Rossi F, Pistoria A, et al. Prognostic factors for radiographic progression, radiographic damage, and disability in juvenile idiopathic arthritis. Arthritis Rheum 2003;48(12): 3509–3517.
63. Guccione AA. Arthritis and the process of disablement. Phys Ther 1994;74:408–414.
64. Eberrhardt K, Larsson BM, Nived K. Early rheumatoid arthritis: some social, economical and psychological aspects. Scand J Rheum 1993;22:119–123.
65. Pincus T, Callahan L. Taking mortality in rheumatoid arthritis seriously. Predictive markers, socioeconomic status and comorbidity. J Rheum 1986;13:841–845.
66. Rojer DE, Goodman SB. Total knee replacement in juvenile rheumatoid arthritis. Orthopedics 2005;28(1): 39–47.
67. Angst F, Pap G, Mannion AF, et al. Comprehensive assessment of clinical outcomes and quality of life after total shoulder arthroplasty: usefulness and validity of subjective outcome measures. Arthritis Rheum 2004;51(5):819–828.
68. Bruce ML, Peck B. New rheumatoid arthritis treatments. Nurse Practitioner: American Journal of Primary Health Care 2005;30(4):28–29,32–37, 39–41.
69. Suarez-Almazor ME, Bennett KJ, Bombardier C, et al. Injectable gold for rheumatoid arthritis. Oxford: The Cochrane Library, 2005:CD000520.
70. Suarez-Almazor ME, Belseck E, Homik JJE, et al. Antimalarials for treating rheumatoid arthritis. Oxford: The Cochrane Library, 2005:CD000959.
71. Ganz SB, Viellion G. Pre- and post-surgical management of hip and knee. In: Wegener ST, Belza BL, Gall EP. Clinical Care in the Rheumatic Diseases. Atlanta: American College of Rheumatology 1996:103–106.
72. Trombley CA. Theoretical foundations for practice. In: Trombley CA, ed. Occupational Therapy for Physical Dysfunction. 4th Ed. Baltimore: Williams & Wilkins, 1995:15–27.
73. Christiansen CH, Matuska KM, eds. Adaptive Strategies for Rheumatic Diseases. In: Ways of Living: Adaptive Strategies for Special Needs. 3rd Ed. Bethesda: American Occupational Therapy Association Press, 2004:191–192.
74. Backman C, Mackie H, Harris J. Arthritis Hand Function Test: Development of a standardized assessment tool. Occup Ther J Res 1991;11:245–256.
75. Poole JL, Gallegos M, O'Linc S. Reliability and validity of the Arthritis Hand Function Test in adults with systemic sclerosis (scleroderma). Arthritis Care Res 2000;13:69–73.
76. Durouz MT, Poiraudeau S, Fermanian J, et al. Development and validation of a rheumatoid hand functional disability scale that assesses functional handicap. J Rheum 1996;23:1167–1172.
77. Beaton DE, Katz JN, Fossel AH, et al. Measuring the whole or the parts? Validity, reliability, and responsiveness of the Disabilities of the arm, shoulder, and hand outcomes measure in different Regions of the upper extremity. J Hand Ther 2001;14:128–146.
78. Chung KC, Pillsbury MS, Walters MR, et al. Reliability and validity testing of the Michigan Hand Outcomes Questionnaire. J Hand Surg 1998;23: 575–587.
79. van Lankveld W, Pad Bosch P, Bakker J, et al. Sequential Occupational Dexterity Assessment (SODA): a new test to measure hand disability. J Hand Ther 1996;9:27–32.
80. Cordery J, Rocchi M. Joint protection and fatigue management. In: Melvin J, Jensen G, eds. Rheumatologic Rehabilitation Series, Vol 1: Assessment and Management. Bethesda, MD: American Occupational Therapy Association, 1998:279–322.
81. Hammond A, Freeman K. One-year outcomes of a randomized controlled trial of an educational-behavioral joint protection program for people with rheumatoid arthritis. Rheumatology 2001;40: 1044–1051.
82. Steultjens EMJ, Dekker J, Bouter LM, et al. Occupational therapy for rheumatoid arthritis: A systemic review. Arthritis Rheum 2002;47:672–685.
83. Harrell PB. Splinting of the hand. In: Robbins L, Burckhardt CS, Hannon MT, et al. eds. Clinical care in the rheumatic diseases. 2nd Ed. Atlanta, GA: Association of Rheumatology Health Professionals, 2001:191–196.
84. Chaney J, Mullins L, Wagner J, et al. A longitudinal examination of causal attributions and depression symptomatology in rheumatoid arthritis. Rehabil Psychol 2004;49(2):126–133.
85. Ewert T, Fuessi M, Cieza A, et al. Identification of the most common patient problems in patients with chronic conditions using the ICF checklist. J Rehabil Med 2004;36(44):22–29.
86. JRA Criteria Subcommittee of the Diagnostic and Therapeutic Criteria Committee of the American Rheumatism Association. Current Rehabil Psychol proposed revisions of the JRA criteria. Arthritis Rheum 1977;20(Suppl):195–199.
87. Ansell BW. Chronic arthritis in childhood. Ann Rheum Dis 1978;37:107–120.
88. Fink CW. Keynote address: arthritis in childhood. Report of the 80th Ross Conference in Pediatric Research, Columbus: Ross Laboratories, 1979:1–2.

Recommended Learning Resources

Consumer and Professional Resources

Health Organizations

Arthritis Foundation (AF)
Tel: 404–872–7100, 1–800–568–4045
www.arthritis.org

American Juvenile Arthritis Organization (AJAO)
Tel: 404–872–7100, 1–800–568–4045
www.arthritis.org

The Arthritis Society (Canada)
393 University Avenue, Suite 1700
Toronto, Ontario M5G 1E6
Canada
Tel: 416–979–7228
Fax: 416–979–8366
www.info@arthritis.ca

Higher Education and Training for People with Handicaps (HEATH)
American Counsil on Education
One Dupont Circle, Suite 800
Washington, D.C. 20036–1193
Tel: 202–939–9320, 1–800–544–3284

The European League Against Rheumatism (EULAR)
EULAR Executive Secretariat
Seestrasse 240
8802-Kilchberg
Switzerland
Tel: +41 44 716 30 30
www.secretariat@eular.org

National Chronic Pain Outreach Association (NCPOA)
P.O. Box 274
Millboro, VA 24460
Tel: 540–862–9437
Fax: 540–862–9485
www.chronic pain.org

Support Groups

Contact the Arthritis Foundation for local groups across the United States of America

Professional Organizations

American College of Rheumatology (ACR)/Arthritis Health Professionals Association (AHPA)
1800 Century Place
Suite 250
Atlanta, GA 30345
Tel: 404–633–3777
Fax: 404–633–1870
www.acr@rheumatology.org
For Juvenile Arthritis Information
www.rheumatology.org/patient/jra.htm

American Occupational Therapy Association (AOTA)
4720 Montgomery Lane
PO Box 31220
Bethesda, MD 20824–1220
Tel: 301–652–7711, 800–377–8555 (TDD), 1–800-SAY-AOTA
www/aota.org

American Physical Therapy Association (APTA)
111 N. Fairfax Street
Alexandria, VA 22314–1488
Tel: 1–800–999–2782, 703–683–6748 (TDD)
www.apta.org

The American Orthopedic Society for Sports Medicine
6300 N. River Road Suite 500
Rosemont, Illinois 60018
Tel: 847–292–4900
www.sportsmed.org

American Podiatric Medical Association, Inc.
9312 Old Georgetown Road
Bethesda, MD 20814–1621
Tel: 1–800-FOOTCARE
www.apma.org

Research Centers and Institutes

Arthritis Center
Boston University
Conte Building
71 E. Newton Street
Boston, MA 02118
Tel: 617–534–5154

Arthritis Center
University of Missouri-Columbia
MA427 Health Sciences Center
1 Hospital Drive
Columbia, MO 65212
Tel: 314–882–8738

Arthritis Research Institute of America
300 South Duncan Avenue
Suite 240
Clearwater, FL 33755
Tel: 727–461–4054
www.preventarthritis.org

Boston University School of Medicine
Arthritis Center
Silvio O. Conte Medical research Center
715 Albany Street
K-501
Boston, MA 02118
Tel: 617–638–5226, 617–638–4310
www.bumc.bu.edu/Dept/Home

Missouri Arthritis Rehabilitation Research and Training Center
Walter Williams Hall
Room 13
Columbia, MO 65211
Tel: 1–877–882–6826
marrtc@missouri.edu

University of Connecticut Health Center
School of Medicine
Division of Rheumatic Diseases
263 Farmington Avenue
Farmington, CT 06030–1310
860–679–3605
www.penguin.uchc.edu/rheum

National Arthritis and Musculoskeletal and Skin Diseases Information Clearinghouse (NAMSIC)
9000 Rockville Pike
PO Box AMS
Bethesda, MD 20892
Tel: 301–495–4484
www.niams.nih.gov/

Adaptive Aids
These companies have catalogs that contain resources for those with arthritis.

AliMed Rehabilitation Products, Inc.
297 High Street
Dedham, MA 02026–9135
Tel: 1–800–255–2160
www.alimed.com

Amigo Mobility International, Inc.
6692 Dixie Highway
Bridgeport, MI 48722–9725
Tel: 1–800–248–9131

info @myamigo.com
DeRoyal/LMB, Inc.
PO Box 1181
San Luis Obispo, CA 93406
Tel: 1–800–541–3992

Independent Living Aids, Inc.
27 East Mall
Plainview, NY 11803
Tel: 1–800–537–2118

Invacare Corporation
899 Cleveland Street
Elyria, OH 44036
Tel: 1–800–333–6900

Lumex Medical Products
100 Spence Street
Bay Shore, NY 11706–2290
Tel: 1–800–645–5272

Maddak, Inc.
PO Box 384
Penquannock, NY 07440–1993
Tel: 1–800–443–4926

North Coast Medical, Inc.
187 Stauffer Boulevard
San Jose, CA 95125–1042
Tel: 1–800–821–9319

S&S AdaptAbility
PO Box 513
Colchester CT 06415–0515
Tel: 1–800–266–8856

Sammons Preston Rolyan
PO Box 5071
Bolingbrook, IL 60440–5071
Tel: 1–800–323–5547

Smith and Nephew, Inc.
Rehabilitation Division
PO Box 1005
One Quality Drive
Germantown, WI 53022–8205

Consumer Information Brochures
Patient, Caregiver, and professional resources are available from the Arthritis Foundation. To order: www.arthritis.org/conditions/onlinebrochures

"... of the many forms of disability which can beset mankind, a severe injury or disease of the spinal cord undoubtedly constitutes one of the most devastating calamities in human life" (1).
—Sir Ludwig Guttmann, pioneer in 20th-century management of spinal cord injury

"The future lies in our own hands, and if a challenge should enter our life, it is important to remember we have tremendous strength, courage, and ability to overcome any obstacle."
—Douglas Heir, Esq., Attorney-at-Law (personal communication, December 1994)

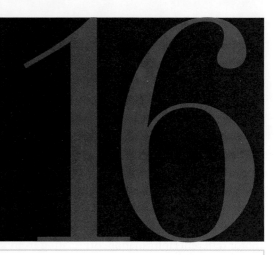

Spinal Cord Injury

Laura V. Miller

Key Terms

Autonomic dysreflexia (hyperreflexia)
Catheterization
Cauda Equina
Credé's method
Decubitus ulcers
Heterotopic ossification
Peristalsis
Reflex arc
Scoliosis
Spinal shock

The full impact of the preceding quotes may not strike the reader unless the whole story is known. The latter author, Doug Heir, sustained a spinal cord injury (SCI) at age 18. He dove into a pool to save a boy who appeared to be drowning. The boy was only playing, but Doug's injury resulted in quadriplegia. Now, nearly two decades later, Doug has become known for being many things, among them an author, U.S. ambassador to the Soviet Union, cover athlete for Wheaties cereal, associate legal editor of the National Trial Lawyer, and a gold medalist in the 1988 Olympics in Seoul, South Korea—an impressive list of accomplishments for someone who sustained "one of the most devastating calamities in human life!"

The goals of the health care team should include empowering clients to take charge of their futures. To accomplish this, the health professional must understand the complexities of the diagnosis. This chapter explores the ramifications of spinal cord injuries, beginning with a brief overview of the central nervous system (CNS) and surrounding structures.

Overview of CNS and Related Structures

The brain and spinal cord make up the CNS. The spinal cord receives sensory (afferent) information from the peripheral nervous system and transmits this information to higher structures (i.e., the thalamus, cerebellum, cerebral cortex) in the CNS. Descending motor (efferent) information, originating from the cortex, also is transmitted by the spinal cord back to the peripheral nervous system.

The consistency of the spinal cord has been compared to a ripe banana, and it is fortunate that the spinal cord and cerebral cortex are protected by bony structures. Whereas the skull protects the brain, the vertebral column protects the spinal cord. The vertebral column is composed of 33 vertebrae, with 7 cervical vertebrae in the neck region (C1 through C7), 12 thoracic vertebrae in the chest region (T1 through T12), 5 lumbar vertebrae in the midback region (L1 through L5), 5 sacral vertebrae (S1 through S5), which are actually fused in the lower back and pelvic region, and 4 fused coccygeal vertebrae that make up the coccyx, or tailbone (Fig. 16.1). There are 31 pairs of spinal nerves, which exit from the spinal cord and branch to form the peripheral nervous system. The nerves exit through the openings formed between each two vertebrae. The spinal nerves are named according to the vertebrae above or below which they exit. Note that spinal nerves C1 through C7 exit above the corresponding vertebrae, whereas the remaining spinal nerves (C8 through S5) exit below the corresponding vertebrae. Thus, although there are seven cervical vertebrae, there are eight cervical spinal nerves. The actual spinal cord ends just below the L1 vertebra. However, some spinal nerves continue, and exit beyond the point where the spinal cord ends. Because of their visual resemblance, this bundle of nerves is referred to as the **cauda equina**, which is Latin for horse's tail (2). The meningeal covering of the spinal cord, which contains the cerebrospinal fluid (CSF) that bathes the structures of the CNS, also extends past the end of the spinal cord to the L4 vertebral level. The CSF-filled meningeal space between L2 and L4, referred to as the lumbar cistern, is the site where spinal taps are performed, because the spinal cord is not present, yet CSF is accessible.

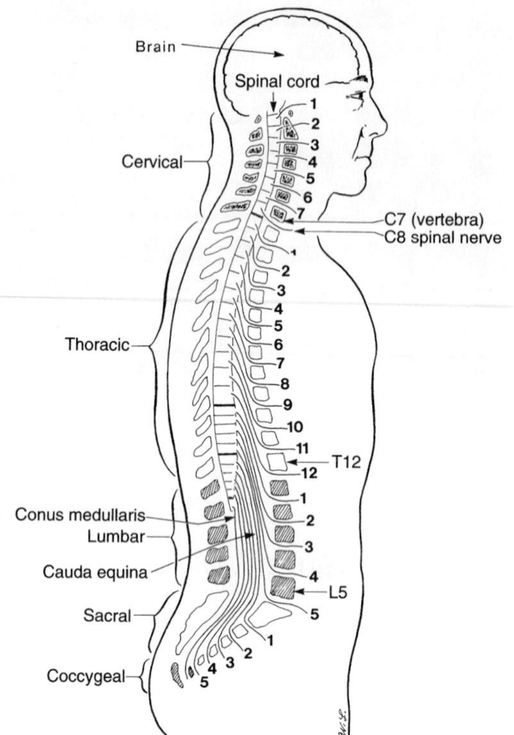

Figure 16.1 The spinal cord, spinal nerves, and vertebral column. (Reprinted with permission from the Rehabilitation Institute of Michigan.)

Sensory and Motor Tracts

The terms tract, pathway, lemniscus, and fasciculus all refer to bundles of nerve fibers that have a similar function and travel through the spinal cord in a particular area. It is important to know the names, locations, and functions of these tracts to understand the possible outcomes of an SCI at a given level.

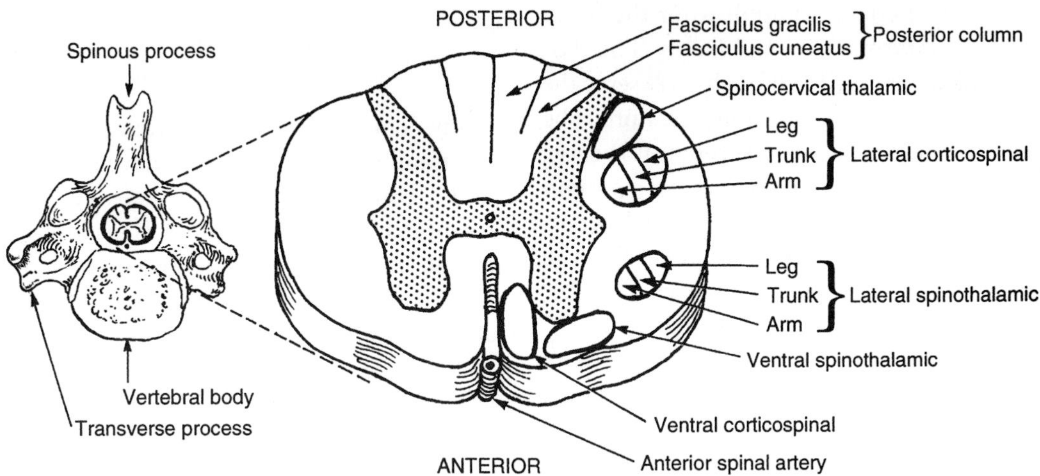

Figure 16.2 Cross-section of cervical spinal cord, shown in relation to surrounding vertebral structures. Selected ascending and descending pathways are illustrated. (Adapted from materials provided courtesy of Rehabilitation Institute of Michigan. Used with permission.)

Figure 16.2 shows the location of major tracts within a cross-section of the spinal cord.

Two basic types of nerve tissue make up the spinal cord. Gray matter is located centrally and resembles a butterfly in cross-sections of the cord. Gray matter is composed of cell bodies and synapses. White matter encompasses most of the periphery of the cord and contains the ascending and descending pathways. Table 16.1 provides a more detailed description of the functions of the various sensory and motor pathways that travel through the white matter of the spinal cord. It may be helpful to remember that many pathways are named according to their origin and the location of their final synapse (e.g., spinocerebellar, corticospinal).

Specific motor and sensory information is carried by each pair of spinal nerves. In general, the cervical nerves (C1 through C8) carry

Table 16.1 NONINCLUSIVE LISTING OF ASCENDING AND DESCENDING PATHWAYS

Ascending afferent (sensory) pathways	Function
Spinocerebellar	Nonconscious proprioception
Lateral spinothalamic	Pain, temperature
Ventral spinothalamic	Touch, pressure
Fasciculus gracilis/fasciculus cuneatus*	Two-point tactile discrimination, vibration, conscious proprioception stereognosis
Spinocervicothalamic	Touch, proprioception, stereognosis, vibration
Descending efferent (motor) pathways	Function
Lateral corticospinal	Movement to extremities
Ventral corticospinal	Movement of neck and trunk
Vestibulospinal	Equilibrium
Reticulospinal	Autonomic functions: motor respiratory functions

*Called the posterior column.

afferent and efferent impulses for the head, neck, diaphragm, arms, and hands. The thoracic spinal nerves (T1 through T12) serve the chest and upper abdominal musculature. The lumbar spinal nerves (L1 through L5) carry information to and from the legs and a portion of the foot, whereas the sacral spinal nerves (S1 through S5) carry impulses for the remaining foot musculature, bowel, bladder, and the muscles involved in sexual functioning. Table 16.2 and Figure 16.3 present a more detailed outline of muscles innervated by each level of the spinal cord and a dermatomal segmentation (sensory map) of the body.

Reflex Arc

Most nerve impulses move up the spinal cord to the brain and back through the cord to the peripheral nerves. However, some impulses merely enter the cord through the dorsal nerve root, synapse, and exit by the ventral nerve root. This causes certain muscle functions or responses without direction from the brain. A simple example of this "looping" can be seen in the knee-jerk reflex. If the knee is tapped with a reflex hammer, the knee will extend without any influence from the brain. The stimulation by the hammer causes afferent impulses to enter the cord, synapse, and exit, causing a contraction of the muscle fibers (Fig. 16.4). This activity is called a **reflex arc.** In persons with an intact spinal cord, afferent nerve impulses also travel to the brain almost instantaneously. This allows an awareness, or "feeling," of the initial stimulation (knee tap) and subsequent response (knee jerk). This concept is important to an understanding of SCIs. It explains why some individuals with SCI continue to have reflexes but do not have voluntary control of their muscles. It also explains why others have no reflexes at all below the level of their injury. This is discussed in much greater detail in the section on classification of injuries.

Etiology

Many demographic sources attempt to count the number of persons who have sustained SCIs. Unfortunately, it has been relatively recent that the United States has made strides in collecting comprehensive data on a national level. In 1985, the Centers for Disease Control and Prevention (CDC) began promoting surveillance mechanisms at state and national levels for the collection and reporting of these data. Nonetheless, current data sources do provide a picture of the etiology and incidence of SCI in this country.

The leading cause of SCI in the United States is motor vehicle accidents, followed by falls and gunshot wounds (Fig. 16.5). Sports-related injuries account for most of the remaining SCIs, with diving being by far the most common (and preventable) cause (Table 16.3).

Analyzing the etiology of SCIs makes for well-targeted prevention programs. Public awareness of the effects of using substances while operating a vehicle is certainly heightened. Tougher penalties for driving under the influence of altering substances have been enacted, and many states have adopted seat belt and child restraint legislation. Grant monies have even been awarded to hospital-based programs that evaluate the home environments of senior citizens. Their recommendations may reduce the risk of falls—a major cause of SCI in the elderly. An innovative program sponsored by the Southeastern Michigan Spinal Cord Injury System tells high-risk youths about the consequences of interpersonal violence and presents strategies to avoid those tragic outcomes. This program is brought to elementary and high schools, where weapons are, unfortunately, too prevalent. Importantly, SCIs as a result of violence have decreased significantly, from a high of 21.8% in the 1990s, to the current level of 16.2% (3).

Table 16.2 SPINAL CORD INNERVATIONS/FUNCTION

Spinal Cord Level	Primary Muscle Groups	Primary Movements
C1–C3	Infrahyoid muscles Head/neck extension` Rectus capitis (anterior and lateral) Sternocleidomastoid Longus colli Longus capitis Scaleni	Depression of hyoid Neck extension, flexion, rotation, and lateral flexion
	Additional Primary Muscle Groups	**Additional Primary Movements**
C4	Trapezius Upper cervical paraspinals Diaphragm	Shoulder elevation, scapular adduction and depression Independent breathing
C5	Rhomboids Deltoids Rotator cuff muscles (partially—some nerve supply is at C6 level) Biceps Brachialis (partially) Brachioradialis (partially)	Scapular downward rotation Weak shoulder external rotation, flexion, and extension Shoulder abduction and rotation Weak approximation of humeral head to glenoid fossa Elbow flexion
C5	Rotator cuff muscles (complete innervation) Serratus anterior (partially) Pectoralis (clavicular segments) Total innervation of elbow flexors Supinators Extensor carpi radialis Flexor carpi radialis	Full shoulder rotation, adduction, flexion, extension Scapular abduction Horizontal shoulder adduction Strong elbow flexion and supination Wrist extension (weak) Tenodesis action of hand Very weak wrist flexion
C7	Latissimus dorsi Pectoralis major (sternal portion) Triceps Pronator teres Flexor carpi radialis Flexor digitorum superficialis Extensor digitorum (partially) Extensor pollicis longus and brevis	Elbow extension Forearm pronation Wrist flexion Finger flexion (trace) Finger extension (weak) Thumb extension (weak)
C8	Flexor carpi ulnaris Extensor carpi ulnaris Flexor digitorum profundus and superficialis	Complete wrist extension, adduction, and abduction Finger flexion (stronger) Thumb flexion, abduction, adduction, opposition

(*Continued*)

Table 16.2 SPINAL CORD INNERVATIONS/FUNCTION (*CONT.*)

Spinal Cord Level	Primary Muscle Groups	Primary Movements
	Flexor pollicis longus and brevis Abductor pollicis longus Abductor pollicis Opponens pollicis Lumbricals (partially)	Weak flexion at MCP with IP extension
T1	Doral interosseal Palmer interossei Abductor pollicis brevis Lumbricals (complete innervation) Erector spinae muscles (partially) Intercostal muscles (partially)	Finger abduction Finger adduction Thumb abduction (strong) MCP flexion with IP extension (strong) Thoracic spine extension Increased respiratory function with presence of intercostalis
T4–8	Erector spinae muscles (partially) Intercostal muscles (partially) Abdominal muscles (beginning at T7)	Stronger thoracic spine extension Stronger respiratory function Thoracic flexion Weak trunk flexion
T9–12	Lower erector spinae muscles Lower intercostal muscles Abdominal muscles Quadratus lumborum (partially)	Strong thoracic spine extension Trunk flexion, extension, rotation, and stability Pelvic control and stability
L1–3	Quadratus lumborum (full innervation) Iliopsoas Erector spinae (lumbar segment)	Pelvic elevation Hip flexion Lumbar extension
L4–5	Lumbar erector spinae Hip adductors Hip rotators Quadriceps Hamstrings (partially) Tibialis anterior	Lumbar extension and stability Hip adduction Hip rotation Knee extension Knee flexion (weak) Ankle dorsiflexion (weak)
S1–2	Hip extensors Hip abductors Hamstrings (complete innervation) Plantar flexors Invertors of ankle Evertors of ankle	Hip extension Hip abduction and stability Knee flexion Ankle plantar: flexion Ankle inversion and stability Ankle eversion and stability
S2–5	Bladder Lower bowel Genital innervations	Genitourinary functions Bowel functions

MCP, metacarpophalangeal; IP, interphalangeal.

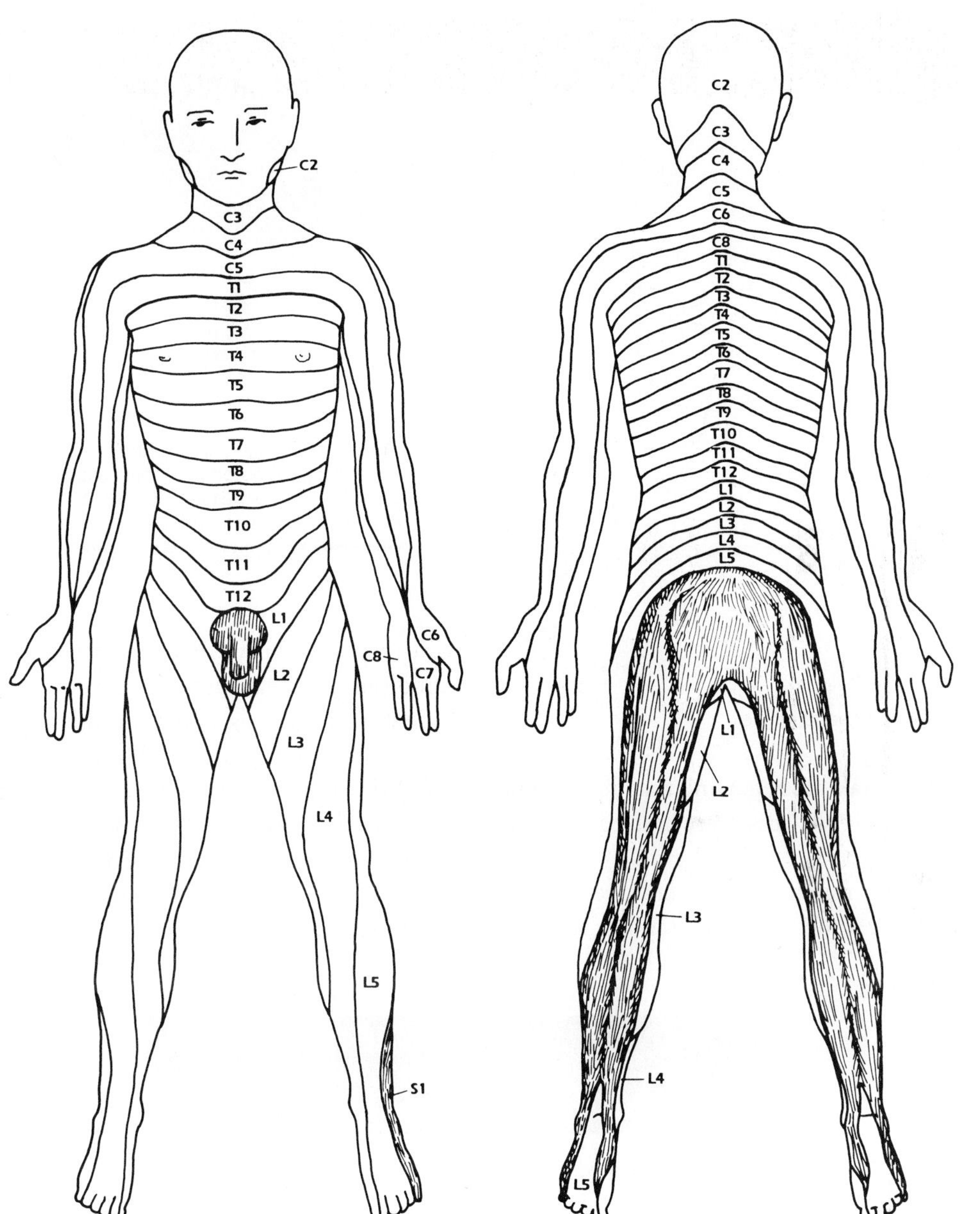

Figure 16.3 Dermatome map. (Reprinted with permission from Hammond M, Umlauf R, Matteson B, et al. Yes, You Can! A Guide to Self Care for Persons with Spinal Cord Injury. Washington, DC: Paralyzed Veterans of America, 1989.)

Incidence and Prevalence

Incidence rates for SCI in the United States are estimated at 40 cases/million population/year, excluding those who die at the scene of an accident (4). This translates to about 11,000 new cases of SCI every year. Who is the average person with SCI? The statistics indicate it is a 38-year-old white male involved in an auto accident, but this can vary widely, both geographically and seasonally. Seasonal sports cause fluctuations in etiology and incidence statistics, and some

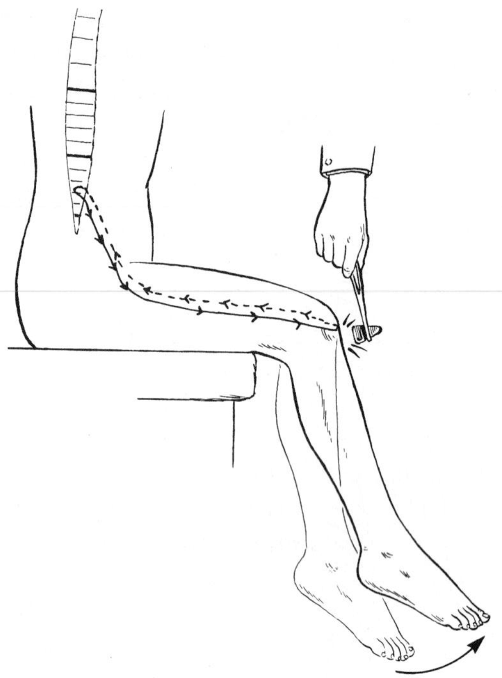

Figure 16.4 Knee-jerk reflex.

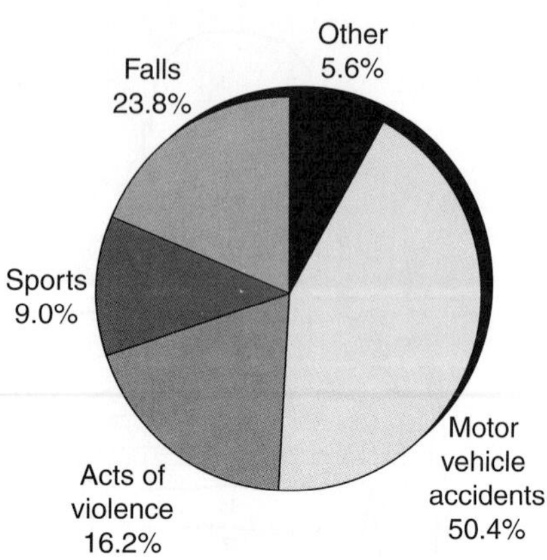

Figure 16.5 Etiologic distribution of spinal cord injury. (Adapted from the National Spinal Cord Injury Statistical Center. 2004 Annual Statistical Report. Birmingham, AL: University of Alabama at Birmingham, 2004.)

urban hospitals are reporting that a predominance of their SCI cases are caused by gunshot wounds.

Although much of the literature focuses on trauma, there are many nontraumatic causes of spinal cord damage. Developmental conditions, such as spina bifida, **scoliosis**, and spinal cord agenesis, may yield the same clinical signs as traumatic SCI. Many acquired conditions, such as bacterial or viral infections, benign or malignant growths, embolisms, thromboses, hemorrhages—even radiation or vaccinations—can lead to damage of spinal cord tissue.

Table 16.3 SPORTS-RELATED SPINAL CORD INJURIES

Sport	Percentage
Diving	66.0
Football	6.1
Snow skiing	3.8
Trampoline	2.6
Other winter sports	2.3
Wrestling	2.3
Gymnastics	2.2
Horseback riding	2.0
Other	9.6

Reprinted with permission from Stover SL, Fina PR, eds. Spinal Cord injury: The Facts and Figures. Birmingham, AL: The National Spinal Cord Injury Statistical Center, University of Alabama at Birmingham, 1986.

Signs and Symptoms

Sensory Functions

The two major classifications of SCI are complete and incomplete. A complete SCI occurs with a complete transection of the cord. In this case, all ascending and descending pathways are interrupted, and there is a total loss of motor and sensory function below the level of injury. The injury also may be referred to as an upper motor neuron (UMN) injury, if the reflex arcs are intact below the level of injury but are no longer mediated by the brain. UMN lesions are characterized by (a) a loss of voluntary function below the level of the injury, (b) spastic paralysis, (c) no muscle atrophy, and (d) hyperactive reflexes (Fig. 16.6).

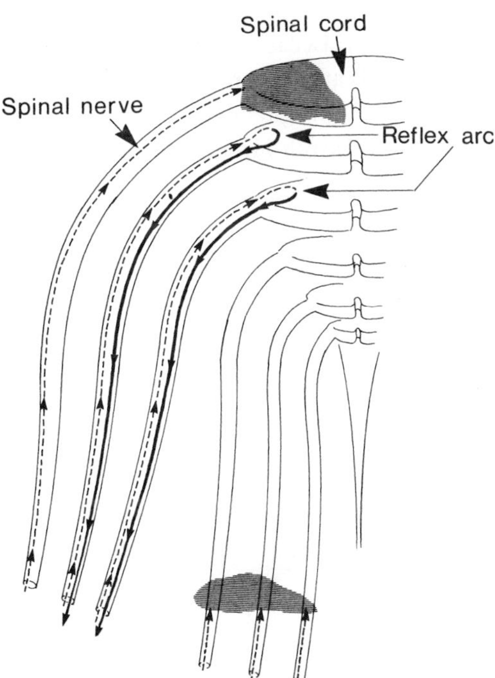

Figure 16.6 A diagrammatic representation of the reflex arc. The shaded lesion above denotes a UMN lesion, with the exception of the spinal nerve entering at the level of the lesion. The shaded lesion below represents an LMN lesion. (Reprinted with permission from the Rehabilitation Institute of Michigan.)

Complete injuries below the level of the conus medullaris (Fig. 16.1) are referred to as lower motor neuron (LMN) injuries, because the injury has affected the spinal nerves after they exit from the cord. In fact, injuries involving spinal nerves after they exit the cord at any level are referred to as LMN injuries. In these injuries, the reflex arc cannot occur, because impulses cannot enter the cord to synapse. As a result, LMN injuries are characterized by (a) a loss of voluntary function below the level of the injury, (b) flaccid paralysis, (c) muscle atrophy, and (d) absence of reflexes.

UMN and LMN injuries may be complete or incomplete. There also may be a mixture of UMN and LMN signs after an incomplete lesion in the lower thoracic/upper lumbar region. The following section discusses incomplete injuries in greater detail.

Incomplete Injuries

If damage to the spinal cord does not cause a total transection, there will still be some degree of voluntary movement or sensation below the level of injury. This is known as an incomplete injury, which may be further categorized according to the area of the spinal cord that was damaged and the clinical signs that are present.

Anterior Cord Syndrome

This syndrome results from damage to the anterior spinal artery or indirect damage to anterior spinal cord tissue (Fig. 16.7). Clinical signs include:

- Loss of motor function below the level of injury. Loss of thermal, pain, and tactile sensation below the level of injury.
- Light touch and proprioceptive awareness are generally unaffected.

Brown–Séquard's Syndrome

This syndrome occurs when only one side of the spinal cord is damaged (Fig. 16.8).

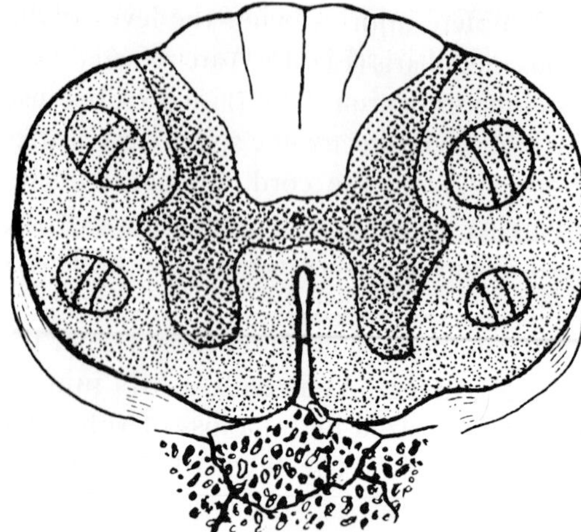

Figure 16.7 A cross-section of the spinal cord illustrating the damage that causes anterior cord syndrome. The anterior artery is involved, resulting in damage to most areas, with the exception of the posterior columns. (Reprinted with permission from the Rehabilitation Institute of Michigan.)

A hemisection of this nature frequently is the result of a stab or gunshot wound. The clinical signs of Brown–Séquard's syndrome generally include:

- Ipsilateral loss of motor function below the level of injury.
- Ipsilateral reduction of deep touch and proprioceptive awareness. (There is a reduction rather than loss as many of these nerve fibers cross.)
- Contralateral loss of pain, temperature, and touch.

Clinically, a major challenge presented by Brown–Séquard's syndrome is that the extremities with the greatest strength have the poorest sensation.

Central Cervical Cord Syndrome

In this lesion, the neural fibers serving the upper extremities are more impaired than those of the lower extremities (Fig. 16.9). This occurs because the fibers that innervate the upper extremities travel more centrally in the cord and, as the name of the syndrome implies, the central structures are the ones that are damaged (Fig. 16.2). Injury to the central portion of the spinal cord is often seen, along with structural changes in the vertebrae. Most commonly, hyperextension of the neck, combined with a narrowing of the spinal canal, results in this type of injury. Because arthritic changes can lead to spinal canal narrowing, this syndrome is more prevalent in aging populations. The signs of central cord syndrome often include:

- Motor and sensory functions in the lower extremities less involved than in the upper extremities.

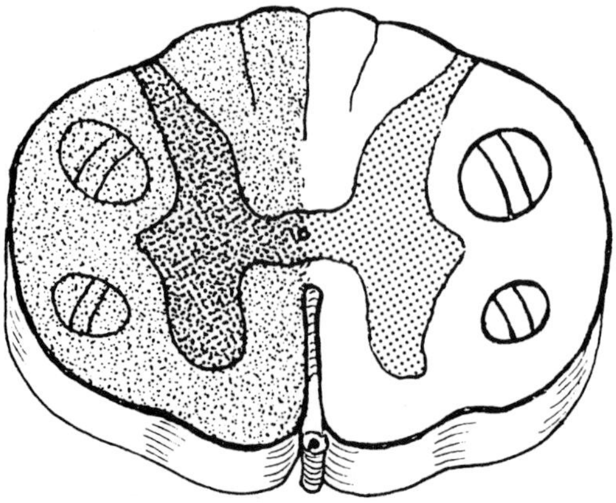

Figure 16.8 Cross-section of the cord, illustrating the damage that results in Brown–Séquard's syndrome. (Reprinted with permission from the Rehabilitation Institute of Michigan.)

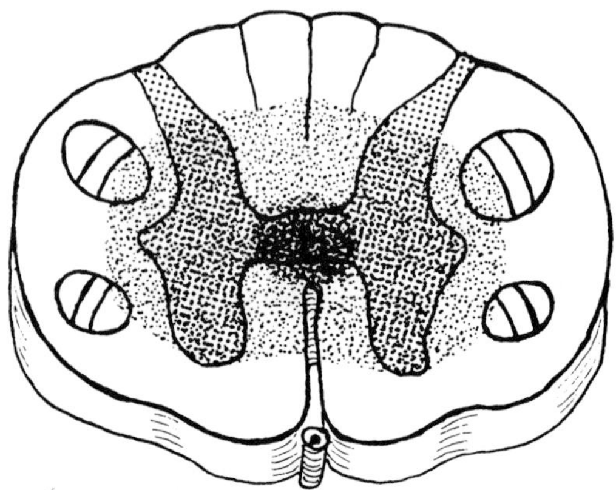

Figure 16.9 Cross-section of the cord, illustrating the damage resulting in central cervical cord syndrome. (Reprinted with permission from the Rehabilitation Institute of Michigan.)

- A potential for flaccid paralysis of the upper extremities, as the anterior horn cells in the cervical spinal cord may be damaged. Because these are synapse sites for the motor pathways, an LMN injury may result.

Cauda Equina Injuries

Cauda equina injuries do not involve damage to the spinal cord itself, but rather to the spinal nerves that extend below the end of the spinal cord (Fig. 16.1). Injuries to the nerve roots and spinal nerves that comprise the cauda equina are generally incomplete. Because this type of injury actually involves structures of the peripheral nervous system (exiting spinal nerves), there is some chance for nerve regeneration and recovery of function if the roots are not too severely damaged or divided. These injuries are usually the result of direct trauma from fracture dislocations of the lower thoracic or upper lumbar vertebrae. Clinical signs of cauda equina injuries include:

- Loss of motor function and sensation below the level of injury.
- Absence of a reflex arc, as the transmission of impulses through the spinal nerves to their synapse point is interrupted. Motor paralysis is of the LMN type, with flaccidity and muscle atrophy seen below the level of injury.

Complete Versus Incomplete Injuries

In both complete and incomplete injuries, the terms quadriplegia, tetraplegia, and paraplegia may be used to further describe the impact of the injury. Quadriplegia refers to lost or limited function of all extremities as a result of damage to cervical cord segments. The American Spinal Injury Association (ASIA) prefers the term tetraplegia over quadriplegia. Tetraplegia refers to impairment or loss of motor or sensory function in the cervical segments of the spinal cord that is the result of damage of neural elements within the spinal canal. Tetraplegia causes impairment of function in the arms as well as in the trunk, legs, and pelvic organs. It does not include brachial plexus lesions or injury to peripheral nerves outside the neural canal (5). Paraplegia, which refers to lost or limited function in the lower extremities and trunk depending on the level of injury, occurs after lesions to thoracic, lumbar, or sacral cord segments.

Spinal cord injuries are frequently classified further, based on the ASIA Impairment Scale (6), which contains the following categories:

A = Complete; no motor or sensory function is preserved in the sacral segments S4 through S5.
B = Incomplete; sensory but not motor function is preserved below the neurological level and extends through the sacral segments S4 through S5.
C = Incomplete; motor function is preserved below the neurological level, and the majority of key muscles below the neurological level have a muscle grade less than 3.
D = Incomplete; motor function is preserved below the neurological level, and the majority of key muscles below the neurological level have a muscle grade of greater than or equal to 3.
E = Normal; motor and sensory function is normal.

A manual muscle test is performed to assess the strength of muscles and aid in the determination of the extent and nature of injury. Usually, strength is graded on a six-point scale (7–10):

0 = Total paralysis
1 = Palpable or visible contraction
2 = Active movement, full range of motion (ROM) with gravity eliminated
3 = Active movement, full ROM against gravity
4 = Active movement, full ROM against moderate resistance

5 = Normal active movement, full ROM against full resistance
NT = Not testable

Posttraumatic Progression

The period of altered reflex activity immediately after a traumatic SCI is known as **spinal shock.** As a result of injury, spinal cord segments below the level of the lesion are deprived of excitatory input from higher CNS centers. What is observed clinically during this phase is a flaccid paralysis of muscles below the level of injury and an absence of reflexes (11). The bladder is also flaccid, requiring **catheterization,** and there is no voluntary control of the bowel. Depending on the level of the injury, the person with an SCI may require a ventilator because of lost or temporarily interrupted innervation to the diaphragm, intercostals, and abdominal muscles.

Spinal shock generally lasts from 1 week to 3 months after injury. Once spinal shock subsides, the areas of the spinal cord above the level of the lesion operate as they did premorbidly. Below the level of the lesion, reflexes will resume if the reflex arc is intact. This is an important concept to understand. Unlike a plant, which may die entirely if its stem is cut in half, the spinal cord is still alive and functional above and below the level of injury. The problem is one of communication; the brain cannot receive sensory information beyond the lesion site and cannot volitionally control motor function below that point.

After spinal shock subsides, there is often an increase in spasticity, especially in the flexor muscle groups. The reflex arc "fires" and the brain is unable to interfere. After this phase, there may be a period of 6 to 12 months after injury when an increase in the spasticity of the extensor groups is common. Usually, after 1 year postinjury, the wide fluctuations in tone will cease.

An array of complications can greatly affect the prognosis of a person who has sustained an SCI. Some of the more common medical complications are addressed in the next section.

Respiratory Complications

Persons with spinal cord injuries at or below the level of T12 generally have a normal respiratory status. Injuries above that level, however, compromise the respiratory system to some degree. The abdominal musculature is innervated by segments T7 through T12, the intercostal muscles are served by segments T1 through T12, and the diaphragm is innervated by C4. Persons with complete injuries above C4 usually need a respirator. Some may be candidates for a phrenic nerve stimulator if the nerve shows the ability to conduct an impulse. Generally, persons with complete injuries at C4 and below do not use respirators, but respiratory complications may persist. Breathing may be shallow, and the ability to cough productively may be weak. Various deep-breathing and assisted-coughing techniques may be taught, along with other procedures to keep the lungs clear. Prevention and early management of respiratory complications is crucial. Currently, respiratory complications are the most common cause of death following SCI.

Autonomic Dysreflexia (Hyperreflexia)

As implied by its name, **autonomic dysreflexia,** or hyperreflexia, involves an exaggerated response of the autonomic nervous system (ANS). It may be recalled that a function of the ANS is the integration of body functions in the fight-or-flight response—heart rate, blood vessel constriction/dilation, regulation of glands, and smooth muscle. The condition usually occurs in persons with spinal cord injuries above the T6 level. Signs to look for include a sudden, pounding headache, diaphoresis, flushing, goose bumps, and tachycardia followed by bradycardia. All of this is caused by an irritation of nerves below the level of injury. Common sources of irritation include an overfull bladder or bowel, urinary tract infections (UTIs), or **decubitus ulcers.** Even irritations such as ingrown toenails can trigger the response. All these would be bothersome to a person with an intact spinal cord—he or she would feel uncomfortable and act to remedy the situation. But the person with a spinal cord injury lacks this feeling, and autonomic dysreflexia is the body's way of warning that something is wrong below the level of the injury.

The most important aspect of managing autonomic dysreflexia is to find the cause and alleviate it. This may require emptying the bladder, checking for blockages or kinks in external urinary drainage tubing, checking for bowel impaction, or evaluating for other factors. It helps to decrease blood pressure if the person assumes an upright position. Most persons with tetraplegia will experience an episode of autonomic dysreflexia at least once, but if the signs of autonomic dysreflexia appear frequently, medication may be indicated. Although autonomic dysreflexia may appear suddenly, it must be managed promptly. Because the blood pressure may elevate dramatically, there is risk of stroke or death if the situation is ignored or mismanaged.

Postural Hypotension

In contrast to autonomic dysreflexia, blood pressure decreases in postural hypotension. This condition, often seen in persons who have sustained cervical or thoracic SCIs, also may be referred to as orthostatic hypotension (12). Blood tends to pool distally in the lower extremities as a result of reduced muscle tone in the trunk and legs. The symptoms of postural hypotension frequently occur when a person attempts to sit up after prolonged periods of bed rest. Symptoms include lightheadedness, dizziness, pallor, sudden weakness, and unresponsiveness. Preventive measures include the use of anti-embolism hosiery and abdominal binders, which externally assist circulation. Also, assuming an upright position slowly can help avoid these symptoms. If symptoms do occur, a semireclined or reclined position should be maintained until the symptoms subside.

Deep Vein Thromboses

Deep vein thrombosis (DVT) can be a serious complication in many types of medical conditions. They are a potential complication in SCI for three main reasons: reduced circulation caused by decreased tone, frequency of direct trauma to legs causing vascular damage (e.g., repeated trauma during transfer or bed mobility activities), and prolonged bed rest. Edema is often seen in SCI for the same reasons. Clinical signs of DVT may include swelling in the lower extremities, localized redness, and a low-grade fever. However, a DVT may be relatively asymptomatic on bedside evaluation. Vigilant medical screenings for DVT should be performed in all cases of SCI. An undetected and unmanaged DVT may result in an embolism and death.

Thermal Regulation

It has already been seen that damage to the spinal cord can disrupt the ANS, possibly resulting in autonomic dysreflexia. Thermal regulation is another function of the ANS that can be disturbed after SCI. Maintaining the appropriate body temperature often is a problem for persons whose injuries are above T6. During the first year after injury, the body tends to assume the temperature of the external environment. This condition is called poikilothermia (13). In time, some adjustment usually occurs. Cold weather often causes discomfort, as blood vessels below the level of injury do not constrict sufficiently to conserve the body's heat. Conversely, excessive sweating may occur above the level of injury in warmer weather but not below, which hampers the body's efforts to prevent hyperthermia. Because of this, extreme temperatures should be avoided, and attention should be given to the extent and type of clothing worn in all conditions.

Musculoskeletal

Spasticity. In persons who have UMN lesions, increased tone appears in muscles below the level of injury after spinal shock subsides. Virtually all individuals with cervical cord injuries experience spasms; 75% of those with thoracic lesions, less than 58% of those with lumbar injuries, and less than 25% of those with cauda equina injuries report spasms (14). An increase in spasticity can be triggered by a variety of factors including infections, positioning, pressure sores, UTIs, and heightened emotional states. Spasms are not necessarily disadvantageous. The ability to trigger their spasms can help some individuals maintain muscle bulk, circulation, bowel and bladder management, transfers, and other activities of daily living (ADL). Excessive spasticity, however, may result in contractures, pain, and a reduced ability to participate in activities. At this point, medical or surgical options may be recommended.

Heterotopic Ossification (Ectopic Bone). Heterotopic ossification (HO) refers to the abnormal formation of bone deposits on muscles, joints, and tendons. It occurs most often in the hip and knee and less frequently in the shoulder and elbow. It has been estimated that 20% of all persons with SCI have some degree of ectopic bone growth (15). Clinical signs of HO may include heat, pain, swelling, and a decrease in active or passive ROM. These signs should always alert the clinician, as they may indicate other serious complications as well, such as DVT. Many facilities that specialize in the care of persons with SCI routinely provide prophylactic medications that have shown promise in halting this abnormal calcification. In extreme cases in which range of motion is permanently and severely limited by HO, surgery may be indicated.

Genitourinary Complications

Urinary tract infections are a common and dangerous complication of SCI. Prior to modern medical management, many persons with SCI who survived the initial trauma died within a few years after injury, with one of the most common causes being kidney failure as a result of chronic UTI. For several reasons, individuals with SCI are prone to UTI or bladder infections. The bladder is composed of smooth muscle, innervated by sacral segments of the spinal cord. As such, it is affected by a loss of sensory and motor function, as are other parts of the body, depending on the level and extent of injury. The nature of bladder function will depend on whether the injury caused LMN or UMN deficits (Fig. 16.10). Injury at point A yields an UMN bladder, also referred to as a reflex or spastic bladder. In this case, the bladder can contract and void reflexively. Although this action is involuntary, some persons with SCI can trigger the reflex through various stimuli, much as the knee-jerk reflex, which is triggered by tapping with a reflex hammer. That is because impulses can still enter the cord below the level of injury, synapse, and exit.

Persons with a UMN bladder may use various types of catheters and additional techniques to ensure that the bladder does not become distended or retain urine. They generally cannot rely on sensation to alert them that the bladder has exceeded its normal capacity; rather, they must rely on an established voiding schedule.

An LMN bladder may also be referred to as a nonreflex or flaccid bladder. This type of

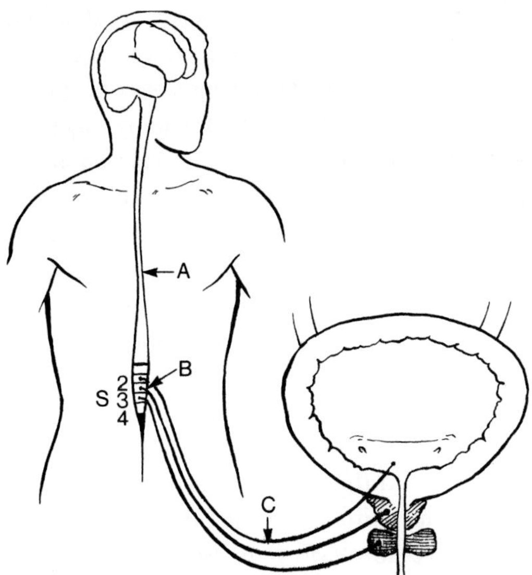

Figure 16.10 Bladder and corresponding spinal segment innervations. Injuries at point A would result in a UMN, or spastic bladder. Injuries at points B or C would result in LMN, or flaccid, bladder function. (Reprinted with permission from the Rehabilitation Institute of Michigan.)

bladder function is usually seen during the spinal shock phase and may remain if the injury has affected the cauda equina area. An injury at point B or C (Fig. 16.10) can result in an LMN bladder. With this type of injury, a reflexive emptying of the bladder cannot occur, as the reflex arc is destroyed. Because the bladder is flaccid and does not spontaneously empty, urine will accumulate continuously. Persons with an LMN bladder must catheterize according to a schedule or must apply external pressure to the abdomen with their fists, which forces urine from the bladder. This application of external pressure is called **Credé's method**.

With either type of bladder (UMN or LMN), voiding must occur routinely and completely. Chronic overstretching of the bladder will reduce its ability to empty adequately. Residual urine is a breeding ground for infections that can spread to all structures in the urinary system, including the ureters and kidneys. Chronic infections can lead to renal calculi (kidney stones), kidney failure, and, potentially, death. Warning signs of a UTI include urine that appears cloudy or has excessive particles, dark or foul-smelling urine, an elevated fever, chills, or an increase in spasticity. The best treatment of UTI is prevention—adhering to an effective voiding schedule, using clean or sterile techniques, maintaining a proper diet and adequate fluid intake, and prompt attention to warning signs.

Complications Associated with the Bowel

Normally, elimination occurs when stool is present in the rectum. Nerves in the rectal musculature are stimulated, triggering a reflexive **peristalsis** and a relaxation of the rectal sphincters. A bowel movement may be prevented at this step of the process if the brain overrides this reflex, sending down an impulse to tighten the sphincter muscles until an appropriate time. We have all experienced the sensation of urgency caused by a full rectum, but perhaps we have not fully appreciated our brain's ability to allow us to forestall the inevitable until a socially acceptable time.

Unfortunately, a SCI can interfere with bowel function in much the same way as it impedes the bladder. The bowel can become spastic or flaccid. A reflex bowel can be caused by a lesion at point A (Fig. 16.11). In this case, stool can be eliminated reflexively if nerves located in the rectum are stimulated. This stimulation may be done manually through digital stimulation or in conjunction with the use of suppositories. Establishing and following a regular schedule for bowel management can reduce occurrences of incontinence.

The bowel is usually flaccid during the phase of spinal shock and may remain in that state if the injury involves the areas illustrated at points B and C (Fig. 16.10). As with the flaccid bladder, the flaccid bowel cannot be stimulated to empty reflexively. Stool may often remain in the rectum after attempts at

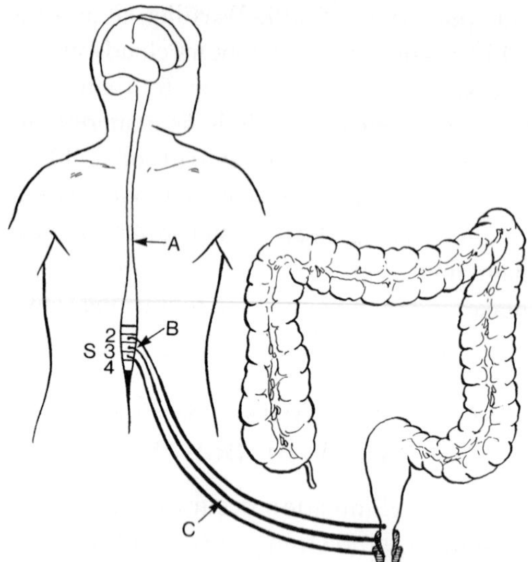

Figure 16.11 The bowel and corresponding spinal segment innervations. Injuries at point A would result in a UMN, or spastic bowel. Injuries at points B or C would result in LMN, or flaccid, bowel function. (Reprinted with permission from the Rehabilitation Institute of Michigan.)

evacuation, and it may be necessary to remove it manually to prevent impaction.

Constipation or impaction may result if elimination does not occur regularly. Aside from the standard discomfort associated with this, autonomic dysreflexia may be triggered in persons with lesions above the T6 level.

Diarrhea is another complication that can be particularly frustrating for the person with a SCI who is trying to establish a set schedule for bowel management. This condition is always frustrating, but the majority of the general population has the benefit of intact sensation to provide a warning. The best prevention for diarrhea in the person with a SCI is to make sure to use (not overuse) laxatives if they are prescribed, eat a proper diet, and follow a scheduled bowel program that reduces the chance of impaction, which can result in diarrhea.

Dermal Complications

The skin is the largest organ of the body, and it performs essential functions in maintaining your health. Skin assists in thermal regulation, insulating us in cold weather and sweating to prevent hyperthermia during hot conditions. Aside from literally keeping the body together, skin acts as a barrier to the external environment. At the cellular level, skin provides the site for O_2/CO_2 exchange through the capillary system. Keeping skin intact is essential and requires conscious effort by a person with a SCI, as sensations that would normally provide warning of potential skin damage, such as pain and extremes in temperature, are not perceived below the level of injury.

Damage to the skin as a result of pressure sores, or decubitus ulcers, is a major reason for hospital re-admissions in SCI populations. The mechanism of injury is continued pressure due to lack of movement. Circulation is impaired because of the pressure, and capillary exchange is impeded. This can result rapidly in tissue necrosis. The severity of pressure sores can be classified in four stages:

Stage I. Clinical signs are reddened or darkened skin. Damage is limited to more superficial (epidermal and dermal) layers. At this stage, tissue breakdown can be halted merely by removing pressure until the skin returns to its normal color.

Stage II. The skin now appears reddened and open. A blister or scab is present. The scab is not a sign of healing; rather, the tissue beneath it is necrotic. This involves the epidermal and dermal layers, as well as deeper adipose tissue. Wound dressings may be involved at this stage, and it is imperative that pressure be kept off the site.

Stage III. The skin breakdown is deeper, and the wound is now draining. Muscle may be visible through the open wound. An ulcer is developing in the necrotic tissue. In addition to wound dressings, surgical intervention may be indicated if more conservative treatment is unsuccessful.

Stage IV. All structures, from the superficial levels to the bone, are destroyed. Infection and bone decay occur. Surgical intervention is likely, and the person with a pressure sore at this stage often must spend weeks after a skin graft with pressure totally removed from the involved site (16).

Pressure sores are preventable with diligent attention and preventative strategies. A person with SCI can use, or instruct another person to assist with, a variety of pressure relief methods. Also, visual skin inspections should be performed at least twice daily, taking particular note of areas most prone to breakdown. These would include areas where bony prominences (e.g., the sacrum, ischium, calcaneus, and scapula) can add to pressure. Proper nutrition also should be heeded, as healthy skin is less apt to break down and is more responsive to healing in early stages of pressure sore development.

Other dermal complications, such as burns or frostbite, are prevented by attentiveness and common sense. Even commonly encountered things, such as space heaters or exposed plumbing under a sink, can cause severe burns to persons with a SCI without their immediate knowledge. It is important to be aware of the environment and to rely on other, intact senses to avoid injury.

Course and Prognosis

A prognosis implies that one can forecast or predict the outcome and chances for recovery from a particular disease or traumatic injury. That is somewhat challenging for SCIs. Although some aspects of SCI are highly predictable (e.g., specific muscle functions impaired with a complete lesion at C5), other aspects are much more vague.

Part of the ambiguity lies in the definitions of the term "recovery." One definition is to get back, or regain, which tends to be the client's focus. Another definition for recovery stresses compensation, which is often the thrust of the health care professional working with SCI. Whereas we will discuss the physiological prognosis of SCI, the clinician should always be aware, and acknowledge the validity, of the client's perspective on recovery. To get back and to compensate for are dramatically different terms. When discussing prognosis with a person who has survived a SCI, the clinician should always be truthful, but must also be acutely aware of the impact of what the client is hearing. Perhaps the most crucial indicators of an individual's functional outcome are personal characteristics such as motivation, use of support systems, and coping mechanisms. The clinician must be skilled at fostering these strengths while at the same time providing accurate information.

Physiologically, although extensive research is ongoing, there has not been independently confirmed, widespread success in inducing functional axonal regeneration within a damaged human spinal cord. Recent research headlines have reported that the use of steroids—specifically, methylprednisolone—may improve neurological outcomes of patients with SCI if administered within the first 8 hours after injury (17). Experimental drugs, such as GM-1 ganglioside and 4AP, are touted as aiding in the preservation of damaged nerves and insulating them from the toxic level of chemicals the body releases during trauma. Another new drug, Sygen, is in clinical trials to determine if it can reduce cell death if administered near the time of injury, thus improving functional outcomes. While fetal stem cell research relating to spinal cord regeneration is prevalent in the media, meaningful functional outcomes have been limited. New research related to stem cells found in a living donor's brain and spinal cord, which may be possible to remove, divide in a lab, and re-inject into a person with SCI may hold promise, and potentially avoid problems of cell rejection (18). Very recently, headlines were made regarding the treatment of spinal cord injuries with the use of stem cells from umbilical blood. This process reportedly resulted in a South Korean woman who had been paralyzed for 20 years being able to perform some level of ambulation with assistance (19). Additional research is being aimed at a variety of strategies, including pharmacologic and enzyme therapy, cloning of nerve cells, fetal tissue transplants, and the highly sophisticated altering of the cellular environment to encourage actual regeneration. As stated earlier, the spinal cord is alive above and below the level of injury; one goal of current research is to encourage functional reconnection of the disrupted pathways.

A different picture is presented with cauda equina injuries or injuries involving the nerve root. These types of injuries carry the potential for regeneration if the nerve roots are not severely damaged or divided. The degree of regeneration that can be expected is very difficult to predict, which must be done on an individual basis after extensive medical testing.

Aside from research on actual spinal cord regeneration, significant work also is being done with highly technical devices to compensate for paralysis. Functional electrical stimulation (FES) is one example. Persons with UMN injuries have experienced increases in their functional abilities (improved upper extremity function, standing ability, ambulation) with the external application of electrodes that stimulate muscle contraction. Although some may feel that the FES apparatus is cumbersome, unsightly, time consuming, and difficult to apply, refinements are ongoing (20). Many persons with SCI feel that, although not ideal, the technology provides an appealing alternative to outcomes from traditional methods of rehabilitation. Recently, the Food and Drug Administration (FDA) approved the Freehand System, a neuroprosthetic device that may be surgically implanted in a person with tetraplegia (21). This system combines internal electrodes, stimulators, sensors, and transmission coils within an external control box. It allows a person with tetraplegia to achieve a degree of prehension function, enhancing such ADL as eating, writing, and phone and computer use.

Overall, although actual regeneration of the cord may not be on the immediate scientific horizon, the advances in all phases of SCI management are promising. Everyone has the right to hope for what is not yet reality, without being said to have unrealistic expectations. Assisting someone to be hopeful, while simultaneously working to maximize today's function, is to truly master the art of the therapeutic relationship.

Impact of Condition on Occupation

Performance in areas of occupation relates to a person's ability to engage in activities that are essential and meaningful. Performance in areas of occupation include ADL, instrumental activities of daily living (IADL), education, work, play, leisure and social participation. Clearly, a SCI can have a catastrophic effect on a person's ability to function in these areas, because it can affect body function categories that support the ability to participate in these activities. Body function categories which may be impacted by a SCI include sensory functions and pain, voice and speech functions, functions of cardiovascular and respiratory systems, genitourinary and reproductive functions, neuromusculoskeletal and movement-related functions, functions of the skin and related structures, and select mental functions. The importance of understanding the theory of occupational performance cannot be overstated. We cannot begin to holistically treat a person with SCI until we can visualize the impact that this diagnosis has on the various aspects of that person's life. The following sections explore occupational performance areas and components to present a comprehensive view of the impact of SCI. Table 16.4 shows generally expected functional outcomes at various levels of complete injuries.

Instrumental Activities of Daily Living

Grooming, Oral Hygiene, Eating, Bathing, Dressing. For a person with quadriplegia, grooming, oral hygiene, and eating may be extremely laborious. The use of extensive adaptive devices or reliance on a caregiver may be necessary because of deficits in sensory and neuromuscular performance components. Persons with paraplegia are generally independent in these tasks, but they must often think ahead, making sure that items are available and sufficient time is allocated.

Bathing and dressing present major challenges for persons with quadriplegia. With higher-level injuries (C1 through C4), total assistance is required. At lower levels of injury, with extensive adaptive equipment and assistance from others in some task components, the person with quadriplegia can be a more active participant. It is extremely important for the person's own goals to be acknowledged. A recent study revealed that a person with a complete C6 injury required from 20 to 60 minutes to dress independently (21), yet none of the 10 patients in the study reported dressing themselves routinely after discharge from the hospital. Assistance was sought from others because of feelings that the task was too time consuming and exhausting. The question becomes, "Is this functional?" If a person is attempting re-entry into the work force or return to school, is it "functional" to spend an entire hour, as well as all the physical energy, in just getting dressed? Or is it a sign of greater autonomy to delegate some tasks to a caregiver to allow participation in activities that are more meaningful?

Secondary conditions aside, individuals with paraplegia are usually independent in bathing and dressing. Many even have the strength to transfer to the bottom of a tub without assistive devices.

Toileting. Managing altered bowel and bladder function is a challenge for everyone with SCI. The two aspects to this challenge are the actual physiologic management and the various techniques and equipment used in the toileting process.

Medications may be required for physiologic management. Stool softeners are used, as well as suppositories to assist in evacuation. A goal of effective bowel management is to eliminate reliance on medications. For persons with injuries at C7 or below, independence in toileting can usually be achieved with an array of equipment that may include suppository inserters, digital stimulators (devices that trigger reflexes to relax the rectal sphincter in UMN injuries), catheterization devices, leg separators, mirrors, and adapted commode chairs that allow access to the peri-anal area for bowel-training procedures.

Aside from medications and equipment, additional strategies include maintaining a specific schedule for elimination, eating a healthy diet that promotes regularity, assuming positions that facilitate elimination, and the use of Credé's method. If toileting appears to be tiring, then it has been portrayed correctly! But many persons with SCI become adept at its management. It may be a very different picture, though, when a person attempts these procedures in a community environment (i.e., rest rooms at work or school).

The person with a higher-level cervical injury faces another scenario. Although the bowel- and bladder-management concepts are the same, neuromuscular deficits limit performance of the tasks, even with adaptive equipment. Generally, persons with injuries above

Table 16.4 EXPECTED FUNCTIONAL OUTCOMES OF VARIOUS LEVELS OF COMPLETE INJURY (NONINCLUSIVE)

Last Spinal Cord Level Intact (Spared)	Expected Functional Outcome
C1–C3	Requires 24-hour availability of caregiver General ventilator-dependent Requires maximal assistance of another for pressure relief, or requires an adapted switch and reclining chair May propel power chair independently with adapted switches (pneumatic, chin, head, mouthstick); requires maximal for set-up Maximal assistance needed for transfers, positioning, bed mobility, dressing, feeding, hygiene, grooming, and bowel/bladder care Dependent with driving
C4	Requires 24-hour availability of caregiver Generally not using ventilation; continued difficulty with productive coughing and deep breathing Pressure relief, wheelchair propulsion, transfers, bed mobility, dressing, hygiene, bowel/bladder care, and driving comparable to C1–C3 level Adaptive feeding and grooming devices are available; they are very time-consuming and exhaustive for a person at this level and generally do not result in task independence
C5	May require 24-hour availability of caregiver Decreased respiratory endurance, but not using ventilator A strong person with a C5 injury may be independent in pressure relief by leaning side to side; a weaker person may require maximal assistance. Independent on level surfaces with a power chair and occasionally wrist/forearm supports; a manual wheelchair with rim adaptations may be used by a strong person for short distances Moderate to maximal assistance is required for all transfers, and generally a sliding board is used Moderate assistance is required for bed mobility A strong person with a C5 injury may assist with some dressing, hygiene, and grooming activities with the aid of adapted equipment. Feeding is generally possible with the use of adapted utensils and set-up. Driving is generally not feasible at this level, but an exceptionally strong person may be able to drive with specially adapted steering, braking and acceleration hand controls
C6	Amount of assistance needed from another person varies from moderate to very limited with just a few specific activities Some decreases in respiratory capacity and productive cough Has potential for independence in pressure relief Independently uses a manual wheelchair on level surface, gradual inclines, and down a curb backward. May require an electric chair for long distances or rough terrain.

(*Continued*)

Table 16.4 EXPECTED FUNCTIONAL OUTCOMES OF VARIOUS LEVELS OF COMPLETE INJURY (NONINCLUSIVE) (*CONT.*)

Last Spinal Cord Level Intact (Spared)	Expected Functional Outcome
	Ability to transfer varies. Some strong persons with C6 injuries are able to transfer independently with the use of a sliding board to a car, chair, bed, commode, or tub seat. Has the potential for independent bed mobility and positioning with rails, power controls, and trapeze With some adapted devices, usually independent with hygiene, shaving, and grooming. Potential for independence in bathing and bowel/bladder care with equipment. Generally independent with upper extremity (UE) dressing, and potential for independence in lower extremity (LE) dressing with adaptive devices. Independent with feeding, although a wrist-hand orthosis (WHO) and set-up may be required Generally able to drive independently using hand controls and adaptive devices
C7–C8	May be able to live independently without attendant care Some decreased respiratory endurance Independent in pressure relief Independently uses manual wheelchair Generally able to transfer without a sliding board; very strong persons may be able to transfer to the floor and tub bottom independently Generally independent with positioning, bed mobility, hygiene, feeding, shaving, hair care, dressing, bathing, cooking, and light housekeeping. (Independent with bowel/bladder care using adaptive equipment/techniques) Drives independently with hand controls/steering adaptations Can stand in parallel bars once assisted to upright position, with the use of a knee-ankle-foot orthosis (KAFO)
T1–T3	Can live independently Respiratory capacity and coughing abilities significantly improved All transfers generally independent Independent with all self-care; may require assistance with heavy household cleaning Finger dexterity, strength, and coordination are functional Drives independently with hand controls. Can get own wheelchair in and out of car Able to stand with minimal assistance, KAFO, and use of walker or parallel bars. Ambulation is generally not practical because of reduced balance and high energy expenditure.
T4–T8	Can live independently Respiratory status stronger than T1–T3 level; only slightly decreased Pressure relief, wheelchair use, positioning, bad mobility, and self-care all independent. May continue to require assistance with heavy cleaning

(*Continued*)

Table 16.4 EXPECTED FUNCTIONAL OUTCOMES OF VARIOUS LEVELS OF COMPLETE INJURY (NONINCLUSIVE) (*CONT.*)

Last Spinal Cord Level Intact (Spared)	Expected Functional Outcome
	Driving: comparable to T1–T3 level Generally able to ambulate short distances with the use of a walker to Lofstrand clutches and KAFO. Can stand independently with the use of a walker. May be able to manage curbs or stairs, but generally requires assistance. Ambulation requires high energy output.
T9–T12	Respiration is functional Pressure relief, wheelchair use, transfers, positioning, bad mobility, self-care, homemaking (except heavy tasks) all independent Able to drive with hand controls Can generally ambulate short community distances with KAFO and Lofstrand crutches
L1–L3	Same as T9–T12 level with the addition of improved ambulation distances; a wheelchair may still be required for long distances
L4–L5	Same as above, with exceptions Driving independent without adaptive devices Generally able to ambulate with ankle foot orthosis (AFO) and canes Wheelchairs generally not needed
S1–S2	A person with a S2-spared injury has the potential to ambulate without devices or orthoses A wheelchair is required. Hip extensors/abductors, knee flexors, and ankle plantar flexors are weak at the S1 level of injury. As with all other preceding levels, bowel and bladder function is impaired but managed independently at the level through adapted devices/techniques

Developed with material from the Rehabilitation institute of Michigan, 1996.

the C6 level require a caregiver to perform functions such as suppository insertion, digital stimulation, catheterization, and general perianal care. The person with SCI must indicate who the caregiver will be, particularly for tasks that are socially sensitive. Even though family members may be willing to assist, it is perfectly justifiable for the person to request someone else as a caregiver. Some persons may have no reservations about who assists them, whereas others may feel strongly that it would negatively affect established roles. Whatever the case, whenever feasible, the preferences of the person should be the deciding factor in selecting caregivers for various tasks.

Personal Device Care. The extent of personal and adaptive devices required by an individual with an SCI can generally be predicted by the level of injury (Table 16.4). Additional complications, such as reduced ROM resulting from contractures, may require use of more extensive devices than are typically seen at a particular level. Usually, personal device care is performed by others for those with injuries at C4 and above. Those with injuries at the C5 level and below have progressively more ability to assist in personal device care and use, but this fluctuates greatly depending on the individual's endurance, motivation, resources, and priorities.

Health Maintenance. Fostering a healthy lifestyle is critical, but often challenging, after a SCI. Most persons with a SCI are advised to follow lifelong exercise programs to preserve and enhance ROM and strength, as well as to promote good cardiovascular fitness and weight management. Many individuals report weight gains in the months after injury, as their energy demands are greatly altered in great part by use of a wheelchair for mobility. Attention also must be given to proper nutrition for weight management, impact on skin integrity, and bowel and bladder management. As mentioned earlier, routine attention to skin condition is crucial to avoiding dermal complications. A health maintenance routine may require the assistance of others, depending on the level of injury, for such activities as setting up weights and equipment, performing passive ROM, and aiding in skin inspection.

Socialization, Functional Communication, and Emergency Response. In pure SCIs, no cognitive deficits can preclude a person from socializing in an appropriate contextual manner. What is challenging, though, are the variety of barriers that may inhibit socialization. Architectural, environmental, and transportation barriers; reduced endurance; and increased reliance on others may discourage or actually prevent someone from traveling to the places where they socialized before their injury. Psychological barriers also may prevent reintegration into a premorbid social support system, and these "barriers" are as real as physical ones.

In all but the highest of injuries, verbal communication is functional. Persons with injuries at C7 or below are generally independent with a variety of forms of communication (e.g., writing, keyboard use, phone use) without the use of adaptive equipment. Above this level, however, adaptive devices are needed.

Requesting assistance in emergencies is possible at virtually all levels of injury, depending on the environment and adaptive equipment available. For persons with higher-level injuries, adaptive phone devices, emergency call systems, and environmental control units make contact with emergency agencies feasible. At the level of C4 and above, however, the availability of a caregiver 24 hours a day remains the most appropriate safety option. Individuals with injury below this level may use a phone independently but may be limited in other emergency responses, such as exiting a dwelling or attending to the physical needs of another injured person.

Functional Mobility. Persons with complete injuries at the T3 level and above usually rely on wheelchairs for household and community mobility. Those with injuries at C6 or above may require additional assistance in wheelchair management, or they may use an electric wheelchair with adapted controls. Acquiring an electric wheelchair may be a function of financial resources, not just need. Persons with complete injuries at T4 and below often can ambulate short distances with ambulation devices (walkers, Lofstrand crutches) and orthotic devices. Persons with sacral injuries often can ambulate community distances without orthoses or devices.

Sometimes it is not so much the ability or inability of the person with SCI but the inaccessibility of the environment that limits functional mobility. Whereas the home environment can be modified through creative thought, planning, and finances, the community environment is much harder to change. Many states have laws related to accessibility, but enforcement and compliance are less than ideal. Many physically challenged persons are fighting discriminatory situations (e.g., inaccessible public transportation, restaurants, offices, classrooms) in court. As these individuals become more numerous and visible, more legislation will be introduced to ensure their rights (22). A lighter side of the inaccessibility issue was recalled recently by Ed Roberts, founder of the first Center for Independent Living. He reminisced that early protestors in the disability rights movement were released from police custody because paddy wagons and jail cells were inaccessible (23)! In the vast majority of situations, however, an inaccessible environment is frustrating, demeaning, and personally violating. The health care team can do its part by helping physically, emotionally, or cognitively challenged persons to be aware of their rights, as well as by providing them with information on advocacy groups.

An extension of the functional mobility category includes driving. A strong C5-injured person may be able to drive with specially adapted low-effort steering, braking, and acceleration hand controls. Usually, those with injuries below the C5 level cannot drive because of physical and respiratory limitations. Persons with C6 injuries and below may be able to drive independently using hand controls and adaptive steering devices. A van with an electric lift may be recommended for someone who has difficulty maneuvering a wheelchair in and out of a car or van. Again, finances more than need may dictate the type of transportation used.

Sexual Expression

As with bowel and bladder function, most persons with SCI experience alterations in their ability to perform sexually as compared with their premorbid status. The nerves that innervate the genital area (both motor and sensory components) originate at the sacral spinal cord levels, so in the great majority of cases, sexual function is affected.

For the most part, the person can participate in a variety of sexual activities despite SCI, although the level of sensation and motor response will vary, depending on the extent and level of injury. Medications, surgical implants, and sexual enhancement devices may be recommended by specialists, but this is highly individualized.

Advances in the field of fertility have improved the chances for a spinal cord-injured male to father a child. Although fertility rates for men with SCI are estimated at less than 10%, techniques such as electrostimulation to induce ejaculation in paraplegics have proven successful in many cases (24). Men may be well advised to delay a decision about surgical penile implants until at least 1 year after injury. This allows time to evaluate the full impact of the SCI on sexual function and to determine the extent, if any, of sensory or motor return in an incomplete injury. The reproductive capabilities of women are generally unaltered by a SCI, and women and their partners should be made aware that the potential for pregnancy exists.

Addressing sexual function should be an integral part of each person's treatment plan, but a distinction should be made between purely physiological sexual performance—arousal, orgasm, ejaculation—and sexuality, which is the totality of a person's attractiveness, personality, and self-perception as a sexual being. Sexuality does not have to rely on physiology. Whereas performance may be hampered as a result of an SCI, one's sexuality can be quite healthy and intact. The health care provider must make accurate information available and identify sources of more detailed information or expertise. It is entirely at the discretion of the person with an SCI to explore, or not explore, options available to them.

Home Maintenance

Tasks such as household maintenance, meal preparation, shopping, cleaning, clothing care, and safety procedures are included within the general category of home maintenance. Usually, persons with a C6-level injury or above require assistance with all of these activities and need some attendant care. Persons with injuries at C7 or lower can live independently (without attendant care) in accessible environments. Heavier home-maintenance tasks may be performed by others, but most routine activities can be accomplished with adaptive techniques and equipment.

Care of Others

An SCI can certainly make caring for others difficult, particularly if the injured person had been the primary care giver for a child, spouse, or parent. Although a major goal of those with SCI is mastering self-care, a concurrent goal may be the introduction of activities (e.g., diapering, bathing a child) that can allow them to assume some premorbid roles. Often, many of these previous responsibilities must be delegated to others. In these cases, it is ideal if the person with SCI retains the responsibility for the verbal direction of care.

Education

Persons with SCI can generally resume educational activities, even while still inpatients in rehabilitation facilities. Many specialty hospitals retain the services of teachers from local school districts, and educational instruction is often scheduled along with other therapies for elementary, secondary, and high school students, allowing smoother reintegration after discharge.

College students would most likely be able to resume their studies. Depending on their level of injury, however, persons may re-evaluate their course of study to prepare for a more feasible career.

Adaptive writing devices, page turners, tape recorders, and computers have made returning to the classroom less intimidating. Laws have also improved the accessibility of public buildings, such as schools. It is challenging for the student to manage bowel and bladder schedules, adjustment of clothing, eating devices, and so forth, but with planning and the assistance of others, if needed, many individuals have successfully returned to the classroom.

Vocational

It is appropriate for a person with any level of SCI to begin to formulate vocational options, even as an inpatient, with the members of the health care team. Individual situations are so variable—premorbid occupation, level of injury, educational level, other vocational interests, family support, cognitive abilities, motivation, financial resources—making it impossible to say whether a person with a certain level of SCI can or cannot be gainfully employed. However, legislation mandates that work sites be accessible, within reason. Also, many employers recognize the importance of a trained employee and will make additional accommodations to return a valued person to the workplace.

As we move from an industrial to an information society, the job market will change, with positions requiring less menial labor (and being better compensated) than previously. Job requirements for this "new society" will include analytical thought, problem solving, and creativity, all of which are certainly intact after a spinal cord injury!

Leisure Activities

For most people, leisure pursuits are an integral part of a meaningful life. Although an SCI can alter the way in which one participates in leisure activities, it does not have to change the intensity of participation.

Sports, both individual and team, are excellent leisure pursuits that are growing in popularity for persons with SCI. Virtually any sport can be undertaken, from basketball to tennis to archery. True, adaptive equipment and modified regulations help make some sports more feasible and competitive for persons with SCI, but most athletes use "adaptive" equipment. How long would a catcher last in baseball without a mitt and a mask? Adaptive equipment need not detract from the legitimacy of the contest. It is heartening to see that, even internationally, the wheelchair athlete is recognized for excellence, with designated events in the Olympic games. Persons with SCI who want to participate have numerous avenues open to them.

Aside from sports, opportunities for social activities from square dancing to traveling abound. Travel agencies and tour groups have recognized the market created by the wheelchair traveler and have responded. Most hospitals with specialized SCI rehabilitation units have well-established programs that help persons get involved with special interest groups. Often, during the acute phase of SCI, persons cannot envision themselves participating again in the things they enjoy. The health care professional must be available for these individuals to encourage renewed interest in favorite leisure activities.

Several resources related to leisure activities, as well as other issues, have been discussed in this chapter. The reader is encouraged to consult the references and suggested readings at the end of this chapter for more information. Additionally, Table 16.4 gives an overview of specific expected outcomes for each level of SCI.

CASE STUDY

Case Illustration

■ CASE 1

M.L. is a 19-year-old woman who sustained an SCI during a motor vehicle accident while on her honeymoon. Her husband was thrown from the vehicle but received only minor injuries. M.L. was transported by emergency medical services (EMS) to the local emergency department. She was diagnosed with a C5 through C6 vertebral subluxation and a C6 crush injury, resulting in a complete C6 spinal cord injury. She also sustained a left clavicular fracture. She received nasal O_2 for respiratory support. Once stabilized, she was transferred to the specialized trauma center near her home. A halo vest was applied, which stabilized her cervical spine. No operative procedures were indicated at that time. After 22 days, her endurance improved so that she could tolerate sitting upright in a chair for up to 1 hour. She was transferred to the nearby rehabilitation facility's SCI unit. During her 12 weeks there, the only complications she experienced were two episodes of autonomic hyperreflexia (apparently secondary to hard stool in the lower rectum) and a mild UTI. Spasticity developed in her wrists, elbows, and lower extremities.

Before her injury, M.L. was a college student in a liberal arts curriculum. She and her new husband had recently signed a 1-year lease on an upstairs apartment close to the university. She had been totally independent in all of her ADL and home-management activities. Her leisure pursuits included recreational team sports (particularly softball) and more sedentary activities like reading and gourmet cooking. She was also involved with her family, particularly two sisters and her parents, who live close by.

Many body functions are significantly affected by M.L.'s injury. Her sensorimotor deficits are consistent with those anticipated for a C6 complete quadriplegia.

M.L. is challenged by the psychosocial/psychological issues facing her as a result of her SCI. She feels that her role has changed significantly, especially in her relationship with her husband. He has been willing to assist her in those activities in which she is physically limited; however, his assistance in some activities—particularly bowel management—has been difficult for her to accept. This has been a source of frustration for her, and she has discussed with him the possibility of hiring an attendant on a limited basis to assist with specific activities. He resists this idea, stating that it is his desire and duty to care for her. He took a temporary leave of absence from the family-owned landscaping company where he is employed when she was discharged 2 weeks ago. There is no definite timetable for his return. M.L. also is concerned about her ability to express herself sexually, as well as her potential to have children in the future. She attended classroom sessions on these topics in the rehabilitation facility, but she did not seek any individual counseling. M.L. states that she probably wasn't ready to hear anything specific then, but she now wishes she has someone to whom she could ask questions.

M.L. has not begun to consider her work activities or return to school. Even before her accident, she had been undecided about a career path. She has expressed interest, however, in exploring possible alternatives.

M.L. has stated that eventually she might like to get involved in team sports again. In the 2 weeks since her discharge, though, her main leisure pursuits have been reading and watching television.

References

1. Guttmann L. Spinal Cord Injuries. Oxford, England: Blackwell Scientific, 1976.
2. Hanak M, Scott A. Spinal Cord Injury: An Illustrated Guide for Health Care Professionals.New York: Springer Publishing, 1983.
3. Spinal cord injury facts and figures at a glance—August 2004. Spinal Cord Injury Information Network. Available at http://www.spinalcord.uab.edu. Accessed November 5, 2004.
4. Woodruff BA, Baraon RC. A description of nonfatal spinal cord injury using a hospital based registry. Am J Prev Med 1994;10:10–14.
5. American Spinal Injury Association/International Medical Society of Paraplegia. International Standards for Neurological and Functional Classification of Spinal Cord Injury. Chicago: American Spinal Injury Association, 1992:5.
6. American Spinal Injury Association/International Medical Society of Paraplegia. International Standards for Neurological and Functional Classification of Spinal Cord Injury. Chicago: American Spinal Injury Association, 1992:27.
7. Aids to Investigation of Peripheral Nerve Injuries. Medical Research Council War Memorandum. 2nd Ed. Revised. London; HMSO, 1943.
8. Brunnstrom F, Dennen M. Round table on muscle testing. Annual Conference of American Physical Therapy Association, Federation of Crippled and Disabled, Inc. New York, 1931:1–12.
9. Hislop H, Montgomery J, Connelly D, eds. Muscle Testing: Techniques of Manual Examination. 6th Ed. Philadelphia: Saunders, 1995.
10. Lovett RW. The Treatment of Infantile Paralysis. 2nd Ed. Philadelphia: P. Blakiston's Son, 1917:136.
11. Yashon D. Spinal Injury. 2nd Ed. East Norwalk, CT: Appleton-Century-Crofts, 1986:35–36.

12. Bloch RF, Basbaum M. Management of Spinal Cord Injuries. Baltimore: Williams & Wilkins, 1983:153–154.
13. Hanak M, Scott A. Spinal Cord Injury: A Illustrated Guide for Health Care Professionals. New York: Springer Publishing, 1983:30.
14. Burke DC, Murray DD. Handbook of Spinal Cord Medicine. New York: Raven Press, 1975:67.
15. Hernandez AM, Fjorner JV, DeLaFuente T, et al. The paraarticular ossifications in our paraplegics and tetraplegics: a survey of 704 patients. Paraplegia 1978;16:272–275.
16. Cassell BL. Treating pressure sores stage by stage. RN 1986;49:36.
17. Bracken M, Holeord TR, Shepard MJ, et al. A randomized, controlled trial of methylprednisolone or naloxone in the treatment of acute spinal cord injury. N Engl J Med 1990;322(20): 1405–1416.
18. Research in spinal cord injury—SCI info sheet #18. Spinal Cord Injury Information Network. RRTC in Secondary Complications of SCI at the University of Alabama at Birmingham, Dept. of PM&R, December, 1998. Available at http://www.spinalcord.uab.edu. Accessed November 5, 2004.
19. Stem cell therapy brings paralyzed to feet. Available at http://chinadaily.com.cn/english/doc/ 2004–11/29/ content_395570.htm. Accessed December 21, 2004.
20. Pipp TL. Mobilizing hope. Detroit News, September 15, 1997:1–2B.
21. Weingarden S, Martin C. Independent dressing after spinal cord injury: a functional time evaluation. Arch Phys Med Rehabil 1989;70:518–519.
22. Price D. Building lives with no barriers. Detroit News Washington Bureau, March 18, 1990:17–23A.
23. Berczeller PH, Bezkor MF. Medical Complications of Quadriplegia. Chicago: Year Book Medical Publishers, 1986:165.
24. Perkash I, Martin D, Warner H, et al. Electroejaculation in spinal cord injury patients: simplified new equipment and technique. J Urol 1990;143:305–307.

Recommended Learning Resources

General Texts/Resources Relating to SCI

American Spinal Injury Association/International Medical Society of Paraplegia. International Standards for Neurological and Functional Classification of Spinal Cord Injury. Chicago: American Spinal Injury Association, 1992.

Berczeller PH, Bezkor MF. Medical Complications of Quadriplegia. Chicago: Yearbook Medical Publishers, 1986.

Buchanan LE, Nawoczenski DA. Spinal Cord Injury: Concepts and Management. Baltimore: Williams & Wilkins, 1987.

National Institute of Neurological Disorders and Stroke. Available at http://www.ninds.gov. Accessed July 22, 2005.

National Spinal Cord Injury Statistical Center (NSCISC). 619 19th Street South, SRC 515, Birmingham, Alabama, 35249–7330. Available at http://www.spinalcord.uab.edu. Accessed August 12, 2005.

Ozer MN. The Management of Persons with Spinal Cord Injury. New York: Demos Publications, 1988.

Treischmann R. Spinal Cord Injuries: Psychological, Social and Vocational Rehabilitation. 2nd Ed. New York: Demos Publications, 1988.

Whiteneck G, Lammertse D, Manley S, et al. The Management of High Quadriplegia. New York: Demos Publications, 1989.

Yashon D. Spinal Injury. 2nd Ed. East Norwalk, CT: Appleton-Century-Crofts, 1986.

Patient/Family Resources

Christopher Reeve Foundation.
P.O. Box 277,
FDR Station, New York,
NY 10150–0277.
www.apacure.com

Corbet B. Options: Spinal Cord Injury and the Future. Denver: A.B. Hirschfield, 1980.

Hammond M, Umlauf RL, Matteson B, et al. Yes You Can! A Guide to Self Care for Persons with Spinal Cord Injury. Washington, DC: Paralyzed Veterans of America, 1989.

Phillips L, Ozer A, Axelson P, et al. Spinal Cord Injury: A Guide for Patient and Family. New York: Raven Press, 1987.

Spinal Cord Injury Information Network. Available at: www.spinalcord.uab.edu. Accessed July 22, 2005.

The Miami Project to Cure Paralysis. University of Miami School of Medicine. P.O. Box 016960, Mail Locator R-48, Miami, FL 33101. Available at: www.miamiproject.miami.edu. Accessed September 4, 2005.

General Neuroanatomy

Barr ML. The Human Nervous System: An Anatomic Viewpoint. 3rd Ed. New York: Harper & Row, 1979.

Liebman M. Neuroanatomy Made Easy and Understandable. 3rd Ed. Rockville, MD: Aspen Publishers, 1986.

Functional Electrical Stimulation

Kralj A, Bajd T. Functional Electrical Stimulation: Standing and Walking after Spinal Cord Injury. Boca Raton: CRC Press, 1989.

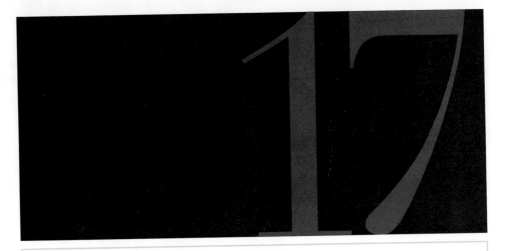

Orthopaedics

Heather (Gallew) Javaherian

Key Terms

- Arthroplasty
- Closed fracture
- Colles' fracture
- Comminuted fracture
- Complex regional pain syndrome (CRPS)
- Compound fracture
- Delayed union
- Disuse syndrome
- Echymosis
- Greenstick fracture
- Malunion
- Nonunion
- Open fracture
- Open reduction internal fixation (ORIF)
- Osteoarthritis
- Osteoporosis
- Pathologic fracture
- Remodeling
- Smith's fracture
- Volkmann's deformity

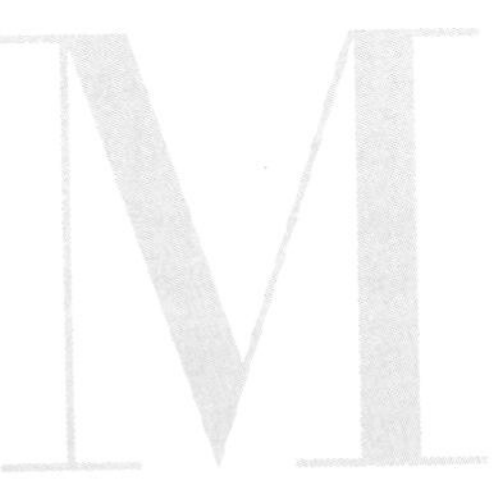

Mary Adda, a 62-year-old married woman, lived with her husband in a small two-story home. Though obese and managing diabetes, Mary Adda was very active. She volunteered at her church and the community hospital. She loved to garden, walk, play cards with her friends, and do crossword puzzles. At home she did most of the cooking but shared the housework with her husband. Mary Adda and her husband also square danced with a local club twice a week—they both liked to stay busy.

Mary Adda had been diagnosed with arthritis several years earlier. She regularly took anti-inflammatory medication to manage her pain and discomfort. However, the past year her right hip had become more and more painful. She had difficulty getting out of bed in the morning and had stopped square dancing because of the pain. Her husband took over the gardening as she could not get down on the ground to do the planting and weeding. Mary Adda's children also noticed her decline in activity. She no longer played out in the yard with the grandchildren and had cut back on her volunteer hours.

Her family encouraged her to talk to her physician about her arthritis.

After several consultations, Mary Adda decided to have an elective total hip replacement (THR). Plain radiographs obtained from the right hip revealed severe arthritic changes. Her physician thoroughly discussed the benefits and risks of the surgery with her and her husband. She was seen for pre-assessment training which involved meeting with several members of the orthopaedic total joint team. During this time she met with both an occupational and physical therapist. The occupational therapist asked her several questions about her postoperative goals, the design of her home, her family support, and the activities in which she liked to engage. The occupational therapist explained that she would receive occupational therapy after the surgery to help her regain independence in daily activities while safely following her hip precautions. The occupational therapist told her that it would take about 6 weeks to recover, and that she should be slow dancing with her husband and back to volunteering within 12 weeks. Both Mary Adda and her husband looked forward to her return to an active lifestyle.

Joint replacements are just one example of an orthopaedic condition that occupational therapy practitioners will commonly come across in their practice. In the late 1960s, Sir John Charnely completed the first successful hip **arthroplasty** (1). The technology of arthroplasties, also known as joint replacements, continues to evolve making them a key to promoting participation in daily activities and improving quality of life in people with severe arthritis. In the United States alone, approximately 500,000 total hip and knee arthroplasties are performed annually with this number expected to rise with the aging of our population (2). Therapists working in acute care, rehabilitation, and long-term care facilities will often be a part of the orthopaedic team. According to the National Board for Certification in Occupational Therapy, registered occupational therapy practitioners work most often with people who have had hip and knee replacements, as well as strokes (3).

Etiology

Orthopaedic conditions involve injury and disease of bones, joints, and their related structures. These conditions may be caused by a traumatic injury such as a fall or motor vehicular accident (MVA), or by diseases such as **osteoarthritis** and **osteoporosis**. Fractures are one of the most common orthopaedic conditions. A fracture is a break in the continuity of the bone. Most fractures result from falls, MVAs, and sports injuries. Falls contribute to a significant number of fractures. It is important to carefully evaluate the nature and circumstances surrounding the fall. This is especially important in children. Children are likely to sustain fractures in their play and sports activities. In some circumstances, however, a fracture may be a result of child abuse. Therefore, it is important to conduct a thorough history of the fall, the developmental level of the child, and a radiologic analysis of the fracture (4).

There are two critical factors involved in the determination of a fracture. They are the amount of force applied to the bone and the strength of the bone (5). Forces can be high energy such as those experienced in a MVA, or low energy such as those experienced in a fall or from continued stress to a bone or joint from running. The bone strength may be normal or weakened from pathological conditions such as tumors, osteoarthritis, and osteoporosis. The age of the person and the size of the bone further influence its ability to withstand a force.

The pathological conditions mentioned above negatively affect bone density, elasticity, and supportive structures, thus making the bone more vulnerable to fracture. The bone is weak and unable to sustain normal forces experienced during daily activities. Thus the bone may fracture while someone simply bends over or gets out of bed. This type of fracture is called a **pathologic fracture**. Osteoarthritis and osteoporosis are common conditions that may lead to a pathologic fracture.

Osteoarthritis, also referred to as degenerative joint disease, is a noninflammatory joint disease that results in deterioration of articular cartilage and the formation of new bone or osteophytes on the joint surface. These changes often result in pain, joint edema, and impaired participation in life activities. Osteoarthritis is the most common joint disease in the upper extremity. In the United States, more than 20 million people have osteoarthritis (6). The most common joints affected are the knee, distal interphalangeal joint, proximal interphalangeal joint, and the first carpal metacarpal joint. Osteoarthritis of the knee tends to cause the most disability. As a result of osteoarthritis, many individuals seek elective surgery for hip and knee replacements to enable them to return to a more active and pain-free lifestyle.

Osteoporosis is a disease characterized by low bone density and deterioration of bone. According to the National Osteoporosis Foundation, 10 million people have osteoporosis and 80% are women (7). It is common in postmenopausal women due to the cessation of estrogen production. A person with osteoporosis may fracture a bone through normal movement such as turning to reach an item of clothing when getting dressed in the morning. The most common sites of these fractures are the neck of the femur, humerus, and distal radius with over 300,000 hip fractures, and approximately 250,000 wrist fractures annually (7). A balanced diet, supplements, weight-bearing exercise, and bone density screenings are measures to decrease osteoporosis.

Incidence and Prevalence

In 2002, the National Center for Injury Prevention (NCIP) reported unintentional falls as the leading cause of nonfatal injury in the United States. This includes all age groups except for the age range of 15 to 24 (8). This is not surprising given the interest in sports activities, high-risk activities such as sky diving, and the number of MVAs. The most common fractures that result from falls are those of the humerus, wrist, pelvis, and hip (9).

Falls are the leading cause of fractures among older adults (10). In 2001, more than 1.6 million older adults were treated for fall-related injuries, which included fractures and other conditions (11). The 2000 census reported that there are 360,000 to 480,000 fall-related fractures in older adults per year (12). These include fractures of the hip, wrist, humerus, vertebrae, and pelvis, with the most serious being a hip fracture. Older adult women sustain approximately 80% of all hip fractures (13). It is expected that by the year 2040, the number of people older than age 65 will reach 77.2 million. Given this significant increase in the older adult population, the number of hip fractures in the United States is expected to exceed 510,000 (14).

Hip fractures are a primary cause of disability and mortality in the older adult. Statistics suggest that one in five people die within the first year of sustaining a hip fracture (15). Other studies report that many patients will not regain their premorbid functional level (16–20). However, in a randomized trial, Hagsten et al. found that occupational therapy intervention increased patient's ability to perform activities of daily living (ADL), sooner than those who did not receive occupational therapy (21). Thus, patients receiving occupational therapy were more likely to return to an independent living situation and require less postoperative care.

This charges occupational therapy practitioners with the role of promoting life participation and well-being among individuals who are recovering from fractures as well as other orthopaedic conditions.

Signs and Symptoms

The general symptoms of a break are localized pain at the fracture site, deformity, edema, and **ecchymosis** (usually after 24 to 48 hours) (22). A physician completes a clinical evaluation obtaining information on the signs and symptoms, and the circumstances surrounding the fracture. The physician then makes a referral to the radiologist to confirm and determine the degree and classification of the fracture. The radiologist also evaluates for other associated findings such as a pathological fracture (bone weakened by a tumor), stress fracture, or other pre-existing conditions that may have affected the integrity of the bone. The diagnosis is commonly confirmed through plain films though other studies may be ordered depending on the physician, suspected injury, and location of the suspected injury.

There are several types of fractures. A **closed fracture** refers to a fracture that has not broken through the skin, whereas in an **open fracture** the bone breaks through the skin surface. Open fractures, also known as **compound fractures**, have an increased chance for infection. The term comminuted is applied to fractures that have two or more fragments. A displaced fracture involves segments that have become separated or shifted from the bone (22). **Greenstick fractures** are often seen in children whose bones are still soft and growing. Rather than snapping into two, the bone breaks on one side and bends on the other. It is similar to how a young twig or tree limb breaks, thus the name greenstick fracture.

Fractures are further described by the type of fracture line. A complete fracture involves a break in the full continuity of the bone. An incomplete fracture involves a partial disruption in the continuity of the bone. Such breaks are often called cracks or hairline fractures (22). A transverse fracture occurs when the fracture line is at a right angle to the longitudinal axis of the bone. An oblique fracture involves a fracture line that is diagonal or slanted. Torsional stress applied to bone causes a twisting fracture line, which is called a spiral fracture.

Hip Fractures

A hip fracture generally refers to a fracture of the proximal femur. It may be intracapsular or extracapsular. Intracapsular fractures involve the femoral neck such as a subcapital or transcervical fracture (Fig. 17.1). Extracapsular fractures involve the trochanters such as a subtrochanteric or intertrochanteric fracture. An individual with a hip fracture may experience referred pain to the knee, be unable to bear weight on the involved lower extremity, and will often have a leg-length discrepancy.

Distal Radial Fractures

Distal radial fractures may cause loss of sensation, strength, movement, and functional use of the hand and possibly the arm. As most of these injuries are caused by a fall on an outstretched arm, the entire upper extremity should be examined for injury. A **Colles' fracture** will reveal "dorsal displacement, dorsal comminution, and radius shortening" (23). This is often referred to as a dinner fork deformity given its resemblance to an upside down fork. A **Smith's fracture** is the reverse of a Colles' fracture, therefore the deformity displaces toward the volar or palmar aspect of the wrist (23). Refer to Figure 17.2 for an illustration of distal radial fractures.

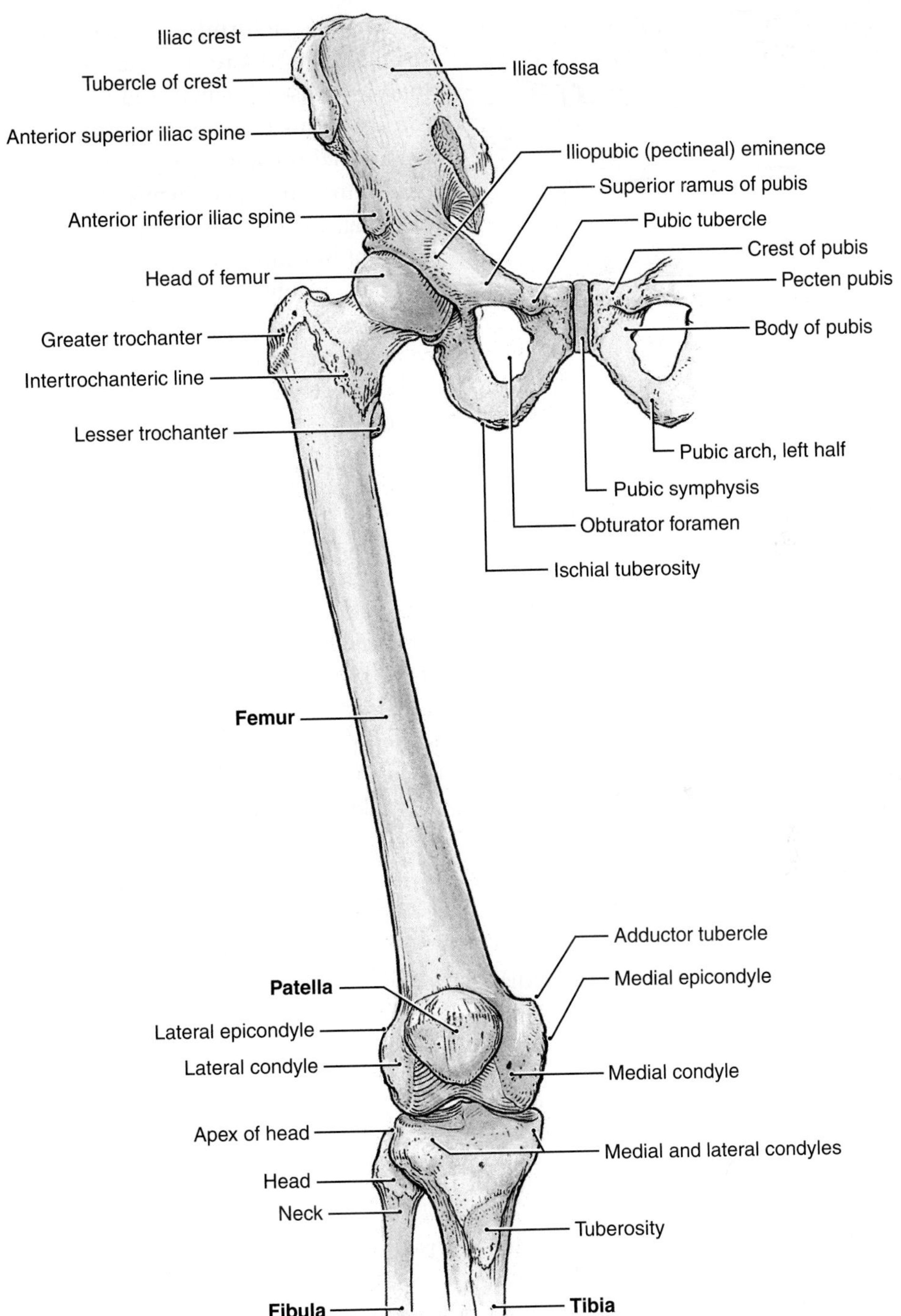

Figure 17.1 Lower extremity, anterior view. (Reprinted with permission from Agur AMR. Grant's Atlas of Anatomy. 9th Ed. Baltimore: Williams & Wilkins, 1991:256).

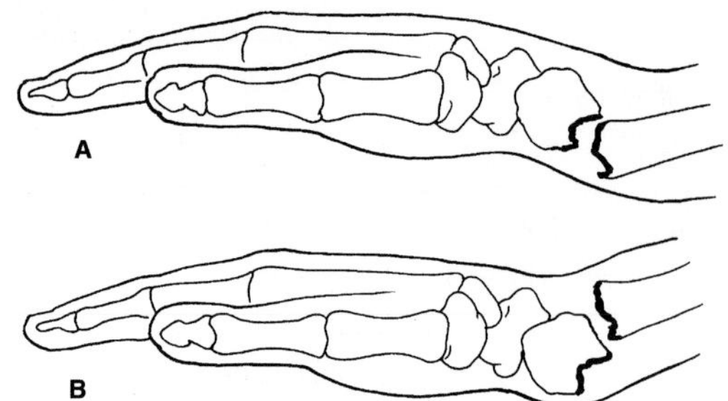

Figure 17.2 Distal radial fractures: **(A)** Colles' fracture and **(B)** Smith's fracture.

Humeral Fractures

The incidence of humeral fractures in the United States has increased as a result of the aging of our population, increased participation in sports, and the rise of osteoporosis (24). A humeral fracture may present with humeral displacement and malposition of the distal limb. Radial nerve injury is found in approximately 18% of humeral shaft fractures (25). A spiral fracture may lacerate the radial nerve or it may be damaged by displaced bony segments. Clinical signs of radial nerve involvement include loss of wrist extension and impaired sensation on the dorsal aspect of the wrist. Seventy-five percent to 90% of individuals who have closed humeral fractures have recovery of the radial nerve in 3 to 4 months (25).

Fractures that occur at the distal end of the humerus just above the medial and lateral condyles are referred to as supracondylar fractures. These fractures are commonly known as elbow fractures. The medial and lateral condyles serve as an origin site for many muscles of the forearm and have bony connections to the radius and ulna of the forearm. Nerves and arteries pass along this area. Therefore, a supracondylar fracture can also result in injury to muscles, nerves, and tissue that further affect the function of the entire arm. Understandably, it is associated with a high risk for complications such as **malunion** and **Volkmann's deformity**. Volkmann's deformity is a condition that results from severe damage to tissues and muscles caused by increased pressure in the forearm compartments (26). Increased compartmental pressures may be caused by several factors such as ischemia, compartmental bleeding, and excessively tight bandages (26). Signs of ischemia include pale or bluish skin, absence of radial pulse, decreased sensation, and severe pain. Suspected cases of increased compartmental pressure should be immediately reported to the physician as it can result in nerve damage and necrosis.

Scaphoid Fractures

The position of the scaphoid in the proximal row of the carpal bones makes it particularly vulnerable to injury. It is the most commonly fractured bone in the wrist with an incidence of 35,000 to 50,000 annually (27). Scaphoid fractures are commonly seen in young males with a sports injury resulting in wrist hyperextension with radial deviation. Fractures of the middle and proximal poles of the scaphoid are susceptible to avascular necrosis because of its poor blood supply (27). Plain radiographs are commonly used to classify the scaphoid fracture. However, other radiographic procedures may be necessary to evaluate its healing.

Course and Prognosis for Fractures

Prognosis and functional outcomes for fractures are dependent upon several factors: age, type of fracture, fracture location, severity of the fracture, and the patient's intrinsic motivation and premorbid health status. Hip fractures; however, are the most serious in that they are the leading cause of morbidity and mortality in older adults (13,16,20). Occupational therapy practitioners should work closely with the referring physician who will identify the precautions and provide the prescription for therapy. For example, the physician may limit the patient's weight-bearing status to partial weight-bearing or nonweight-bearing, or request a customized splint to protect and/or immobilize a fracture.

The way in which the bone heals will also influence the patient's course and prognosis. There are two types of bone: cancellous and cortical. Cancellous bone is the spongy inner layer, while cortical bone is the hard outer layer. The periosteum consists of connective tissues and elastic fibers which adhere to the surface of most bones. Bone contains many vessels that travel through the periosteum to reach cortical bone (28). A fractured bone normally takes 6 to 12 weeks to heal (5). The healing process is influenced by the type of fracture, location, severity, and premorbid health status of the individual. To achieve optimal healing it is important that the fracture site receive adequate circulation and immobilization. The healing process involves five stages (5). First, a hematoma forms, sealing off damaged blood vessels. Osteoclasts begin to resorb the damaged bone and tissue. The second stage is the formation of a granular or fibrocartilage tissue that increases the stability of the bone fragments. The third stage involves the formation of callus. This takes place between 2 to 6 weeks. The formation of the callus has a significant influence on the outcome of the fracture. The fourth stage is ossification and the formation of a bony union. The final stage is often referred to as consolidation and **remodeling** occurring between 6 weeks and 1 year. The bone is reshaped and remodeled to return to its original form or to perform its intended function as optimally as possible.

In some instances, the bone heals abnormally. Abnormal healing can be caused by several factors including open fractures, severe soft tissue damage, infection, poor vascularization, nerve damage, phlebitis, or compartment syndrome. Such complications can result in **delayed union**, malunion, and **nonunion**. A delayed union may be suspected if significant pain persists three months to one year after the initial fracture. A delayed union takes more time to heal than is typically expected. A delayed union may be suspected when pain and tenderness persist at the fracture site 3 months to 1 year after the injury (5). It may be caused by several factors including infection, poor vascularization, or inadequate immobilization. Once the causing factor is identified, the bone will typically heal. In a malunion fracture, the fracture heals in an abnormal or deformed position. Factors that may contribute to malunion include muscle imbalance and inadequate protection of the fracture (22). This abnormal position may limit range of motion (ROM), strength, and function use of the involved extremity. Nonunion fractures refer to a fracture that has not completely healed within the expected timeframe. A nonunion fracture may be caused by several factors such as vascular and tissue damage, poor alignment, stress to the fracture site, and infection (22).

Occupational therapy practitioners should be aware of signs of **complex regional pain syndrome** (CRPS) also known as reflex sympathetic dystrophy. CRPS may be a complication in fractures. This syndrome is characterized by disproportionate pain, stiffness, edema, loss of ROM, changes in vasomotor activity (temperature), sudomotor activity (edema, sweating asymmetry), and trophic changes (hair, nails, and skin) (29). Osteopenia is noted in 70% to 80% of patients on plain radiographs (30). CRPS results after a trauma or noxious event. The pain, atrophy, and loss of movement cause significant impairment of the ability to carry out normal daily activities. CRPS may affect anyone who has had a noxious injury though it is most commonly seen in Caucasian, adult females who smoke cigarettes (30).

Medical Management

Hip Fractures

Most hip fractures require surgical intervention. The type of procedure "depends on the fracture, preference of the surgeon, severity of the injury, the age of the patient, the presence or absence of comorbid conditions, and the prognosis for recovery during rehabilitation" (31). The goal of the intervention is to align and immobilize the fracture site to allow for normal healing. Hip fractures are treated with closed reduction and immobilization or **open reduction and internal fixation** (ORIF). Closed reduction involves realigning the fracture fragments through manual manipulation or traction, which may be done under general or local anesthesia (5). Immobilization can be accomplished through casts, traction, splints, or braces. Open reduction on the other hand, involves surgically opening and reducing the fracture site. Internal fixation is commonly done after an open reduction to secure the fracture. Internal fixation involves securing the fracture site with pins, rods, plates, and screws. This promotes healing and allows for early mobilization, which can reduce complications often associated with immobility.

Some hip fractures such as an intracapsular femoral neck fracture, may be treated with hemiarthroplasty or a THR (31). A hemiarthroplasty is a partial joint replacement in which the femoral head and neck are replaced by a metal prosthesis. A total hip arthroplasty or THR may be necessary when the femur and acetabulum are damaged from the injury or a pre-existing disease.

Total Hip Replacements

Total hip replacements (THRs) are typically indicated for those who have severe arthritis that causes pain, stiffness, and significantly limits functional activities. THRs are most commonly seen in individuals older than age 55 years. The procedure involves replacement of the acetabulum and ball of the femur with artificial implants. These may be secured by bone cement or a cementless prosthesis, which allows for bone growth. Hip replacements or arthroplasties generally last for 10 to 25 years (32), though researchers continue to evaluate implant wear. The National Institutes on Health (NIH) provided grants to researchers between 2001 and 2004 to study orthopaedic implant wear in an attempt to achieve health promotion and disease prevention as outlined by Healthy People 2010 (2). It is hoped that as technology improves, implants will last longer.

Following a THR, there are several precautions that a patient must follow for 6 to 8 weeks after the surgery. These precautions include no hip adduction and rotation of the operated leg, and no bending forward beyond 90 degrees of the operated leg (Table 17.1). If the surgeon uses an anterior approach, the patient must also avoid hip extension. Oftentimes, therapists will encourage their clients to avoid hip rotation in general to ensure that the surgical hip is protected. These precautions have functional implications for the person in

Table 17.1 TOTAL HIP PRECAUTIONS

1. Avoid hip flexion beyond 90°
2. Avoid hip rotation of operated leg
3. Avoid hip adduction of operated leg (avoid crossing legs)

regard to sitting, dressing, bathing, and reaching. These precautions are currently the standard of care. However, recent research suggests that an anterolateral surgical approach rather than adherence to traditional hip precautions was more likely to be associated with a low rate of dislocation. In regards to driving, patients are to avoid driving for 4 to 6 weeks following surgery (33). At this time most patients have reached their pre-operative driving reaction time and continue to show improvements in reaction time for up to one year. Depending on the severity of the condition, the surgical procedure, and the orthopaedic surgeon, there may be weightbearing (WB) precautions for THRs and ORIFs. Common WB statuses include nonweightbearing, touch-down weightbearing, partial weightbearing, weightbearing as tolerated, and full weightbearing (Table 17.2).

Total Knee Replacements

As discussed earlier, severe osteoarthritis in the knee may also warrant a total joint replacement. The person may present with pain and stiffness in the knee that significantly limit their participation in daily activities. If conservative treatment is not an option, the surgeon will perform a total knee replacement (TKR). A TKR involves resurfacing the knee joint with metal prosthetic components. The procedure typically involves the use of a femoral component, tibial plate, and a patellar button (32) and may be done unilaterally or bilaterally.

After surgery, the patient will need to be instructed on several precautions including to avoid putting a pillow under the knee while in bed, to rest both feet on the floor when sitting to increase knee ROM, and to wear an immobilizer as instructed by the physician (34). The physician may prescribe a knee immobilizer to protect the operated knee until the thigh muscle is strong enough to support it. The immobilizer may be required when walking, while in bed, or at all times. A continuous passive motion (CPM) machine may also be prescribed. This may be used while in the hospital or at home to help improve circulation and movement at the knee joint. Kneeling should be avoided. Other considerations include not driving, running, and jumping until cleared by the physician (34). Generally, patients are able to return to most of their normal daily activities after 3 to 6 weeks (35). Driving may be resumed around 4 to 6 weeks as long as the patient is able to bend his or her knee enough to get in and out of the car and operate the pedals and have appropriate muscle strength and control to operate the pedals (35).

Table 17.2 WEIGHTBEARING STATUS

Weightbearing status	Percentage and Description
Nonweightbearing	0%. No WB on the operated leg, it should not touch the floor
Touchdown or toe-touch weight bearing	10%–15%. Foot of operated leg may rest on floor
Partial weightbearing	30%–50%. May put 30%–50% of weight through the operated leg
Weightbearing as tolerated	Patient may put as much weight through operated leg as tolerates without unnecessary pain or discomfort
Full weightbearing	75%–100%. Patient bears full weight on the operated leg

Modified from Goldstein TS. Geriatric Orthopaedics: Rehabilitative Management of Common Problems. 2nd Ed. Gaithersburg, MD: Aspen, 1999.

Distal Radial Fractures and Humeral Fractures

It is necessary that distal radial and humeral fractures be reduced or realigned. Closed fractures may be reduced manually and immobilized with a cast. If the fracture is unstable or cannot be manually reduced, surgery may be required. This procedure is called an ORIF and it secures the fracture site with screws, pins, plates, and rods. Open and **comminuted fractures** often require ORIF. Some distal radius fractures may occasionally require a long arm cast to prevent forearm rotation which could result in displacement as a result of the articulations of the ulna and radius with the humerus (23). A cast is worn approximately 4 to 6 weeks depending upon the physician, type of fracture, and healing process. Following bone healing, external fixators are often removed at 6 to 8 weeks dependent upon fracture consolidation. Some fractures that are relatively stable may require splinting for as little as 3 weeks (23).

Scaphoid Fractures

A nondisplaced scaphoid fracture is typically immobilized with a thumb spica cast for approximately 8 to 10 weeks (27). Proximal scaphoid fractures may require a long arm-thumb spica cast followed by the use of a short-arm-thumb spica cast to promote healing for as long as 6 weeks to 6 months. Displaced or unstable scaphoid fractures require an ORIF with a compression screw (27). Following the ORIF, a wrist splint should be used for 2 to 6 weeks or until the bony union is formed. A percutaneous fixation technique using a Herbert screw is a common and effective approach used in the treatment of acute scaphoid fractures. This technique has been found to be associated with a more rapid return of hand function, higher satisfaction and minimal complications (36). The physician and therapist should closely monitor the fracture to ensure proper vascularization.

Impact of Conditions on Client Factors

Orthopaedic conditions may compromise participation in several areas of occupation which include ADL, instrumental activities of daily living (IADL), education, work, play, leisure, and social participation (37). The degree of impairment depends upon the severity of the injury, location of the injury, and the client's premorbid health status. Several client factors may be compromised by orthopaedic conditions (Table 17.3). The main client factors that will affect one's participation in occupation are neuromusculoskeletal and movement-related functions and structures, and sensory and pain functions and structures. Joint mobility and stability will be directly affected by a fracture or a condition such as osteoarthritis. The stability or alignment of the joint will be immediately affected by a fracture. This is why it is necessary that a fracture be reduced or realigned. Limited joint mobility may affect an individual's ability to participate in daily activities such as dressing, cooking, and cleaning. This in turn can affect one's role performance. For example, a woman with a distal radius fracture may have difficulty fulfilling her caregiver and worker roles.

Muscle strength and endurance are often affected by orthopaedic conditions as a result of immobilization of a joint during recovery. These limitations may also be caused and worsened by disuse of the involved extremity. **Disuse syndrome** refers to holding the involved extremity in a dependent or guarded position and refraining from using it (38). This further compounds the patient's symptoms and often leads to involvement in other related joints and musculature. Impairments in muscle strength and endurance directly impact one's performance and participation in daily activities. A person recovering from a humeral fracture may find it difficult to golf

Table 17.3 CLIENT FACTORS: PRACTICE FRAMEWORK (AOTA, 2002)

Body Function Categories

- ■ Neuromusculoskeletal and movement-related functions
- o Mobility of joint
- o Stability of joint
- o Mobility of bone
- o Muscle power
- o Muscle endurance
- ■ Sensory functions and pain
- o Vestibular function (balance)
- o Sensations of pain
- ■ Skin and related structure functions
- o Protective functions of the skin
- o Repair function of the skin
- ■ Mental Functions
- o Orientation
- o Energy and drive

or may find that his or her arm tires easily when painting or doing household chores.

Orthopaedic conditions may affect sensation function and pain in the areas of balance, sensation, and pain. When recovering from a THR or hip fracture an individual may struggle with balance as he or she tries to walk, move around in the bathroom, and get dressed while following WB precautions. As a result, the individual may need to modify how he or she does certain activities in order to prevent a fall. Sensation may be affected if there is nerve involvement at the fracture site. Depending on the degree of sensory involvement, an individual may have difficulty picking things up. Pain, as noted earlier in the discussion, is a common sign of an injury. Pain will vary depending on the person, severity of the injury, and complications. Sharp or continuous pain may affect an individual's ability to complete daily tasks. The pain experienced by people who develop CRPS can be so overwhelming that it affects their ability to work and carry out their life roles.

In addition, functions of the skin and related structures and mental functions may be impacted by orthopaedic conditions. Compound fractures that break through the skin will result in a wound and be at risk for infection. This type of fracture will involve more medical management and may consequently limit an individual's ability to participate in a variety of daily occupations due to pain, wound care procedures and the type of fixator.

Mental functions such as one's self-concept, motivation, and interests may be impacted by an orthopaedic condition. For example, a distal radius fracture may present with skin changes, edema, and severely limited movement in the fingers. As a result, the individual may have difficulty doing many tasks such as dressing, grooming, and writing. The inability to perform these daily tasks that we often take for granted may impair one's self-concept. Therefore, the person may have decreased motivation and withdraw from activities that he or she is normally interested in.

Summary

Orthopaedic conditions involve injury and disease of bones, joints, and their related structures. Common orthopedic conditions with which occupational therapy practitioners will work include hip fractures, THRs, distal forearm fractures, humeral fractures, and scaphoid fractures. Such fractures, along with associated conditions such as osteoporosis, impact an individual's engagement in meaningful life occupations. The role of occupational therapy is to promote rehabilitation of the fracture or condition through a variety of interventions with the outcome directed at individualized functional goals. As a result of complex and evolving changes in technology, occupational therapy practitioners should seek more in-depth information on specific interventions and protocols for orthopaedic conditions.

CASE STUDY

Case Illustrations

■ CASE 1: TOTAL HIP REPLACEMENT

As noted in the introduction to this chapter, Mary Adda had an elective right THR. After surgery, Mary Adda was confused and very agitated. She did not recognize her husband and was combative toward the staff. Her husband was frightened to see his wife in this condition. He spoke to the nurse who explained to him that Mary Adda had delirium as a result of the medications and surgery. The physician and nursing staff addressed the delirium through medications and monitoring fluids. Within 2 days Mary Adda was alert, oriented, and back to her normal self. However, she complained of feeling tired and having little strength.

Mary Adda had a difficult time adjusting to the new environment and roommate. She longed to be home with her husband and hated when he left in the evenings. After a week, Mary Adda became more withdrawn and depressed, feeling that she had lost her sense of identity. The occupational therapist noted these changes and talked to her about her feelings, interests, and goals. The therapist drew upon Mary Adda's interests to design occupation-based interventions that helped her to interact with other clients in small group formats. Mary Adda soon developed relationships with other residents at the SNF and was motivated to actively participate in therapy to help her return home.

Questions

1. Prior to surgery, what areas of occupation were affected by the osteoarthritis in Mary Adda's hip?
2. What factors contributed to Mary Adda's sense of lost identity and depressive feelings after the surgery?
3. List at least four client factors that the occupational therapist would need to closely assess in this scenario.
4. Describe several occupation-based activities that the therapist could use during treatment sessions with Mary Adda.

■ CASE 2: COLLES' FRACTURE

Joe was doing some home repair when he fell off of his ladder and fractured his left distal radius. The fracture was surgically reduced and stabilized with an external fixator to prevent the bone from collapsing because of the pull of the extrinsic muscles of his forearm. One week after his surgery, Joe went see his physician. His physician wrote him a prescription for occupational therapy. Upon evaluation, the occupational therapist noted that Joe's fixator was held in place by four external screws and a cross bar that extended approximately two

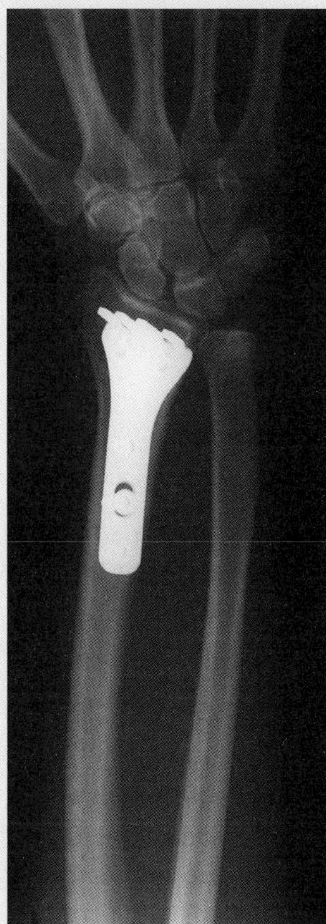

Figure 17.3 External fixator.

inches above the lateral radial border of the forearm and hand (Fig. 17.3). His wrist was in a slightly flexed and ulnarly deviated posture, with moderate edema in his fingers and wrist area. The therapist also observed that Joe held his arm in a dependent position. His shoulder was internally rotated, his humerus adducted, and his elbow pronated. Joe complained of pain and stiffness in his elbow, shoulder, and neck.

The occupational therapist conducted an occupational profile in which he gathered the following information. Joe reported that he was having more and more difficulty completing self-care tasks and simple household chores. Being left-hand dominant he was frequently frustrated with computer and paperwork. The occupational therapist continued the evaluation which involved identifying the limitations and precautions prescribed by the physician.

Questions

1. Describe signs of disuse.
2. What emotional issues may Joe have to deal with as a result of his fracture?
3. List Joe's roles that were affected by his injury.
4. List 3 client factors that you would assess.

■ CASE 3: SUPRACONDYLAR FRACTURE OF THE HUMERUS

Betty is a 52-year-old woman who fractured her humerus in an MVA. She was taken to the emergency room (ER) where the physician conducted a clinical assessment and ordered x-rays to confirm the suspected fracture. The radiologist report confirmed that there was a closed transverse fracture of the middle third of the right humeral shaft. The physician was able to reduce the fracture without surgery. He immobilized the arm in a sling. Four weeks later, Betty still had significant pain and tenderness in her upper arm. Radiological tests revealed that the bone was forming a malunion. The physician determined that it was necessary to surgically reduce the fracture and stabilize it with internal fixation. Radiologic studies showed signs of healing six weeks after the second reduction as well as signs of osteopenia. The physician wrote a prescription for occupational therapy.

The occupational therapist evaluated Betty. He noted that she held her arm in a dependent position and was very hesitant to move it or let him examine it. She reported significant pain and had atrophy of her upper arm and forearm muscles. Her skin appeared shiny in comparison to her left arm. Betty had limited movement and reported that her husband had to help her with everything. She had been unable to return to work as an office manager because the pain was just too great.

Questions

1. List two clinical signs of a humeral fracture.
2. What causes CRPS?
3. List four signs of CRPS.
4. Describe the normal healing process of a fractured bone.
5. Describe three client factors that may be affected by CRPS.

Acknowledgement:

I would like to extend a special thank you to Chris Bochenek, OTR/L, CHT, Lisa Mason, OTR/L, and Hamid Javaherian, MD for their assistance, support, and careful review of this chapter.

References

1. Utah Hip & Knee Center. History of total joint replacement. Utah Hip & Knee Center n.d., Available at http://www.utahhipandknee.com/history.htm. Accessed February 6, 2005.
2. National Institutes of Health. Orthopaedic implant wear. PA Number: PA-01–141, 2001.
3. National Board Certification for Occupational Therapy. Final report of 2003 practice analysis of occupational therapy entry-level practice. Gaithersburg, MD: National Board for Certification of Occupational Therapist, 2003.
4. American Academy of Pediatrics. Diagnostic imaging of child abuse. Pediatrics 2000;105:1345–1348.
5. Kunkler CE. Fractures. In Maher AB, Salmond SW, Pellino TA; eds. Orthopaedic Nursing. Philadelphia: Saunders, 2002.
6. National Institutes of Health. Osteoarthritis. NIH Publication No. 02–4617. United States Department of Health and Human Services: Public Health Service, 2002.
7. National Osteoporosis Foundation. Disease statistics fact sheet. 2004; Available at http://www.nof.org/osteoporosis/stats.htm. Accessed June 21, 2004.
8. National Center for Injury Prevention and Control. Ten leading causes of nonfatal injury, United States. Office of Statistics and Programming, NCIP, CDC, 2002. Available at http://www.cdc.gov/ncipc/wisqars/nonfatal/quickpicks/quickpicks_2002/allinj.htm. Accessed June 21, 2004.
9. Rothstein J, Roy S, Wolf, S. The Rehabilitation Specialist's Handbook. Philadelphia: FA Davis, 1997.
10. Bell AJ, Talbot-Stern JK, Hennessy A. Characteristics and outcomes of older patients presenting to the emergency department after a fall: A retrospective analysis. Med J Aust 2000;173:176–177.
11. Centers for Disease Control and Prevention. Web-based injury statistics query and reporting system. 2003. Available at http://www.cdc.gov/ncipc/wisqars. Accessed June 21, 2004.
12. National Center for Injury Prevention and Control. Falls and hip fractures among older adults. 2004. Available at http://www.cdc.gov/NCIPC/factsheets/falls.htm. Accessed June 15, 2004.
13. Stevens JA, Olson S. Reducing falls and resulting hip fractures among older women. National Center for Injury Prevention and Control. 2000. Available at http://www.cdc.gov/mmwr/preview/mmwrhtml/rr4902a2.htm. Accessed June 21, 2004.
14. Cummings SR, Rubin SM, Black D. The future of hip fractures in the United States: Numbers, costs, and potential effects of postmenopausal estrogen. Clin Orthop Relat Res 1990;252:163–166.
15. Gillespie W. Hip fractures. Clin Evid 2002;8:1126–1148.
16. Hall SE, Williams JA, Senior JA, et al. Hip fracture outcomes: Quality of life and functional status in older adults living in the community. Aust N Z J Med 2000;30:327–332.
17. Jette AM, Bette AH, Clearly PD, et al. Functional recovery after hip fracture. Arch Phys Med 1994;68:735–740.
18. Meadows SE, Zuckerman JD, Sakales SR, et al. Ambulatory ability after hip fracture: A prospective study of geriatric patients. Orthopaedica Transplant 1991;15:700.
19. Morrottoli RA, Berkman LF, Cooney LM. Decline in physical function following hip fracture. J Am Geriatr Soc 1993;289:166–169.
20. Wolinsky FD, Fitzgerald JF, Stump TE. The effects of hip fractures on mortality, hospitalization, and functional status: A prospective study. Am J Public Health 1997;87:398–403.
21. Hagsten B, Svensson O, Gardulf A. Early individualized postoperative occupational therapy training in 100 patients improves ADL after hip fracture. Acta Ortho Scand 2004;75:177–183.
22. Altizer L. Fractures. Ortho Nurs 2002;21:51–59.
23. Laseter GF. Therapist's management of distal radius fractures. In: Mackin EJ, Callahan AD, et al., eds. Rehabilitation of the Hand and Upper Extremity. 5th Ed. St. Louis: Mosby, 2002.
24. Gill M. Managing distal and humeral shaft fractures. Journal of the National Association of Orthopaedic Technologists 2002;4:1–4.
25. Wheeless CR. Humeral fractures. Duke Orthopaedics—Wheeless' Textbook of Orthpaedics. 1996. Available at: http://www.wheelessonline.com. Accessed June 21, 2004.

26. Kare JA. Volkmann contracture. Available at http://www.emedicine.com/orthoped/topic 578.htm. 2004 April. Accessed June 30, 2004.
27. Dell PC, Dell RB. Management of carpal fractures and dislocations. In: Mackin EJ, Callahan AD, Skirven TM, et al. eds. Rehabilitation of the Hand and Upper Extremity. 5th Ed. St. Louis: Mosby, 2002.
28. Lewis WH. Bone. In: Gray H. ed. Gray's Anatomy. New York: Bartleby.com, 2000. Available at http://www.bartleby.com/107/18.html. Accessed June 22, 2004.
29. Aronoff GM, Harden N, Stanton-Hicks M, et al. American Academy of Disability Evaluating Physicians position paper: Complex regional pain syndrome I(RSD): Impairment and disability issues. Pain Med 2002;3:274–288.
30. Koman LA, Smith BP, Smith TL. Complex regional pain syndrome associated with fractures of the distal radius and ulna. Orthopaedic Care Textbook. Orthopaedic Care.net. J South Orthop Assoc. 2002. Available at http://www.orthopaediccare.net/view/templates/. Accessed DATE. Chapter_Entry.asp?uniqueid=7538810&chapterid=hnfxrupna§ionid=536675628§ionname=Hand. Accessed September 13, 2004.
31. Brunner LC, Eshilian-Oates L. Hip fractures in adults. Am Fam Physician 2003;67:537–542.
32. Roberts D. Degenerative disorders. In: Maher AB, Salmond SW, Pellino TA, eds. Orthopaedic Nursing. Philadelphia: Saunders, 2002.
33. Ganz SB, Levin A, Peterson, MG, et al. Improvement in driving reaction time after total hip arthroplasty. Clin Ortho 2003;413:192–200.
34. Health Alliance. Total knee replacement: Activities? Restrictions? Incisions? Diet? Medications? Cincinnati: Alliance Primary Care, 2001.
35. Mayo Clinic. Knee replacements: Surgery can relieve pain. Available at: http://www.mayoclinic.com/health/knee-replacement/HQ00977. Accessed January 5, 2006.
36. Jeon IH, Oh CW, Park BC, et al. Minimal invasive percutaneous Herbert screw fixation in acute unstable scaphoid fractures. Hand Surg 2003;8:213–218.
37. American Occupational Therapy Association. Occupational therapy practice framework: Domain and process. Am J Occup Ther 2002;56:609–639.
38. Jagmin, MG, Assessment and management of immobility. In: Maher AB, Salmond SW, Pellino TA, eds. Orthopaedic Nursing. Philadelphia: Saunders, 2002.

Recommended Learning Resources

Bonder BR, Wagner MB. Functional Performance in Older Adults. 2nd Ed. Philadelphia: FA Davis, 2001.

Hunter JM, Mackin EJ, Callahan AD. Rehabilitation of the Hand. In: Mackin EJ, Callahan AD, Skirven, TM, et al. eds. Rehabilitation of the Hand and Upper Extremity. 5th Ed. St. Louis: Mosby, 2002.

Maher AB, Salmond SW, Pellino TA, eds. Orthopaedic Nursing. Philadelphia: Saunders, 2002.

Rothstein J, Roy S, Wolf S. The Rehabilitation Specialist's Handbook. Philadelphia: FA Davis, 1997.

Glossary

Affect—Observable facial expressions of a feeling or emotion. Patients may be described as having a flat or blunt affect.

Agnosia—Inability to recognize the import of sensory impressions despite being able to recognize the elemental sensation of the stimulus. Language deficits must be absent for this diagnosis. Various agnosias correspond to several senses and may be distinguished as auditory, gustatory, olfactory, tactile, and visual. Specific sensory agnosias can occur when the connections are disrupted between the primary cortical receptor region for a stimulus and the memory of prior stimuli. For example, the inability to recognize familiar objects by sight or touch.

Agoraphobia—"a mental disorder characterized by an irrational fear of leaving the familiar setting of home, or venturing into the open; often associated with panic attacks." Commonly referred to as fear of the marketplace.

Algorithms—A step-by-step approach to treatment based upon controlled clinical trials.

Alogia—Absence of speech because of mental illness.

Ambiguous hand preference—Absence of a dominant hand preference; the switching of hands within the same activity.

Amotivation—Lacking in motivation.

Amygdala—A structure that is part of the limbic system and is involved in the emotions of aggression and fear.

Analgesic—A pain medication.

Aneurysm—Localized abnormal dilatation of the wall of a blood vessel, usually an artery, or in the heart, resulting in the formation of a sac. Usual causes are the weakness of the vessel wall, resulting from atherosclerosis, or a congenital defect. However, any injury to the middle or muscular layer of the arterial wall can predispose the stretching of the vessel wall.

Anhedonia—Reduced ability or inability to experience pleasure.

Anomia—Inability to name objects.

Anterograde amnesia—The inability to learn new long-term declarative information.

Anticholinergic side effects—Most commonly dry mouth or constipation.

Antipsychotic medications—Medications designed to reduce positive and negative symptoms.

Anxiety—"apprehension of danger, and dread accompanied by restlessness, tension, tachycardia, and dyspnea unattached to a clearly identifiable stimulus."

Anxiolytic—A sedative or mild tranquilizer used to treat anxiety or alcohol withdrawal.

Apathy—An absence or suppression of emotion, feeling, or concern.

Aphasia—Difficulty with expressive and/or receptive language.

Apraxia—Loss of skilled purposeful movement that cannot be attributed either to deficits in primary motor skills or problems in comprehension. It can affect ideation and concept formation as well as programming and planning of movement.

Arteriovenous—Referring both to an artery and a vein. An arteriovenous malformation, or AVM, is a congenital malformation characterized by an abnormal collection of blood vessels near the surface of the brain. AVM can lead to subarachnoid hemorrhage.

Asperger's Disease—A neurobiologic disorder of unknown etiology in which cognitive and communication skills develop normally or nearly normally during the first few years of life. However, social impairment is evident, repetitive and stereotypical behaviors are observed, and communication, though not delayed, is marked by unusual topics of interest and rigidity.

Aspiration—Pathological inhalation of food or mucus into the respiratory tract.

Associated reactions—Involuntary movements or reflexive increases in tone on the affected side of individuals with hemiplegia. These movements replicate synergy patterns and often appear when the individual is trying new or stressful activities, e.g., a resisted grasp by the noninvolved hand causes a grasp reaction in the involved hand.

Astereognosis—Inability to recognize objects by touch (also called tactile agnosia; see Agnosia).

Asterixis—A hand-flapping tremor.

Ataxia—Inability to coordinate muscle activity during voluntary movement. In posterior column damage of the spinal cord, incoordination and a loss of proprioception is caused by misjudgment of limb position with balance problems. Cerebellar ataxia produces a reeling, wide-based gait.

Atheromas—An abnormal mass of fatty or lipid material with a fibrous covering, which forms a discrete raised plaque within the inner layer (intima) of an artery.

Atherosclerosis—A widespread form of arteriosclerosis in which deposits of plaques (atheromas) containing cholesterol and other lipid material are formed within the inner layer (intima) of large- and medium-sized arteries.

Athetoid (dyskinetic)—Resembling athetosis or repetitive involuntary, slow, sinuous, writhing movements. Classification of cerebral palsy in which involuntary purposeless movement occurs when an individual attempts purposeful motion. The abnormal movements may not only occur in the limb being moved but also involve an "overflow" of activity to all the other limbs with an exaggeration of reflexes.

Auditory processing—The process of the brain recognizing and interpreting sounds in the environment. This process is responsible for the comprehension of language.

Autistic disorder—A neurobiologic disorder with an unknown etiology, characterized by significant delay or deviation in social interaction, communication, and repetitive or stereotyped behaviors.

Autonomic dysreflexia (hyperreflexia)—An uninhibited and exaggerated reflex of the autonomic nervous system to stimulation. The response occurs in about 85% of all patients who have spinal cord injury above the level of the 6th thoracic vertebra. It is potentially dangerous because of attendant vasoconstriction and immediate elevation of blood pressure, which in turn can bring about hemorrhagic retinal damage or cerebrovascular accident. Less serious effects include severe headache, changes in heart rate, sweating and flushing above the level of the spinal cord injury, and pallor and goose bumps below that level.

β-amyloid plaques—Insoluble shards of β-amyloid that stick to dead and dying neurons.

Babinski's reflex—Dorsiflexion (extension) of the great toe and outspreading of the outer toes when the sole of the foot is stroked. Normally present in infants under the age of 6 months, in adults this reflex occurs in lesions of the pyramidal tract.

Bradykinesia—Slowness of all voluntary movement and speech.

Brain attack—Synonym for stroke, or cerebrovascular accident.

Casein—A protein found in cow's milk. A theory in the field of autism suggests that children with autism do not digest this protein appropriately, leading to a buildup of morphine-like substances in the body and causing social withdrawal and abnormal behaviors.

Catatonia—Extreme psychomotor agitation or retardation.

Catheterization—Passage of a catheter into a body channel or cavity, especially introduction of a catheter via the urethra into the urinary bladder.

Cauda equina—The collection of dorsal and ventral nerve roots descending from the lower spinal cord and occupying the vertebral canal below the cord at the L1 region.

Cerebellum—A region of the brain that is found at the rear of the head and is above the brainstem. It has been traditionally known for its role in the coordination of movement, but recent research suggests the cerebellum may also have a role in cognitive, sensory, language, and abstract-thinking skills.

Cerebrovascular accident (CVA, stroke, brain attack)—Disorder of the blood vessels serving the brain, resulting in disruption of blood flow to parts of the brain leading to neuronal death. Impact of CVA varies according to the cause of the disruption (blockages or hemorrhages) and location of the insult, as well as a variety of premorbid and psychosocial conditions.

Childhood disintegrative disorder—A rare neurobiologic disorder that develops in children who had appeared completely normal during their first few years of life. Following its onset, language, social interaction, and self-care skills are lost and autistic-like symptoms appear.

Chronic obstructive pulmonary disease (COPD)—A term that includes chronic bronchitis, asthma, emphysema, and bronchiectasis. The condition is irreversible and characterized by progressive limitation in the flow of air in and out of the lungs.

Circumlocution—The use of pantomime, nonverbal communication, or word substitution to avoid revealing an inability to say or remember a word.

Clonus—Alternate involuntary muscular contraction and relaxation in rapid succession.

Cogwheel rigidity—Stiff movement in one direction in small evenly spaced segments. The tension in muscle gives way in little jerks when the muscle is passively stretched.

Collateral circulation—Secondary circulation that continues to an area of the brain following obstruction of a primary blood vessel and may prevent major ischemia.

Coma—A nonsleep loss of consciousness associated with unresponsiveness to touch, pain, sound, or movement that lasts for an extended period.

Compulsion—"uncontrollable impulses to perform an act, often repetitively, as an unconscious mechanism to avoid unacceptable ideas and desires which, by themselves, arouse anxiety; the anxiety becomes fully manifest if performance of the compulsive act is prevented; may be associated with obsessive thoughts."

Concrete thinking—Literal interpretation of words without understanding abstract meanings.

Congestive heart failure—The inability of the heart to function as a pump, which results in a decreased blood flow to the tissues and congestion in the pulmonary and circulatory systems.

Constructional apraxia—Apraxia caused by loss of visuospatial skills; for example, difficulty drawing a clock face.

Contracture—Abnormal shortening of muscle tissue that renders the muscle highly resistant to stretching, which can lead to permanent disability. In many cases, contractures can be prevented by range of motion (ROM) exercises (active or passive) and by adequate support of the joints to eliminate constant shortening or stretching of the muscles and surrounding tissue.

Crede's method—Use of manual pressure on the bladder to express urine, particularly in bladder training for individuals with paralysis. The hands are held flat against the abdomen, just below the umbilicus. A firm downward stroke toward the bladder is repeated six or seven times, followed by pressure from both hands placed directly over the bladder to manually remove all urine.

Cyclothymia—Characterized by a chronic course of hypomania and mild depression, this disorder presents as a mild form of bipolar disorder (BPD).

Decerebrate rigidity—An extensor posture of all limbs and/or the trunk.

Decorticate rigidity—Flexion of the upper, but extension of the lower, limbs.

Decubitus ulcers—An ulcer caused by local interference with the circulation, usually occurring over a bony prominence at the sacrum, hip (trochanter), heel, shoulder, or elbow. It begins as a reddened area and can quickly involve deeper structures and become an ulcer, also called a bedsore or a pressure sore. Individuals most at risk for the development of decubitus ulcers are those who are emaciated, obese, or immobilized by traction or some other form of enforced immobility, and those who have diabetes mellitus or some type of circulatory disorder. Because urine and feces contribute to skin breakdown, incontinent patients are at high risk for pressure sores. Two major factors in their development are prolonged pressure on a part caused by the weight of the body or an extremity, and a shearing force that exerts downward and forward pressure on tissues beneath the skin. The shearing action can occur when a patient slides downward while sitting in a bed or chair, or when bedclothes are forcibly pulled from under a patient.

Decussation—An X-shaped crossing, especially of nerves or bands of nerve fibers, connecting parts on opposite sides of the brain or spinal cord.

Deep vein thrombosis (DVT)—A thrombosis, commonly seen in the legs or pelvis, that results from phlebitis, vein injury, or prolonged bed rest.

Deformity—Distortion of any part or general disfigurement of the body.

Delusions—Atypical and well-organized beliefs not explained by evidence or culture.

Delusions of grandeur—Self-inflated views usually present in conversation.

Delusions of persecution—Individuals have consistent and organized beliefs about other people intending to harm them.

Demyelination—Destruction, removal, or loss of the myelin sheath of a nerve or nerves.

Diabetic foot—A person who has diabetes is at increased risk for slow-healing injuries to distal extremities. It is caused by decreased vascularization; the risk of an infection that does not heal is higher. One possible intervention is limb amputation.

Diabetic ketoacidosis—State of medical emergency; life-threatening condition caused by a state of relative insulin deficiency, characterized by hyperglycemia, ketonemia, metabolic acidosis, and electrolyte depletion. Often the first presenting sign of type 1 diabetes.

Diastolic blood pressure—The pressure in the arteries when the heart is at rest.

Diplegia—Paralysis of like parts on either side of the body. In cerebral palsy, diplegia describes involvement of the lower extremities predominantly, with only mildly affected upper extremities.

Disinhibition—Loss of inhibition, or the cultural and social sense of self restraint.

Dysarthria—Imperfect articulation of speech caused by disturbances of muscular control resulting from central or peripheral nervous system damage.

Dysesthesia—Impairment of any sense, especially of the sense of touch; a painful, persistent sensation induced by a gentle touch of the skin.

Dysgraphia—Inability to write a sentence.

Dysosmic aphasia—Difficulty naming objects.

Dysphagia—Difficulty in swallowing, which may range from mild discomfort to a seriously compromised ability to control the muscles needed for chewing and swallowing. Dysphagia may seriously interfere with a patient's nutritional status. Interventions, such as positioning the patient during feeding and use of foods of the proper consistency, are widely used.

Dyspnea—Difficult, labored, or painful breathing.

Dysthymia—Unlike individuals with depressive disorders, people with dysthymia report that they have always been depressed. Characterized by insidious onset frequently beginning in childhood, a persistent or intermittent course, and ongoing feelings of depression over a period of at least 2 years.

Echolalia—The automatic and meaningless repetition of another's words or phrases. In autism, this repetition may be either immediate or delayed, and often does not appear appropriate to the conversation or activity.

Electroconvulsive therapy—The induction of a brief seizure by passing electric current through the brain. This treatment is used mostly for depression.

Electroencephalogram—The record obtained during the amplification, recording, and subsequent analysis of the electrical activity of the brain using an instrument called an electroencephalograph.

Embolism—Sudden blockage of an artery by a moving clot of foreign material (embolus) lodged in place by the blood current. Emboli usually lodge at divisions of an artery, where the blood vessel narrows, and are typically blood clots. However, they may also be formed from globules of fat, air bubbles, pieces of tissue, or clumps of bacteria.

Emotional lability—Inability to regulate emotions appropriately, typically resulting in laughing or crying in unsuitable contexts.

Emphysema—The destruction of the walls of the bronchioles and alveoli, which results in abnormal and enlarged air spaces.

Endarterectomy—Excision of thickened atheromatous areas of the innermost layer of an artery (intima) to improve circulation.

Euphoria—A feeling or state of well-being or elation.

Euthymia—Normal range of mood.

Executive functioning—A broad band of skills that allow an individual to engage in independent, self-directed behavior. Includes volition, planning, purposeful action, and self-awareness. Executive functions involve the ability to formulate context-appropriate goals and to initiate, plan and organize, sequence and adapt behavior based on anticipated or actual consequences of actions.

Extrapyramidal symptoms—Involuntary movement, changes in muscle tone, and abnormal posture.

Fixed ideas—An individual holds an unchangeable idea.

Flaccidity—Abnormally low muscle tone, which is felt as too little resistance to movement. Also known as hypotonus.

Flight of ideas—Accelerated speech with rapid changes in subject. Associations are understandable unlike the lack of connections that are associated with looseness of associations.

Frontal lobes—Region of the brain located at the front of the cerebrum. This region is responsible for social behavior, spontaneous production of language, initiation of motor activity, processing sensory stimuli and then planning reaction as a result of the input, abstract thinking, problem solving, and judgment.

γ Aminobutyric acid (GABA)—"a constituent of the central nervous system; quantitatively the principal inhibitory neurotransmitter."

Gastrointestinal disorder—A disorder of the digestive system.

Genes—A region of DNA that carries the genetic instructions for a cell.

Generalized anxiety disorder—Chronic, repeated episodes of anxiety or dread accompanied by autonomic changes.

Genotype—Genetic makeup of a living organism.

Gluten—A protein found in wheat products. A theory in the field of autism suggests that children with autism do not digest this protein appropriately, leading to a buildup of morphine-like substances in the body and causing social withdrawal and abnormal behaviors.

Graphesthesia—The ability by which outlines, numbers, words, or symbols traced or written on the skin are recognized.

Hallucinations—Disorders of perception. Atypical auditory, visual, and/or olfactory sensory perceptions.

Hematoma—A localized collection of extravasated blood, usually clotted, in an organ, space, or tissue. Familiar, typically benign forms of hematoma include contusions (bruises) and black eyes. Hematomas can occur almost anywhere in the body and are especially serious when they occur inside the skull, where they may produce pressure on the brain. The most common types affecting the brain are epidural (above the dura mater, between it and the skull) and subdural (beneath the dura mater, between the touch casing and the more delicate membranes covering the tissue of the brain, the pia-arachnoid).

Hemianopsia—Defective vision or blindness in one half of the visual field, usually referring to bilateral defects resulting from a single lesion, often as the result of a cerebrovascular accident (CVA). The individual is unable to perceive objects to the side of the visual midline. Visual loss is contralateral, i.e., it is on the side opposite the brain lesion.

Hemiparesis—Paresis or weakness affecting one side of the body.

Hemiplegia—Paralysis of one side of the body, usually caused by a brain lesion, such as a tumor, or a cerebrovascular accident. Paralysis occurs on the side opposite the lesion, or infarct, because of decussation of most of the fibers in the motor tracts of the brain. For example, damage to the right hemisphere of the brain affects motor control of the left half of the body.

Hemorrhagic stroke—A type of stroke resulting from blood that has escaped the normal vessels and entered brain tissue or the subarachnoid space. Intracerebral hemorrhage is a type of hemorrhagic stroke that occurs when blood leaking from a cerebral vessel directly enters the brain tissue.

Heterotopic ossification—The formation of bone in soft tissue and periarticular locations. Early clinical signs include warmth, swelling, pain, and decreased joint motion. Common joints for heterotopic ossification are the shoulder, elbow, hip, and knee.

Hippocampus—A structure that is part of the limbic system and is involved in long-term memory functions.

Homonymous hemianopsia—Loss of one half of the visual field, on the same side, in both eyes.

Hydrocephalus—The abnormal accumulation of cerebrospinal fluid (CSF) in the brain.

Hyperflexia—Overflexion of a limb.

Hyperglycemia—An abnormally high concentration of glucose (115 to 139 mg/dL) in the circulating blood, especially with reference to a fasting level.

Hyperlexia—The ability to read words above age-level expectation. Usually, children with this ability have difficulty understanding the meaning of the words they read.

Hyperorality—Excessive overeating.

Hypersexuality—Disinhibition in regard to sexual impulses.

Hypertension—Persistent blood pressure measurements above the normal systolic (140 mm Hg) or diastolic (90 mm Hg) pressures.

Hypertonicity (spasticity)—Abnormal muscle tone felt as too much resistance to movement as a result of hyperactive reflexes and loss of inhibiting influences from higher brain centers.

Hypoglycemia—An abnormally small concentration of glucose in the circulating blood, i.e., <50 mg/dL in men and <45 mg/dL in women.

Hypomania—An episode of manic symptoms that are not severe enough to meet the criteria for mania listed in *DSM IV-TR*.

Hypoxemia—Insufficient oxygenation of the blood.

Ideas of reference—Individuals believe that others are talking about or referring to them.

Incentive spirometry—A machine that measures the amount (volume) of air inhaled. This machine is used to validate chronic obstructive pulmonary disease (COPD) as a diagnosis.

Inferior olive—Region of the brainstem that transmits error signals to the cerebellum.

Ischemia—Deficiency of blood resulting from the functional constriction or actual obstruction of a blood vessel, often leading to the death (necrosis) of the surrounding tissue.

Joint attention—The ability to use eye contact and gestures in order to share experiences with others.

Kernicterus—A form of hemolytic jaundice of the newborn. The basal ganglia and other areas of the brain and spinal cord are infiltrated with bilirubin, a yellow-pigmented substance produced by the breakdown of hemoglobin. Develops during the second to eighth day of life.

Kinesthesia—The ability and sense by which position, weight, and movement are perceived.

Kyphosis—Abnormally increased convexity in the curvature of the thoracic spine viewed from the side, resulting from an acquired disease, an injury, or a congenital disorder or disease.

Lability—Rapidly shifting or changing emotions.

Limbic system—This group of subcortical structures is involved in various emotions and memory functions.

Long-term memory—The ability to recall information for long periods of time without effort.

Lordosis—Forward curvature of the lumbar spine.

Melancholia—This term dates back to the fourth century and continues to be used in *DSM IV-TR*. Refers to the following signs: anhedonia, early morning awakening with depression worse in the morning, psychomotor agitation or retardation, weight loss and feelings of guilt.

Mental Disorders—*DSM IV-TR* characterizes a mental disorder as "a clinically significant behavioral or psychological syndrome or pattern that occurs in an individual and that is associated with present distress or disability or with significantly increased risk of suffering death, pain, disability, or an important loss of freedom."

Mild TBI—Clinically identified as a loss of consciousness for <10 minutes or amnesia, a Glasgow Coma Scale (GCS) rating of 13 to 15, no skull fracture on physical examination, and a nonfocal neurological examination.

Moderate TBI—Hospitalization of at least 48 hours, an initial GCS rating of 9 to 12 or higher.

Mutism—Inability to speak.

Myelin—The lipid substance forming a sheath around the axons of certain nerve fibers, occurring predominantly in the cranial and spinal nerves that compose the white matter of the brain and spinal cord. The myelin sheath is formed by a glial cell, either an oligodendrocyte (in the central nervous system) or Schwann cell (in the peripheral nervous system).

Myelogram—A graphic representation of the differential count of cells found in a stained representation of bone marrow.

Myocardial infarction (MI)—Is caused by a lack of blood supply to the heart muscle and tissue death occurs.

Myoclonus—Spasm of a muscle or group of muscles.

Negative symptoms—Decreases or deficits in typical behaviors, seen in mental illness.

Nephropathy—Any disease of the kidney.

Neurobiologic—Of or relating to the biologic study of the nervous system. The cause of autism is considered to be an abnormality in the structure or function of the brain.

Neurofibrillary tangles—Contaminated tau protein that becomes twisted and causes eventual cell death.

Neurogenic bowel/bladder—Dysfunction resulting from congenital abnormality, injury, or disease process of the brain, spinal cord, or local nerve supply to the urinary bladder or rectum and their respective outlets. The dysfunction may manifest as partial or complete retention, incontinence, or frequency of elimination.

Neuroleptic—A medication having antipsychotic action, affecting sensorimotor, cognitive, and psychological functions.

Neuron—A nerve cell that is specialized in transmitting and receiving electrical signals to communicate information between different regions of the body.

Neuropathy—Pathology of the nervous system.

Neurotransmitters—Chemical transmitters, such as dopamine and glutamate, secreted by neurons that bind receptors on nearby cells.

Nonreflex neurogenic bladder or bowel—Also called autonomic bladder/bowel. A neurogenic bladder/bowel resulting from a lesion or injury in the sacral portion of the spinal cord that interrupts the reflex arc that controls the bladder/bowel. The lesion may be in the cauda equina, conus medullaris, sacral roots, or pelvic nerve. It is marked by loss of normal bladder/bowel sensations and reflex activity, inability to initiate urination/elimination normally, and stress incontinence.

Nystagmus—Involuntary, rapid, rhythmic movement (horizontal, vertical, rotatory, or mixed, i.e., two types) of the eyeball.

Obsession—"a recurrent and persistent idea, thought, or impulse to carry out an act that is ego-dystonic, that is experienced as senseless or repugnant, and that the individual cannot voluntarily suppress."

Obsessive-compulsive disorder—"a type of anxiety disorder whose essential feature is recurrent thoughts, impulses or images or compulsions (repetitive, purposeful, and intentional behaviors performed in response to an obsession) sufficiently severe to cause marked distress, be time consuming or interfere significantly with the individual's normal routine, occupational functioning, or usual social activities or relationships with others."

Optic neuritis—Inflammation of the optic nerve, affecting the part of the nerve within the eyeball (neuropapillitis) or the part behind the eyeball (retrobulbar neuritis), usually causing pain and partial blindness in one eye.

Orthostatic intolerance—An inability to tolerate sitting upright or standing, related to a fall in blood pressure that causes dizziness, syncope, and blurred vision.

Oxygen transport—The delivery of fully oxygenated blood to peripheral tissues, the cellular uptake of oxygen, the utilization of oxygen from the blood, and the return of partially desaturated blood to the lungs.

Panic—"extreme and unreasoning anxiety and fear, often accompanied by disturbed breathing, increased heart activity, vasomotor changes, sweating and a feeling of dread."

Panic attack—"sudden onset of intense apprehension, fear, terror or impending doom accompanied by increased autonomic nervous system activity and by various constitutional disturbances, depersonalization, and derealization."

Paraphasia—A language disorder in which a person hears and comprehends words but is unable to speak correctly.

Paratonia—Involuntary resistance to passive movement of the extremities.

Parkinsonism—Characterized by tremor, muscle rigidity, slow shuffling gait, and other classic symptoms of Parkinson's disease.

Peristalsis—The wormlike movement by which the alimentary canal or other tubular organs with both longitudinal and circular muscle fibers propel their contents, consisting of a wave of contraction passing along the tube.

Perseverative—Pertaining to the involuntary and pathologic repetition of verbal or motor response.

Phenotype—Genetic markers that show in observable characteristics in organisms.

Phobia—"any objectively unfounded morbid dread or fear that arouses a state of panic."

Physiatrist—A physician specializing in rehabilitation medicine.

Pneumonia—An inflammation of lung tissue, where the alveoli in the affected areas fill with fluid. The condition is caused by bacteria, viruses, aspiration, or immobility.

Polydipsia—Excessive thirst that occurs frequently.

Polyphagia—Excessive eating.

Polyuria—Excessive excretion of urine.

Positive symptoms—Observable behaviors of psychosis such as hallucinations and delusions.

Posttraumatic stress disorder—"development of characteristic symptoms following a psychologically traumatic event that is generally outside the range of usual human experience; symptoms include numbed responsiveness to environmental stimuli, a variety of autonomic and cognitive dysfunctions and dysphoria."

Primitive reflexes—Innate primary reactions found in newborns and indicative of severe brain damage if present beyond their usual time of disappearance. Adult patients with closed head injury or stroke may manifest these signs; absence on reevaluation is a sign of progress in recovery. Examples include placing reactions, Moro reflex, grasp reflex, rooting reflex, and sucking reflex.

Procedural learning—The ability to learn new motor, perceptual, or basic cognitive behaviors.

Psychomotor agitation—Repetitive and nonproductive motor activity. May present as pacing or fidgeting.

Psychomotor retardation—Movements, reactions, and speech that are slowed.

Psychosis—The inability to distinguish fantasy from reality; delusion or hallucinations that may be mood-congruent or mood-incongruent. Presence of psychotic features in major depressive disorders (MDDs) indicates a poor prognosis.

Pulse oximetry—Measures the oxygen concentration in arterial blood. The normal range is 95% to 100%. Measurements are taken to prevent hypoxia and to evaluate treatment.

Purkinje cells—Cells that form a layer near the surface of the cerebellum and convey signals away from the cerebellum.

Quadriplegia—Paralysis of all four limbs (e.g., tetraplegia).

Rapid-cycling—Four or more episodes of some type of mood disturbance within the past year; episodes meet criteria for either mania, hypomania, mixed or depressed episodes as identified in *DSM IV-TR*.

Reflex arc—A reflex, which is built in and does not need conscious thought to take effect, is the total of any particular automatic response mediated by the nervous system. A reflex arc is usually a simple reflex such as a knee jerk, which involves only two nerves and one synapse. Other arcs may involve an interneuron. When the sensory nerve ending is stimulated, a nerve impulse travels along a sensory (afferent) neuron to the spinal cord. An association neuron or interneuron then transfers the impulse to a motor (efferent) neuron, which carries the impulse to a muscle, which then contracts and moves a body part.

Relapse—Return of symptoms, resulting in rehospitalization for mental illness.

Retinopathy—Noninflammatory degenerative disease of the retina.

Retrograde amnesia—Loss of memory of events that occurred prior to the injury.

Rett's disorder—A rare neurobiologic disorder that primarily affects females and is caused by a deviation on the methyl-CpG-binding protein 2 (MECP2) gene. This disorder has a distinctive course since early development in children is typical, followed by the deceleration of head growth, loss of purposeful hand movements, and appearance of autistic-like symptoms.

Rote memory—The process of memorizing and using language overheard from others rather than producing spontaneously generated language.

Scoliosis—Lateral curvature of the vertebral column. This deviation of the normally straight vertical line of the spine may or may not include rotation or deformity of the vertebrae.

Semantic memory—Ability to remember the name of an object.

Severe TBI—Loss of consciousness and/or posttraumatic amnesia for more than 24 hours, a GCS rating of 1 to 8.

Short-term memory—The ability to recall information after a short period of time.

Social phobia—"a persistent pattern of significant fear of a social or performance situation, manifested by anxiety or panic on exposure to the situation or in anticipation of it, which the person realizes is unreasonable or excessive and interferes significantly with the person's functioning."

Spasticity (hypertonicity)—Abnormally high muscle tone, i.e., tone which is felt as too much resistance to movement, resulting from hyperactive reflexes or the loss of inhibiting influences from higher brain centers.

Sphygmomanometer—The instrument used to measure blood pressure.

Spinal shock—Result of an acute transverse lesion of the spinal cord that causes immediate flaccid paralysis and loss of all sensation and reflex activity (including autonomic functions) below the level of injury. On return of reflex activity, there is increased spasticity of muscles and exaggerated tendon reflexes.

Stereotyped behavior—A pattern of behavior, such as hand flapping or nonproductive exploration of objects, that is often seen in autism.

Strabismus—Deviation of the eye in which the visual axes assume a position relative to each other different from that required by the physiological conditions; also called squint.

Stretch reflex—Reflex contraction of a muscle in response to passive longitudinal stretching.

Subdural hematoma—An accumulation of blood in the subdural space of the brain, usually caused by an injury.

Sundowning—A condition in which a person with cognitive impairment becomes confused or disoriented at the end of the day.

Systolic blood pressure—The amount of force used to pump blood out of the heart into the arterial circulation.

Tactile defensiveness—A type of sensory defensiveness in which a person overreacts or avoids touching certain textures.

Tangential thinking—Rapid shifting from one thought to a closely related thought.

Tangentiality—Pattern of communicating in which the person moves off the central point and, unlike circumstantiality, is unable to return to the point.

Tau—A type of protein.

Temporal lobes—This region of the brain is located at the side of the cerebrum, below the frontal lobe. Its functions include auditory processing, comprehension, naming, verbal memory, and high-level visual processing including object and facial recognition.

Theory of mind—The ability to understand another person's thoughts, feelings, or intentions.

Thrombus—A blood clot comprising such blood factors as platelets and fibrin; frequently the cause of obstructions in the vascular system resulting in medical problems such as stroke.

Topagnosia—Loss of ability to localize site of tactile sensations.

Topographic orientation—Orientation of the self within the environment.

Transient ischemic attacks (TIA)—A sudden episode of temporary symptoms, typically due to diminished blood flow through the carotid arteries or sometimes related to impaired circulation through the vertebrobasilar vessels. TIA is a powerful warning sign of stroke, and symptoms can range from obvious loss of sensation or motor function to more subtle signs. See Cerebrovascular accident.

Tuberculosis (TB)—A bacterial infection that affects the lungs, and sometimes the kidneys and bones. The bacteria that causes TB is spread by airborne droplets.

Type 1 diabetes—A disease in which the pancreas stops producing insulin as a result of autoimmune destruction of β cells.

Type 2 diabetes—A disease where the body cells are insulin resistant.

Unilateral spatial neglect—Inattention to visual stimuli presented on the individual's side contralateral to a cerebral lesion. It may occur independently of visual deficits or with hemianopsia.

Unipolar—Refers to the syndrome that consists only of major depressive episodes without manic episodes.

Utilization behavior—Touching, grasping, or manipulating anything that is within sight.

Vegetative signs—Physiologic signs that develop in the areas of sexual activity, sleep, appetite, and other biologic rhythms.

Visuospatial—Pertaining to the ability to comprehend visual representations and their spatial relationships.

Index

Page numbers followed by *f* or *t* refer to illustrations or tables, respectively.